VALIDATE YOUR PAIN!

Exposing the Chronic Pain Cover-Up

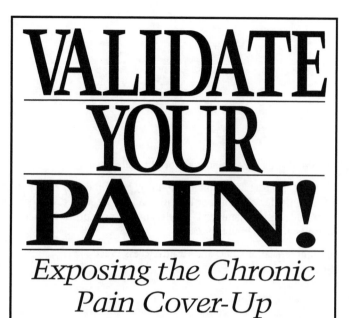

VALIDATE YOUR PAIN!

Exposing the Chronic Pain Cover-Up

by

Allan F. Chino, Ph.D.

Corinne Dille Davis, M.D.

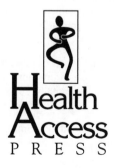

Health
Access
P R E S S

InSync Communications LLC and Health Access Press
2445 River Tree Circle
Sanford, FL 32771
e-mail trivia@magicnet.net
http://www.insynchronicity.com

ISBN 0-9673439-2-5

First Health Access Press Edition
10 9 8 7 6 5 4 3 2 1

Any references to patients/clients in this work are composites of many individuals drawn from the clinical work and life experiences of the authors. Names and details have been changed to protect confidentiality, unless prior permission was granted by those so named.

This publication was designed to provide information in regard to the subject matter covered. It is sold and distributed with the understanding that the publisher is not engaged in rendering legal, medical, or counseling services. If appropriate expert assis-tance is required, the services of a qualified and competent professional should be sought. — This statement is adapted from a Declaration of Principles by a Committee of the American Bar Association and a Committee of Publishers and Associations.

Health Access Press books are available at special discounts when purchased in bulk for use in seminars, as premiums, or in sales promotions. Special editions or book excerpts can also be created to specifications. For details, contact InSync Communications LLC at the address above.

Editorial Direction & Typesetting by Sandy Pearlman
Cover Design by Jonathan Pennell

Printed in the United States of America

To my mother, Bonnie Marie Dille, who taught me early on in life that "books are my friends," and to my father, Major Donald E. Dille, M.D., who inspired me to go to medical school. To my beloved husband and soul mate, Dave, and to the apples of my eye, my children, Natalie and Trevor.

—CDD

To Fred and Florence Chino, who gave me a solid start in life. To Audrey, Ben, and Allison Chino, whose relentless demands for me to be a husband and father kept me from finishing this book sooner, but whose joy and steadfast love made me not care.

—AFC

And most of all, to God Almighty for providing us with all of the things we needed to tell this story.

—CDD & AFC

Contents

Foreword

If you suffer from chronic pain, then chances are you have read one or more of the "pain management" books on the market. Even so, you have never read a book like *Validate Your Pain! Exposing the Chronic Pain Cover-Up*. In *Validate Your Pain!* Drs. Chino and Davis have boldly departed from business as usual for pain books.

First of all, although there are many well-written pain books, it seems that many are written in a rather sterile and antiseptic style. I guess you could argue that these books help you manage your pain by putting you to sleep. *Validate Your Pain!* is just the opposite. Drs. Chino and Davis are not afraid to spice up the presentation through the use of humorous vignettes, colloquialisms, rhythmic sentence construction, running gags, slang, puns, and the like. This writing style brings the information to life. *Validate Your Pain!* is like talking with an old friend who also happens to be an expert in the field of chronic pain.

Second, *Validate your Pain!* dares to takes the position of patient advocate. The authors not only do an excellent job of covering the "how to" aspects of pain management, Drs. Chino and Davis also deal with controversial topics that are of the utmost concern to those who suffer from chronic pain:

♦ Doctors who actually work against you as a patient

♦ How doctors will assume the pain is "all in your head" if a straightforward cause can't be found

♦ The role of narcotic medications

♦ How managed care will often keep the solution to your chronic pain out of reach

As stated in the introduction, the goal of *Validate Your Pain!* is to "arm you with 'insider' information that will help you to maneuver through the healthcare mine field so that you do not become yet another victim of the abuse that is going on" while helping you take control of your pain. *Validate Your Pain!* achieves this goal and more.

> **William W. Deardorff, Ph.D., ABPP**
> Fellow, American Psychological Association
> Past President, American Academy of Health Psychology
> Assistant Professor, UCLA School of Medicine
> Co-author:
> *Back Pain Remedies for Dummies*
> *Win the Battle Against Back Pain*
> *Preparing for Surgery: A Mind–Body Approach to
>   Enhance Healing and Recovery*
> *The Practice of Clinical Health Psychology*
> *Clinical Psychology in Medical Settings*

Introduction

There is something very troubling going on in healthcare when it comes to addressing the problem of chronic pain. Perhaps you know about it. Perhaps you don't. No one really talks about it very much — because it's not very nice. The problem has nothing to do with the latest approaches to diagnosis or treatment. It has nothing to do with discovering a way to ease human suffering and restore quality of life. We already know how to do that. Rather, it has to do with something far more basic: *compassion and the desire to help.* There simply is not enough to get the job done. But what's worse is that there are forces at work which, under the guise of healthcare, actively *undermine* efforts to help people with pain. And these forces are making lots of money in the process. We feel that it is time to expose these dirty little secrets.

Our qualifications to write about this problem have less to do with our training as doctors than they do with our training as human beings. The lessons we have learned from our patients and others about the value of caring and compassion are the foundation upon which our professional lives rest. We are human beings who happen to be doctors. As specialists in chronic pain management, we have had the opportunity to get an insider's view of what's going on. And we don't like what we see.

From the thousands of people we have seen who suffer from chronic pain, we have heard the same things over and over:

- ♦ "Nobody seems to be taking my pain seriously."
- ♦ "I have been to so many doctors, but they don't know what's wrong with me."

♦ "They say that I shouldn't be hurting this much."

♦ "They think I'm faking."

♦ "They say I'm 'addicted' to pain medications — *but they really do help me!*"

♦ "They say it's 'just' muscle pain."

♦ "My insurance company denied my treatment plan."

♦ "I was loyal to my employer for all those years, but now that I got hurt, they just want to get rid of me."

♦ "My doctor won't listen to me."

♦ "Nobody believes me."

♦ "They want me to see a psychiatrist."

♦ "Maybe it *is* all in my head."

Do any of these hit home? If you suffer from chronic pain, some, if not all, probably do. The attitudes among healthcare professionals that are implied by these statements not only do severe damage to already suffering human beings, *they also happen to be just plain wrong!* While some practitioners hold these beliefs out of ignorance, others hold them out of arrogance — and even greed. Yes, there are doctors who will, for example, purposely lie about a patient's true condition in order to keep the business rolling in. There are insurance companies that reward physicians and case managers for denying needed care while enjoying federally sanctioned immunity from legal liability. While these are some of the more egregious examples, abuses of subtler proportion are happening in clinics and offices around the world each and every day. Without exception, they stem from the same human failing: lack of compassion and caring.

There are several excellent books on managing chronic pain. Unlike the others, however, *Validate Your Pain! Exposing the Chronic Pain Cover-Up* exposes the tricks and traps that, through ignorance, arrogance, and greed, sabotage sincere efforts to make things better. It's a story that needs to be told.

Overall, our intent is to arm you with "insider" information that will help you to maneuver through the healthcare mine field so that you do not become yet another victim of the abuse that is going on. While the topic is one of utmost seriousness, there is, as with everything in life, a humorous side to it as well. In the end, we hope that the information provided in this book will assist you in taking control of your pain. And, as we shall see, taking control begins with validating your pain.

Acknowledgments

We wish to thank our colleagues Drs. Bill Deardorff, Jim Lowrance, John Kenny, Gary Whitehead, Lin Zhang, Mark Kabins, and Lou Damis, as well as Judge Lee Wilbur, for their time and expert advice in putting this book together. We are also grateful for the insights provided by Patti Wright. The guidance, support, and encouragement of our publisher, Dennis McClellan of Health Access Press, and our expert editor, Sandy Pearlman, were invaluable. And finally, we are especially grateful to our courageous patients who, through their own painful trials, have given us the gift of an invaluable education.

The Authors

Allan F. Chino, Ph.D., ABPP, is board certified in Clinical Health Psychology and is president of the American Academy of Clinical Health Psychology. He set up and directed two CARF-accredited hospital-based pain rehabilitation programs in northern California (most recently with Dr. Davis) prior to moving to Las Vegas, where he now has a private practice in behavioral pain management. Dr. Chino conducts biobehavioral research in the area of fibromyalgia. In addition to being a father (of two) and a husband (of one), he is a musician and the moderator of the board of deacons at his church.

Corinne Dille Davis, M.D., is board certified in Pain Medicine, Physical Medicine and Rehabilitation, and Electrodiagnostic Medicine. With Dr. Chino, she developed and directed a CARF-accredited hospital-based pain rehabilitation program in northern California. Having had her fill of practicing in a corporate hospital setting, she moved to Las Vegas, where she provides medical pain management services in her private practice. In addition to serving on the Prescription Controlled Substance Abuse Task Force for the State of Nevada, she is a devoted wife, mother, and piano accompanist at her church.

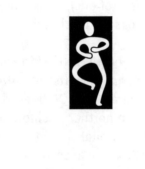

The Power
of Validation

When you were born, what was the first thing you did? Sleep? Eat? Coo at your mother's bosom? Probably not. If you are like just about everyone else on the face of this planet, you *cried*. Remember? (Yes, it was a long time ago, but we're willing to go out on a limb and stand by our assertion.) You cried. So what? What's so profound about that? Well, two things:

1. The fact is that, barring major medical complications, all of us cried within moments of our birth. It is a universal phenomenon. It is in the human blueprint.

2. It started each of us on an important — indeed, *crucial* — journey toward learning how to improve the chances for our personal survival in this world.

While we are not likely to get an argument about our first proposition — that crying at birth is built into us, you may be less likely to put your stamp of approval on the second one. What does crying at birth have to do with personal survival? In a word, *everything*.

Okay, let's all recall the first few days of our lives. There was probably a lot of crying going on. Now, what happened when your mother detected your crying? Hopefully, she would rush to your crib and you would suddenly experience a lot of holding, rocking, soothing, and feeding. A feeling of calm contentment soon washed over you. Your breathing slowed, your blood pressure returned to normal, and your brain stopped pouring large quantities of stress hormone into your bloodstream. The world became your oyster once again. Those were the days, weren't they?

Now, consider that this pattern occurred not once, not twice, but *zillions* of times. (Anyone who has taken care of a newborn can attest that we're not exaggerating — much.) Uncomfortable internal feelings would spark a rise in blood pressure, breathing rate, biochemical changes such as stress hormone production, muscle tension, emotional outrage, and, finally, vigorous verbal protestation. Time and again, all of this was followed by acts of caring from an important person, leading to an immediate soothing of all those dreadful physical and emotional feelings. Get the picture? Discomfort...emotional distress...cries for help...mom's validating response...physical and emotional stress reduction...bliss restored. So, through countless additional instances of this pattern, you learned that, when feeling poorly, a cry for help would lead to feeling a whole lot better — not only emotionally, but physically as well.

What's more, and quite apart from your inborn crying reflex at birth, your nervous system started to learn the same lesson. Through repetition, it automatically began associating internal discomfort and distress with *attention-grabbing* vocal utterances. This behavior was then strengthened by the cavalry arriving on the scene (i.e., mom showed up) and the welcome relief that came therewith. The frontal lobes, or thinking part of the brain, were bypassed. There was no conscious awareness of these connections. Hence came the development of a key survival mechanism: communicating distress.

Consider what would happen if a baby failed to communicate distress by crying or engaging in some other attention-grabbing action. The caretaker would have to guess when the baby was hungry, wet, tired, cold, or hurt. Chances are, that baby's fundamental needs would be overlooked more often than those of his or her more vocal contemporaries. Assuming that he or she continued to experience the disequilibrium that comes with feeling hungry, wet, tired, cold, or hurt, we can surmise that the nervous system would be in a chronic state of stress. As we shall discuss later in more detail, we know that chronic physical and emotional stress greatly suppresses immune function and the body's natural ability to heal itself. Not good odds for survival.

Psychologists understand that this help-eliciting behavior is developed and maintained by *negative reinforcement.* Often confused with punishment, the process of negative reinforcement involves strengthening a given behavior by removing an aversive stimulus (something bad or unpleasant) after the behavior has occurred. For example, have you ever been the victim of nagging? (Who hasn't?) We can probably all agree that nagging is a particularly obnoxious behavior (unless, of course, we, ourselves, happen to be the nagging party, in which case we usually relabel our nagging as merely providing helpful sequential reminders). If we are the "nagee," we can understand our "giving-in" behavior as stemming from the relief we experience when the nagging stops. We give in and the obnoxious stimulus ceases. Thus, our giving-in behavior is negatively reinforced, and we are more likely to give in under similar circumstances in the future. Likewise, our own anxiety serves as a negative stimulus to get things done. When we follow through and accomplish our task, the anxiety goes away and our future efforts are strengthened. We are also more likely to follow through the next time something comes up. Oh, and want someone to try green eggs and ham? Try negative reinforcement ("Sam I am!").

Note the similarity between one's adult anxiety and the discomfort felt by the baby. In both cases, the action (productive behavior for the adult and crying behavior for the baby) stimulated by the noxious feeling state resulted in a lessening of something bad. Thus, the same principles of learning that were in operation when you entered this world continue to operate until you leave it. In fact, unless you happen to be in a coma (and if you are, we recommend that you put down this book and save it for a time when you're feeling more alert), your responses are shaped by positive and negative reinforcement every day. The phone rings...you answer it...the ringing stops. Boom. Your answering-the-phone behavior is strengthened via negative reinforcement. Things can, however, get complicated: The phone rings...you answer it...the ringing stops...but it's a pesky telemarketer. Well...we'll save our discussion of punishment for another time.

Bottom line: We are all biologically and behaviorally programmed to seek comfort when we are in physical or emotional distress. Why else would we be inclined to talk to a co-worker about the boss's latest rampage? Why else would we suddenly strike up a conversation with a total stranger immediately after experiencing or witnessing a traumatic event, such as an earthquake or traffic accident? Or why else would we seek out others who understand and validate our experience of pain? Our genes and experiences in life lead us in this direction. And it produces profound emotional — as well as *physical* — benefits that help us to survive.

Validation, Breast Cancer, and Survival

Several years ago, Stanford psychiatrist and researcher Dr. David Spiegel conducted an important study in which women with metastatic breast cancer were divided into two groups. Both received standard medical treatment, but half also attended support groups in which they discussed their struggle with the disease. They talked. They cried. They laughed. Through this, they formed trusting and caring relationships with one another. In essence, they shared the experience of facing a mortal challenge together. While the original intent of the study was to examine the effect of support groups on *coping* with breast cancer, Dr. Spiegel and his colleagues were surprised, on follow-up, to find that the women who participated survived *twice* as long as those who did not. Indeed, the survival rate for those who dropped out of the groups was similar to that of those who never participated: They died sooner.

As a careful and respected clinician and researcher, Dr. Spiegel tried to account for these incredible findings by examining other possible explanations. None were supported. This study was later carefully replicated by independent researchers, and essentially the same results were found: For women with metastatic breast cancer, meaningful and regular participation in support groups leads to living substantially longer.

But how could this be? We might easily understand this remarkable finding if the "survivors," in addition to receiving standard medical treatment, were given a new, powerful drug or even a special diet. That might make sense. But participation in a support group? What could be happening within these women to result in extending their lives by a factor of two? The leading theory is that exposure to a caring environment, in which one expresses feelings and provides others with support, leads to significantly reduced emotional and physiological stress. And recent research clearly shows that such stress responses can devastate the body's immune system. Reduce the stress by participating in the support group and the immune system gets stronger. It becomes much better able to fight off the invading cancer. Notice the link between biology and behavior? It is real. And it is more powerful than we had ever imagined.

Validation and Chronic Pain

In our many years of experience treating human beings suffering from chronic pain, we have observed some remarkable parallels to Spiegel's findings. While people with nonmalignant chronic pain are not necessarily facing physical death from their condition, they often are facing vocational, social, and emotional "death." We see people who have given up hope. In addition to hurting all the time, they have lost contact with the positive things in life, which give all of us the strength to cope with the negative things. In addition, the impact of pain and subsequent disruption to their lives messes up their biochemistry. Important neurotransmitters become depleted. In response to all the life disruption going on, the brain works feverishly to produce and deliver massive quantities of stress hormone into the bloodstream. (It's that "anxiety...action...mission accomplished" thing again, only this time the "action...mission accomplished" part gets disconnected, leaving the "anxiety" part free to run amok.) This biochemical disruption leads to all kinds of additional bad stuff:

1. **Chronic stress.** There is no control over the pain and disruption to life that are occurring. And there seems to be no light at the end of the tunnel.

2. **Insomnia.** Hey, with all that pain and stress, who can sleep? And we all know that getting enough sleep is essential for the body and mind to operate properly.

3. **Depression.** Tired and hurting all the time, without anyone who really understands, who wouldn't feel depressed?

4. **Muscle tension and spasm.** In addition to the decreased blood flow and subsequent pain produced by chronically contracted muscles, bones and nearby nerves can be pushed and pulled, thus aggravating pain.

5. **Altered neurological functioning.** Research evidence shows that uncontrolled pain can actually produce permanent damage to the nervous system.

6. **Suppressed immune function.** Chronic physiological stress severely inhibits the body's natural ability to heal itself.

Given this rather impressive list, we can see how the deck gets stacked in favor of a vicious cycle of emotional suffering, biochemical disruption, and additional pain. For many, the body simply is not able to overcome this onslaught. The moral of the story is that unless chronic pain is properly managed — both physically and psychologically, it is likely to get worse over time.

Paying Attention to the Human Being with Chronic Pain

In his keynote address to the American Pain Society in 1995, Rabbi Harold Kushner, author of the best-seller *When Bad Things Happen to Good People,* offered a valuable message to clinicians and scientists specializing in chronic pain: When we cannot cure, we must heal. When we cannot eliminate the disease, we must heal the *person* with the disease. In a culture enamored with high-tech approaches to solving all our problems, it is sometimes the seemingly unglamorous, *low*-tech solutions that are most needed. For chronic pain, it starts with sincere, compassionate caring. No lasers, no microchips, and no DNA splicing required.

We are in full agreement with Rabbi Kushner. Quite aside from considering the intricate interaction of biomechanical, biochemical, and biobehavioral variables, it so happens that paying attention to — and *validating* — the human experience of chronic pain will bring about a significant healing effect. Outcome from "proper" physical treatment administered by an unfeeling, uncaring, dispassionate robot will be far inferior to that provided within the context of a caring, compassionate team of human beings. And while we don't know many mechanical robots treating individuals with pain, we do know plenty of human ones. And they tend not to be very good at that healing thing.

"Fluff"

Unfortunately, many doctors focus strictly on the biomechanical aspects of pain while ignoring the impact of the biochemical and biobehavioral elements listed above. A few years ago, as co-directors of a hospital-based pain program in northern California, we were asked by our nurse case manager, Connie, to contact the medical director of an insurance plan. Previously, we had been given the go-ahead by the insurance company to provide an interdisciplinary evaluation for a young woman, Erica, who had a severe and very complex chronic pain condition. From our evaluation, we developed a treatment plan designed specifically for her. Connie sought authorization for the proposed treatment program, but an insurance nurse case manager denied it. Thus, we were appealing the decision to the insurance company's medical director.

Erica had had a very hard life. She had never married and did not have a supportive family to help her cope with the pain and disruption in her life that came with her diagnosis of reflex sympathetic dystrophy.

Moreover, she was saddled with substantial pain and fatigue from fibromyalgia. At 23, she was unable to work. She shared a rented room with all her worldly possessions. She was a good person but rarely met with good fortune. The combination of chronic pain, lack of emotional support, financial stress, and hopelessness led her to contemplate suicide at times, though she had never actually attempted it. Erica needed help. And we believed that we could help her.

Upon phoning the insurance company medical director to explain Erica's complex pain condition, it became clear that it would be a hard sell for us. We carefully described our interdisciplinary treatment plan, which consisted of a three-week inpatient program that included appropriate medical management, pain medications, specialized physical and occupational therapy, biofeedback, and individual and group behavioral pain treatment. Pretty standard stuff in accredited pain centers.

He expressed skepticism regarding the need for such intensive treatment. It seemed to us that he was unfamiliar with the field of chronic pain management and that we had some rapid, yet diplomatic, educating to do. After some discussion, he reluctantly agreed to authorize the program, but with several restrictions. First, Erica could only participate for *one* week, not three. Second, physical therapy was okay, but he wasn't sure about the need for occupational therapy. Third, there would be no biofeedback or psychological treatment whatsoever. As he put it, "We all have to be more efficient these days, and I'm not going to authorize that kind of *fluff*." When we patiently explained Erica's need for these elements, especially given her depressed state and thoughts of suicide, all bets were off. He said, "She's suicidal? Then she needs to be admitted to a psychiatric unit. I certainly wouldn't want her on *my* unit." When we protested that an inpatient pain program, not a psychiatric unit, was the most appropriate clinical choice for Erica, he simply said, "Well then, you can go ahead and treat her if that's what you think she needs. We're just not going to pay for it." He had finally found a reason to deny the total program. And he did.

Now, the skeptical reader may be thinking that we have slanted this account to portray a true villain, a cad, a scoundrel; that there must be more to the story to account for his actions. Maybe Erica's condition was not severe enough to require an expensive inpatient pain program. Perhaps the insurance company medical director's clinical judgment was more objective than ours, given his "distance" from the case. The answers to these propositions are, in order, no, no, no, and *no*!

He was clearly looking for a reason to deny Erica's program. And he did so, in part, by relying on his ignorance of how biomechanical, biochemical, and biobehavioral aspects of human pain interact. He referred to the behavioral treatment elements, especially the group sessions, as "fluff." Translate this to mean "irrelevant," "unimportant," "superfluous," and "an expensive and unneeded luxury." He could see the value in physical therapy, given its obvious biomechanical basis. But how could he justify paying good money for something as "frivolous" as behavioral treatment which, after all, was aimed only at making the patient feel better emotionally; it had nothing to do with the patient's physical pain problem, in his narrow view. For him, it all fit neatly together: Be fiscally "responsible" by cutting out the "fat" from a "bloated" pain program, and make the stockholders happy in the process. He probably slept well that night.

As for Erica, we, rather ironically, took the insurance medical director's advice. We went ahead and treated her anyway — but within the context of an interdisciplinary program that validated her experience of pain. We (the hospital and doctors) picked up the tab. Thankfully, she got better.

The Power of Validation

There will be critics of our message. From a cursory examination, they will see us as encouraging people with chronic pain to feel victimized and to remain in a sick role. While we agree that reducing victimization and adherence to a sick role is an important goal in pain management, we do not agree that our approach contributes to furthering these unfortunate states. To the contrary, our experience and our objective data have shown, time and again, that appropriately validating a human being's experience of pain and suffering will, in most cases, bring about more rapid *positive* changes:

◆ Changes in emotions

◆ Changes in outlook

◆ Changes in the belief that things will get better

◆ Changes in putting forth effort to get better

◆ Changes in biochemistry

◆ Changes in conditioned biobehavioral responses

◆ Changes in physical, emotional, social, and occupational functioning

Far from "fluff," clinical validation of one's experience of pain and suffering is an active, and effective, form of treatment, when properly administered and when combined with other appropriate therapies. It is, indeed, powerful.

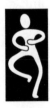

A Tale of Chronic Pain

Sarah is a 38-year-old housewife who lives in northern California. She is married to a truck driver who is on the road for days at a time. Most of the responsibility — or, as Sarah would say, the burden — of parenting their three children falls on her shoulders. Like her mother before her, Sarah suffers from migraine headaches.

Sarah has noticed that increased stress seems to be a trigger for bringing on the headaches. And there has been plenty of that around the house lately. As a matter of fact, ever since Tammy and Michael, her two oldest, hit adolescence, it's been pure hell. They demand an explanation for every decision Sarah makes. They question everything she says or does. They routinely disobey her. And now that they've both begun dating, Sarah is at her wit's end. The fact that Michael towers over her by half a foot has rendered the difficult challenge of commanding respect from her children almost impossible. Her husband, Jerry, although a nice enough guy, isn't around half the time to defend her.

Sarah frequently wishes that she were the breadwinner of the family. She finds herself fantasizing about driving down the road in a big old 18-wheeler, hauling a load and loving every minute away from all the noise and the mass confusion. She smiles in a moment of unsuppressed glee as she envisions Jerry, wearing an apron, left behind to attend to the mundane tasks of housecleaning and child rearing, as she cheerfully waves good-bye.

There are times when Sarah nostalgically longs for bygone days, when her kids were sweet, lovable, and lap size. They were obedient and cute then. She sighs. At other times, she yearns for the day when they will be away at college or off to the army. The operative word is *away*. Then, maybe, just maybe, she could have a minute's peace.

Another trigger for Sarah's headaches is hormones. Her headaches are predictably more frequent, more severe, and longer in duration around the time of her period. And, of course, her mood is usually at an all-time low. "Maybe a hysterectomy would be helpful," thinks Sarah. "I've had my kids. Let's just cut the darn thing out!"

The final trigger that Sarah has identified is exposure to bright sunshine. She has learned the hard way about the importance of wearing dark glasses and a hat pulled down over her brow. "So I look like a sleuth! So what?" she thinks. "Anything to protect me from the glaring sun and the horrible migraines that follow."

Sarah's headaches aren't just simple headaches. The throbbing pain associated with them is excruciating. The slightest sound — a sneeze, a cough — feels like a time bomb going off inside her head. Because her vision blurs, attempts to read result in guaranteed nausea and occasional vomiting.

She heads for the bedroom at the first inkling of a headache. She turns off the lights, lies down, and tries to relax. That's usually about the time Tammy decides to turn her stereo on full blast and listen to the noise she calls music. If she only knew.

Sarah feels guilty because the headaches often interfere with her ability to fulfill her roles and responsibilities as a wife and mother. She firmly believes that her husband and children are suffering as a result. Getting a simple meal on the table has become a real chore. Dirty laundry is piling up all over the place. It's pitiful. And sex? Forget it. That's the last thing on her mind. She is depressed and suffers from feelings of hopelessness and loss of self-esteem. Both the pain and the depression interfere with her sleep. Clearly, Sarah is on a downward spiral.

She turns to her new physician, Dr. H. Emmo, for help. In the six or seven minutes they have together, he expresses little concern about the frequency and the intensity of her headaches. He tells her that certain diagnostic tests, such as an MRI (magnetic resonance imaging) or an EEG (electroencephalogram), might be in order "sometime down the road if things don't improve." What Sarah does not know is that Dr. Emmo has been "counseled" by his employer, a health maintenance organization (HMO) for *"overutilizing"* medical resources such as expensive diagnostic tests and consultations from medical specialists within the system. She also is unaware that his annual bonus is tied to the "savings" he achieves by "managing" the use of these resources. And speaking of savings, Jerry's employer recently switched to this HMO in order to reduce its health insurance costs. Although reluctant to sever their relationship with Dr. Welby, their family physician of many years, who, unfortunately, is not a provider for this HMO, Sarah and Jerry initially supported the change because the HMO would cover such things as medications and required less out-of-pocket expenses overall. It sounded good at the time. But now Sarah needs more help, and she has the strong sense that, for some reason, Dr. Emmo is withholding it. She feels that she is already "down the road" and that the time for further diagnostic testing and treatment is *now*! Yet she sees no change in her treatment course. No further action is forthcoming. So her sense of hopelessness deepens. She feels stuck. Maximal headaches. Minimal help. The bowl of cherries Sarah had envisioned for her life is now nothing but the pits.

Sarah tries a long list of medications, but none of them work. Her medicine cabinet is filled to overflowing with perfectly useless drugs. Then Dr. Emmo has the audacity to advise her to simply "ignore" her headaches. It's as if he were saying, "It's all in your head." Sarah is livid. Her own physician does not take her pain seriously. Nevertheless, she tries to comply. She sings songs, plays solitaire, chats with the neighbors — all in vain. It's like trying to ignore a hot poker against her skin. In the end, she is hurting and depressed. She is furious, too. All she can think about is the pain.

What Is Pain?

Pain has been defined as an unpleasant sensation that occurs in response to tissue injury. It produces a heightened awareness of arousal in the nervous system and motivation to escape from the offending stimulus or agent. Pain is a *subjective* experience that cannot be measured directly by another individual.

What Is Suffering?

Pain and suffering are not synonymous. The degree to which an individual suffers depends on the meaning or significance he or she ascribes to the pain. Sound confusing? Just a bunch of medical mumbo jumbo? Perhaps the best way to explain the difference is by example.

Let's say that our friend Sarah is having a severe migraine headache today, and Dr. H. Emmo asks her to rate the severity of the pain on a numerical scale, from zero (the absence of pain) to ten (excruciating pain that would warrant a trip to the emergency room). Sarah rates the pain intensity of her headache as seven.

Gloria, the next patient that Dr. Emmo sees that day, coincidentally is also suffering from a headache. In her case, however, the headache is not due to a migraine but rather stems from a growing malignant tumor. Gloria is told that this tumor will, in all probability, eventually take her life. Unless, that is, she happens to be hit by a Mack truck first. Dr. Emmo asks Gloria to rate the intensity of her headache pain on the same numerical scale, and she, like Sarah, rates it as seven.

So, both women rate the intensity of their headache pain as seven. Which one do you suppose is suffering more: Sarah, who will, in all likelihood, fully recover from her headache, as awful as it is, or Gloria, who has just been told that her headache condition will lead to certain death? The answer is self-evident. Gloria not only suffers from the headache pain, but she must now contemplate what it means to have all the meaningful connections in her life severed in the near future.

Let's consider another example of how two people can have the same amount of pain but experience different degrees of suffering. Don is a successful landscape designer who has developed his own business and works out of his home. Ron works as a staff nurse in the local hospital. They both incurred low-back injuries which resulted in chronic pain. Although both men are in much discomfort, Don's income is unaffected by his physical limitations, whereas Ron is placed on probation for having missed too many days of work due to his pain condition. Don's wife and kids are very supportive and understanding when it comes to his limitations. Ron's family is becoming increasingly annoyed and irritated at his inability to do the things he used to do. Ron becomes worried that his wife might leave him. Don has no such worries. Ron is afraid of losing his job. Don sees bright horizons in store for his business. Ron cannot even afford to buy a lottery ticket. Ironically, Don just won the lottery! Despite having the same amount of physical pain, we would award Ron first prize in this contest of suffering.

The moral of the story? There are at least two. Number one: If you purchase a lottery ticket, be sure to win. Number two: Factors other than pain intensity can greatly contribute to how much one suffers. It is important to consider what is happening to the *person* with the pain, rather than just the pain itself. The unfortunate fact is that our healthcare system generally attends only to the biomedical aspects of pain while largely ignoring the person in whom the pain resides. We need to treat pain within the context of suffering. This means paying attention to how pain affects the sufferer's life and how the sufferer's world treats him or her as a result. If we don't do this, suffering can continue unabated, *even if pain is reduced.*

Acute Pain

Acute pain is a normal protective mechanism that signifies physical trauma or a disease process. It serves a useful purpose by alerting the organism that trouble is brewing. Speaking of brewing, consider this example. You place a full, uncovered cup of scalding hot coffee between your legs while driving in rush-hour traffic. Unfortunately, it sloshes over into your lap when you hit the brakes to avoid rear-ending the two guys in the white Ford Bronco in front of you. The subsequent sensation of pain is nature's little wake-up call that you should not be such a complete idiot in the future (e.g., by using a cup holder or perhaps switching to iced tea for a potentially more *interesting* sensation). In short, acute pain is good. It gives us valuable feedback about our environment and our behavior in relation thereto. It protects us. Unlike chronic pain, acute pain generally correlates with the degree of tissue damage and diminishes in intensity as healing progresses.

Inadequate treatment of acute pain can lead to permanent changes in your body that place you at increased risk for developing chronic pain. Patients who receive epidural analgesia before undergoing amputation of a limb for vascular insufficiency, for example, are less likely to develop chronic phantom limb pain (pain perceived as occurring in the absent limb), in contrast to those who are treated conventionally.

Research indicates that, even after a brief painful stimulus, long-lasting changes occur within the spinal cord. Sensory input from the injured tissue reaches spinal cord neurons, which, in turn, worsen subsequent physiological responses. Pain receptors in the extremities become sensitized as well. Simply put, sensitivity to pain increases. Injured tissues release substances that bring about a stress hormone response. This "fight-or-flight" reaction is associated with a rapid heart rate and negative emotions, as well as an increase in metabolism, blood clotting, and water retention. In addition, it impairs the body's ability to fight off infection. Pain's adverse impact on the immune system is becoming clearer as more research results are reported. And once pain becomes established, it becomes increasingly more difficult to alleviate.

Clinical studies indicate that effective postoperative pain management results in improved recovery. Among the benefits are earlier mobilization, shorter hospital stays, and reduced costs overall. Inadequately treated acute postop pain, on the other hand, may lead to shallow breathing and "guarding" of the injured site, which can, in turn, lead to the development of pneumonia.

Patients should be told that they have a right to both adequate prevention and treatment of pain. Effective pain management before, during, and after surgery (or acute injury) is associated with both short- and long-term benefits. It is a well-established fact that patients who undergo cesarean section under epidural analgesia request less postoperative pain medication in the following three days compared with those who receive general anesthesia. We also know that when patients are given the opportunity to control their pain medications after surgery, they do better. For example, those who self-administer pain medications intravenously with a programmable pump (patient-controlled analgesia, or PCA pump) report less pain and greater satisfaction with their pain management, compared with those who receive the same drug on an as-needed or "prn" schedule (i.e., medications administered by the nurse upon complaint of pain by the patient). In addition, they are usually discharged earlier from the hospital.

Over 23 million operations are performed in the United States each year. Unfortunately, more than half of postoperative patients will suffer from unrelieved pain due to undermedication. We hope you will not be one of them. Remember, you have the *right* to adequate pain control. Inadequate treatment of acute pain increases your chances of developing chronic pain. Talk to your doctor before surgery to allay your concerns about pain control. If he or she does not promise to effectively address the pain to your satisfaction, find a more enlightened and compassionate doctor who will.

Chronic Pain

Chronic pain has been defined in a number of ways. Some have defined it as *pain that persists beyond six months in duration*. A better definition is pain that persists beyond tissue healing. Unlike acute pain, chronic pain is *not* a normal protective mechanism and does *not* correlate with the degree of tissue damage. Furthermore, it does *not* diminish in intensity as healing progresses and does *not* serve a useful protective purpose. Chronic pain is *not* acute pain that has lasted a long time.

Despite these facts, chronic pain is too often treated as if it *were* the result of ongoing tissue damage, as if the healing process were *still* under way, as if it *will* diminish as healing progresses, as if it *does* provide a protective purpose, and as if it *were* just like acute pain that has simply lasted for a longer period. The unfortunate result is that treatment based upon these erroneous assumptions actually can contribute to one's progression toward increased pain and suffering!

Chronic Pain Syndrome

While acute and chronic pain primarily represent conditions of the body, chronic pain *syndrome* encompasses the effects of chronic pain upon the sufferer and the environment in which he or she lives. Hence, chronic pain syndrome is less a medical disease than an intertwined cluster of changes in psychological, social, and occupational functioning, resulting from chronic pain and, often, its treatment.

If you think about the suffering experienced by those with chronic pain conditions, you may wonder how much is due to physical pain and how much is a result of the impact of the pain on their lives. Imagine a person with chronic, unrelenting pain who is nonetheless able to succeed in his or her roles as spouse, parent, church member, volunteer, employee, breadwinner, taxpayer, and active community member. In other words, nothing has changed in his or her ability to function in the world. Overall, how much is this person suffering? Now contrast this scenario with another person with the same degree of physical pain but who has lost his or her ability to function in all of these areas. While both suffer from the same amount of physical pain, the latter clearly has a more pronounced case of chronic pain syndrome. As in our previous example of Ron, the nurse with back pain, suffering advanced from that attributable to physical pain to that stemming from the loss of identity in the many life roles he once enjoyed.

As you can see, such losses, superimposed upon preexisting physical pain, lead to a further loss of contact with sources of positive reinforcement, that is, the good things in life. This starts to feel like being in solitary confinement. What happens to a human being when he or she is cut off from the positive aspects of life? Profound sadness, depression, anxiety, irritability, hopelessness, and withdrawal are likely to set in. These are normal human reactions to such limiting life circumstances. Hence, suffering takes on a whole new, more aggressive dimension.

There is a great deal of confusion when it comes to treating individuals suffering from chronic pain syndrome. Probably 95% of the effort goes toward treating the physical pain, while the chronic pain syndrome is largely ignored. If you have elements of chronic pain syndrome and have undergone more kinds of treatment than you care to remember, consider how much of it was oriented toward pain reduction. Probably most, if not all, of it. If your pain was relieved and you are able to function better as a result, then your particular treatment was successful and appropriate. But if you have had many types of interventions and received little in the way of pain relief and/or an improvement in your ability to function, you have probably been treated for the wrong thing.

The fact is that the healthcare system equates treatment of chronic pain syndrome with interventions that potentially yield pain reduction. Spinal surgery, spinal cord stimulators, implanted narcotic pumps, and nerve blocks are all examples of such interventions. Unfortunately, these invasive procedures have a higher failure rate than we would like to think. Not everyone obtains significant and lasting pain relief. And even if they do, it does not ensure that they will subsequently function any better.

What is the reason for the failure? The answer is often tragically simple: Doctors are not asking themselves what, other than physical pain, might account for the patient's suffering and debilitation. Recall our friend Ron, who had chronic back pain and lost his capacity to participate in almost all of the activities he previously enjoyed. In all likelihood, even a 25% reduction in physical pain would not yield a corresponding reduction in overall suffering if attention were not also paid to helping him function better. Yet, physicians and patients and their families are often bewildered when procedures designed to achieve pain reduction fail to relieve suffering. The reason suffering goes unrelieved despite the doctor hitting a bull's-eye in his or her treatment is that *the intervention is too often aimed at the wrong target*! The unfortunate result is that the patient, not the doctor, frequently is blamed for the treatment failure. We have heard such false accusations time and again. What is needed is for our healthcare system — from doctors to insurance companies to patients themselves — to take aim not only at chronic pain but chronic pain *syndrome* as well.

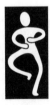

3

Anatomy of Pain 101

James, a 44-year-old carpenter, woke up one morning with severe right shoulder pain. He had been working for months on a crew building residential homes and had noticed mild, then progressive, shoulder pain as the weeks passed. That was before he fell off a ladder and landed on his right side. The pain was so unbearable at that point that he could hardly get up off the ground. Never one to complain, James did his level best to work the remainder of the shift. Since then, excruciating pain has been his constant companion. As much as James hated to go to the doctor, he finally decided to, as much to rid himself of the constant nagging of his adoring wife, Dora, as to seek relief from the pain. He got into his car and headed down the road to Dr. Dille's office, gnashing his teeth under his breath. "Oh! My aching shoulder," he thought. "I don't have time for injuries and pain. I have houses to build."

When James arrived, the receptionist handed him the usual forms to complete. Given the fact that he was right dominant, this task, naturally, required the use of his right hand. Every blank he filled in reminded him of the reason for this office visit. Then he sat impatiently in the waiting room. After what seemed to be an interminable length of time, he at last heard his name called. With great difficulty, James arose from his chair, supporting his right arm with his left. Slowly and carefully, he followed the nurse into the exam room. At her direction, he took off his shirt and changed into a blue gown, grunting and groaning as he did so. Just as he finished, Doctor Dille entered the room and extended his hand in welcome. James tried to do likewise, but the shoulder pain was unbearable. Instead, he smiled weakly and said, "Sorry. I'm an injured worker."

Dr. Dille didn't smile back. He proceeded to take a history and to perform a physical examination. Then he said, "It's possible that you are experiencing shoulder pain because your shoulder is fractured (broken) or dislocated (out of the joint). That was a pretty tough fall you took. Let's start by getting an X-ray." Dr. Dille wrote out an order for the X-ray and handed it to James.

"Do you know which radiology group is on your plan?" asked Dr. Dille.

"No, I don't. I've never thought about it," replied James, wincing with pain.

"Well, you'll have to check," replied Dr. Dille. "We can't keep track of all the insurance plans, HMOs, and PPOs. There are over 75 in this area, all with restrictive provider lists. We have already had to triple our staff to keep up with the requirement that we obtain approval for office visits, tests, and procedures. It's the responsibility of the patient to know the names of the various providers on his or her plan. If the patient doesn't want to assume this responsibility, he or she can find another doctor. You'll have to check your provider book or call your claims adjuster for assistance."

James was in no mood for a delay in treatment. He hurt like crazy. Unfortunately, he had no idea where on God's green earth his provider book was as he had never once needed it during his three years of employment with the company. It was, no doubt, collecting dust somewhere. But where? That was the question of the hour. Could be at home in the desk. Could be on the bookcase. Could be under the bed. Could be in the trunk of the car or in the glove compartment. Could be anywhere. James was in no condition to search, so he decided to call the number on his membership card. Fortunately, the card was in his wallet. He took the telephone receiver off the hook and laid it down on the counter. Then he dialed the number with his left hand. Seconds later, he heard a recorded voice say, "Your call is important to us. All representatives are busy. Please stay on the line and we'll be with you in just a moment."

James waited and waited. Ten minutes went by and still no representative. The pain in his shoulder was sharp and stabbing. James began to sweat. Agitated, he paced the short length of the telephone cord. Back and forth. Back and forth. At long last, a female voice came on the line.

"Yes. How may I help you?"

James provided a brief explanation regarding his shoulder pain. Then he asked what radiology group was approved by the plan.

"Tropicana Radiology," she replied.

"But that's all the way over on the other side of town," James protested. "It's a 30-minute drive, and I'm in pain. Why can't I go to Sunkist Radiology? It's right down the street in that orange building."

"Sorry sir," said the representative. "Sunkist is not on the plan. If you are unhappy with the selection, you may file a formal complaint. Have a nice day."

Beaten to a pulp (sorry), he peeled out (totally unintentional — we swear) of the parking lot and made the trip across town. Three miserable hours later, James was back in the doctor's office with the X-rays in hand. Dr. Dille held them up to the view box.

"Well, the good news is that you don't have a fracture or dislocation. But I do see signs of degenerative arthritis."

"Degenerative what?" asked James, with a confused look on his face.

"Degenerative arthritis. *Arthritis* means inflammation of the joint. There are many different types of arthritis. The type you have is the most common. It is called osteoarthritis and is characterized by progressive loss of irreplaceable cartilage."

"What is cartilage?"

"*Cartilage* is a part of the skeletal system that is softer than bone. It covers the ends of bones where they come together to form joints. Since cartilage itself has no nerve supply, it is insensitive to pain. But as the cartilage is lost, the joint space between the two bones is diminished and the joint works less efficiently. Over time, joint enlargement, pain, stiffness, and limitation of movement occur."

"I see," said James, scratching his head with his left hand.

"I also see evidence of calcific tendonitis of the supraspinatous muscle," said Dr. Dille as he studied the X-ray.

"What does that mean?" asked James with a bewildered look. "It's Greek to me."

"Let me explain," said Dr. Dille. "*Tendons* are tough fibrous bands that attach muscles to bones. Tendonitis means inflammation of the tendon. The term calcific tendonitis means that calcium had been deposited. It indicates that the process is chronic rather than acute. And yet we know that you are experiencing acute pain."

"Great," said James. "Just what I wanted to hear."

"Another possibility," Dr. Dille went on, "is a bursitis."

"Another Greek word. What's a bursitis?" asked James.

"Well, *bursae* are fluid-filled sacs found in and around joints. Their job is to lubricate the space between tendons and bones and tendons and ligaments, thereby reducing friction. Bursae, like tendons, can become inflamed. This condition is called bursitis."

"I see," said James. "It's all becoming clear to me now. My shoulder pain could be caused by a fracture of the bone, a dislocation of the joint (where any two bones meet), arthritis (inflammation of a joint), tendonitis (inflammation of the tendon), or bursitis (inflammation of the bursae). Any other possibilities, Doc?"

"Sure. Lots of them. You could have a sprain."

"You mean like a sprained ankle or something?"

"Yes. A *sprain* is a sudden twist or wrench of a joint with stretching or tearing of the ligaments. The signs of a sprain are swelling, discoloration, disability, joint instability, and pain."

"Sounds like you're describing my shoulder."

"It does, doesn't it."

"So, what's a ligament?"

Dr. Dille paused for a moment and pondered the question. Then he said, "You've heard the song 'the hipbone's connected to the thighbone'?"

"Sure. But what's that got to do with my aching shoulder?"

"Well, the way 'the hipbone's connected to the [pause] thighbone' is by ligaments. And the way 'the shoulder bone's connected to the [pause] arm bone' is also by ligaments. *Ligaments* are dense bands of connective tissue that connect one bone to another. They may serve to either facilitate or restrict the motion of a joint. Some ligaments have pain receptors and, as such, may be a potential source of pain, while others do not."

"This is a real medical education. I've never had a doctor teach me so much."

"Well, that's because the reading audience of this book wants to learn something too. Just think, James, your aching shoulder is benefiting millions."

"Oh!" replied James. "I didn't notice all those readers when I came in. Hi everyone."

"Anyway, you could have a sprain or tear of the ligaments," continued Dr. Dille. "You could also have a strain of the muscles of the shoulder."

"Uh-huh."

"A *strain* is an irritation, slight swelling, or microscopic tearing of muscles. Skeletal muscle is composed of contractile fibers that cause movement of body parts. The unique characteristic of muscle is its ability to shorten or contract. The biceps muscle, for example, contracts and shortens, resulting in flexion of the elbow. Muscles are composed of thousands of individual muscle fibers. When these fibers are strained or torn, pain results. Speaking of muscles, we may have to get an MRI of your shoulder to rule out rotator cuff tear or rupture."

"What's that?"

"The rotator cuff includes four key muscles that support the shoulder joint: the supraspinatous, infraspinatous, subscapularis, and teres minor."

"The teres minor. Yes, of course."

"These muscles can be injured slowly over time from repetitive use or can be injured acutely. The supraspinatous is the one most frequently affected. In a rupture of the rotator cuff, active abduction of the shoulder and rotation are markedly limited, while passive range of motion is full. The best way to determine whether the rotator cuff is causing your shoulder pain is to order an MRI."

"Whatever you say, Doc."

"Another possibility is that you are experiencing referred pain, although I doubt it based on your history. In other words, the pain experienced in the shoulder is due to pathology somewhere else in the body. The shoulder is a common site of pain referral from cervical (neck), intrathoracic (chest), and diaphragmatic lesions."

"Really? I never thought of that," said James.

"Ever have any neck problems?" asked Dr. Dille.

"Why do you ask?"

"Because shoulder pain can actually result from pathology in the neck. That's one type of referred pain. If, for example, you had a herniated disc of the cervical spine that put pressure on the C5–6 nerve root which innervates the muscles of the shoulder and gives rise to the suprascapular nerve which supplies the sensation to the shoulder joint, shoulder pain could result."

"Interesting. Very interesting."

"Although neck pain may radiate to the shoulder, it is typically brought on by neck motion, not shoulder motion, and is not affected by shoulder position."

"Is that so? Well, I'll be."

"James, you said you had a history of gallbladder disease. Right?"

"Doc, I'm here about my shoulder, not my gut!"

"Well, James, did you know that inflammation of your gallbladder can cause shoulder pain?"

"Yeah, right," mumbled James, rolling his eyes.

"No, I'm serious. You have several of the five F's for gallbladder disease. While you are obviously not female, you are in your forties, fat, fertile, and flatulent. All are risk factors associated with gallbladder disease."

"Gee, thanks, Doc."

"Any clay-colored stool?"

"Well, now that you mention it."

James and Dr. Dille continued their briefing session regarding possible causes of the shoulder pain for another 15 minutes. Then, Dr. Dille prescribed a nonsteroidal anti-inflammatory medication and a short course of physical therapy. James was advised not to return to work for several weeks. Fortunately for James, he fully recovered and was able to return to his beloved vocation. But unfortunately for Dr. Dille, his predilection for taking the time required to educate his patients was "rewarded" with a terse termination letter from the HMO. You see, he was spending "excessive" time with his patients. This was "inefficient" and simply not "cost effective." For Dr. Dille, there was no appeal process, no recourse; there was nothing he could do. He had to accept this bitter pill. Now, Dr. Dille is working for James as a carpenter's apprentice.

The Anatomy of Pain: A Quick Tour

The sources of chronic pain are too numerous to count. Name a body part, any body part, and as long as there are pain receptors in that site, there is the potential for acute as well as chronic pain. Pain receptors are found in the head, neck, torso, arms, hands, legs, and feet. They are located in the skin, teeth, bones, joints, muscles, nerves, tendons, ligaments, bursa, blood vessels, and internal organs such as the heart and the appendix.

Perhaps it would be easier to list body parts that are not potential sites of chronic pain. Anyone who has had a haircut can attest to the fact that no physical pain occurs during the process (although our respective toddlers might disagree). And even those of us who are not nail biters know through personal experience that fingernails do not hurt when you bite them. But many people are surprised to learn that the brain itself is practically devoid of pain receptors. Only the meningeal blood vessels supplying the outermost cortical layer of the brain contain pain-sensitive nerve fibers. Stick a needle directly into the brain tissue of a smiling individual and he or she will keep right on smiling (well, maybe). No report of pain will be proffered as a result of the needlestick.

Equally surprising is the little known fact that the infamous intervertebral disc, a structure located between two vertebrae of the spine, is essentially without sensation with the exception of the very outermost layer. "No," you say, "couldn't be. I've been hearing about ruptured discs all my life and I've been told repeatedly that it hurts big time."

While it is true that herniated discs are associated with severe pain, it is not because of the disc itself. Rather, it is the result of the pressure that the ruptured disc places on nearby pain-sensitive structures and the release of chemicals that sets up a localized inflammatory response.

Well, enough about structures in the body that don't hurt. What about the structures that do? Let's begin by discussing one of the more infamous sources of pain and discomfort: the spine. While the purpose of this book is to address general features and characteristics of chronic pain rather than to cover details of specific pain syndromes, a discussion of the anatomy and physiology of this notorious culprit will be instructive and will shed light on the complexities of pain problems overall.

The Spine

The spine is a magnificent piece of machinery with multiple interconnecting parts. It is a system composed of bones, discs, muscles, ligaments, and nerves. This complex architectural masterpiece must be very strong in order to support the human body. At the same time, it also must be extremely flexible, allowing for rotation and bending. A built-in lubrication system is necessary in order to assure smooth functioning of its many components (we don't want squeaks and catches). The spine must be able to withstand bouncing and jostling, which is the task of shock-absorbing discs that are sandwiched between the many bony building blocks of the spine. In addition, the spine is wired with an integrated intercom system so that messages can be sent to and received from the brain to assure coordinated operation.

The individual bones of the spine are called *vertebrae*. These vertebrae vary in size and other characteristics at different levels of the spine. The size of the vertebral bodies increases as one descends down the spinal column because of the increasing weights and stresses borne by successive segments. As an example, the cervical vertebrae of the neck are smaller than the lumbar vertebrae because their job is to support the weight of the head. The task of the lumbar vertebrae, on the other hand, is to support not only the head but also the entire torso. There-fore, greater size is necessary.

Shaped like drums, vertebrae have flat surfaces on the top and bottom. They are stacked on top of each other to form the spinal column. What is known as the "functional spinal unit" is composed of two adjacent vertebrae and their associated ligaments, muscles, and discs. The ante-rior (forward) portion of this functional unit is essentially a weight-bearing, shock-absorbing structure. The posterior (rear) portion, on the other hand, is a nonweight-bearing structure. It is called the neural arch and forms the outer walls of the spinal canal, which houses the all-important *spinal cord,* the main highway that transports messages back and forth between the body and the brain. The various bony pro-jections of the neural arch serve as levers for the muscles and liga-ments attached to them. In addition, paired *facet joints* at the rear of each vertebra act as hinges. These facet joints lie in the vertical plane and restrict rotation and lateral (sideways) flexion of the spine while allowing flexion and extension. As helpful as these joints are, they can be every bit as troublesome because they are potentially subject to a whole host of arthritic conditions. Part of their lining is composed of *synovium,* a very sensitive tissue that lubricates and nourishes the joints. The synovium, however, can become inflamed and irritated, caus-ing severe back pain.

From the base of the skull to the tip of the tailbone are 33 vertebrae contained in five regions. The upper three regions are mobile, provid-ing flexibility for the spine, whereas the lower two regions are fixed or fused, providing stability for the spine.

The upper region, the neck, is called the *cervical spine.* In all, there are seven cervical vertebrae designated, from top down, C1 (C is for cervi-cal), C2, C3, and so on to C7. The cervical vertebrae can be readily distinguished by their small size relative to the vertebrae of other re-gions and by the fact that there is a hole (foramen) in their transverse processes, which are winglike projections that extend sideways. Through these holes, the vertebral artery travels on its way to supplying blood, nutrients, and oxygen to a large portion of the spinal cord, the brain stem, and the posterior part of the brain. This is the key reason why many medical doctors fear spinal manipulation of the cervical spine because of the theoretical possibility of causing a stroke or quadriplegia in a patient with an unstable or severely arthritic spine.

Of the seven cervical vertebrae, the first two are decidedly unique. The first cervical vertebra is called the atlas, named after the mythical giant who carried the earth on his shoulders. Likewise, the cervical atlas supports the "globe" of the skull. For starters, the atlas is distinguished by the absence of a vertebral body. Rather, it consists of a ring with rudimentary projections that connect with other structures. Above, the atlas articulates (joins) with the occiput, that is, base of the skull, while below, it articulates with the second cervical vertebra, the axis. In fact, the atlas rotates about the odontoid process, a toothlike projection that extends upward from the body of the axis through the ring of the atlas. In essence, the odontoid process is the pivot about which the atlas and skull rotate.

The second region is the upper back and is called the *thoracic spine*. There are 12 thoracic vertebrae. The first thoracic vertebra, T1, is located just below C7. The thoracic vertebrae are numbered, from top down, T1 to T12. The distinguishing feature of the thoracic vertebrae is that ribs are attached to all 12 of them. In addition, the upper ribs articulate with the breastplate (sternum) in the front of the torso, which has a stabilizing effect on the upper back, allowing for much less mobility compared to the neck and low-back area.

The third region is the lower back or *lumbar spine*. There are five lumbar vertebrae, predictably numbered L1 at the top, located just below T12, down to L5. The lumbar vertebrae are more massive and heavy relative to the other vertebrae and are designed to bear weight.

The fourth region of the spine is the *sacrum,* a triangular bone which forms the back of the pelvis. The joint where the sacrum joins the [pause] hipbones (…sorry) is called the sacroiliac joint. Like the facet joints, this is a synovial joint, which has an exquisitely pain-sensitive membrane that is susceptible to inflammation and irritation. It can therefore be affected by any kind of arthritis and can be the source of significant pain. Prior to birth, the sacrum is composed of five individual vertebrae, but by the time of birth, those five bones have fused into a single bone.

The final region of the spine is the *coccyx* (pronounced "cock-six"), which is Latin for cuckoo, since it resembles a cuckoo's bill. The coccyx is the tailbone. Like the sacrum, the coccyx contains four or five vertebrae that are fused.

Intervertebral Discs

The intervertebral disc is a spongy, oval-shaped cushion sandwiched between two vertebrae of the spine. Its primary purpose in life is to function as a shock absorber. The disc is composed of three parts: the nucleus pulposus, the annulus fibrosus, and cartilaginous end plates. The nucleus pulposus is a gelatinous substance located in the center of the disc that is encased in the tougher, outer annulus fibrosus. The nucleus contains up to 88% water, although the percentage decreases over the course of a lifetime. The intervertebral discs constitute about 25% of the length of the vertebral column above the sacrum. Progressive dehydration accounts for the loss of height most individuals undergo between youth and old age. As the discs degenerate, the facet joints become more tightly joined and can be a source of pain due to increased friction. The end plates of a disc consist primarily of cartilage and serve as a transition zone between the bony vertebral bodies and the other components of the disc.

The intervertebral discs are reinforced by the anterior and posterior longitudinal ligaments that run the length of the spinal column. These ligaments adhere to the cortex of the vertebral body and essentially comprise the outer layer of the annular fibers of the disc. The posterior longitudinal ligament is broad in the cervical region but tapers as it descends the spinal column. At the level of the lumbar spine, it is only half its original size and thereby provides less support and stability to the disc. This is one of the main reasons that discs of the lumbar spine most commonly herniate in a posterolateral direction.

While most vertebrae are separated by discs, there are important exceptions. There is no disc between the first and second cervical vertebrae, that is, between the atlas and the axis. The first disc of the spine is between C2 and C3. The last normal disc of the spine is between L5 and S1. The fused vertebrae of the sacrum contain no discs; nor do the fused vertebrae of the coccyx. However, there is a small, rudimentary disc connecting the sacrum and the coccyx.

Muscles of the Spine

The back muscles are complex. While there are well over 100, they can be divided into two main groups: the extensors and the flexors. The *extensors* (also known as the erector spinae muscles) hold the spine erect. They can also cause the spine to return to an erect position after bending over. These muscles attach to the back part of the spinal column. Each individual extensor muscle is relatively short and spans only two to three vertebrae.

The *flexor muscles* are in front of the spine. The major players are the abdominal and iliopsoas muscles. The abdominal muscles are crucial in providing spinal stability. They allow us to bend over but also play a significant role in lifting because they control the amount of spinal curvature. The iliopsoas muscles begin in front of the lumbar spine, traverse the hip joint, and insert on the thigh bone (femur). Their main job is to move the legs forward and to support the spine.

All of these muscles are covered with a specialized fibrous tissue called *fascia*. It is the belief of some that fascia may be a key source of back pain. In fact, surgeons in Japan have performed fasciectomies (removal of part of the fascia) with the hope and intention of alleviating back pain. So far, the procedure has not caught on in the United States.

Ligaments of the Spine

Most people know that "the hipbone's connected to the [pause] thighbone," but did you know that the backbone is connected to the [pause] backbone? (Feel free to sing along!) Just how does this wondrous fact occur, you may ask. The answer is by ligaments. Each vertebra is connected to the next by several ligaments. Ligaments are composed of tough fibrous tissue that connects bone to bone. A joint is found where any two bones meet. Ligaments may serve to either facilitate or restrict the motion of a joint. Some ligaments have pain receptors and as such may be potential sources of pain. Other ligaments are devoid of such pain receptors and therefore cannot function as pain generators.

We have already talked about the pain-sensitive anterior and posterior longitudinal ligaments which run the length of the vertebral column, adhere to the cortex of the vertebral body, and compose the outer layer of the annular fibers of the disc. Among the many other ligaments connecting vertebra to vertebra is the ligamentum flavum, which connects the laminae of adjacent vertebrae. This ligament has no nerve supply and is insensitive to noxious stimuli. On the other hand, the intertransverse ligaments, which connect the transverse processes, and the supraspinal and interspinal ligaments, which connect the spinous processes of adjacent vertebrae, are pain sensitive.

Innervation of the Spine

Nerves are the bane of those who suffer from back pain. If it weren't for those pesky nerves, there wouldn't be any pain whatsoever. But the other side of the coin is that if there were no nerves, no one would have much fun. There would be no walks in the summer rain. No overindulging on pralines-and-cream. And, of course, no hugs and kisses. Bummer.

In any event, the *nervous system* is comprised of the central and peripheral nervous systems. The central nervous system includes the brain and the spinal cord. The peripheral nervous system, in contrast, includes all neural tissue outside the brain and spinal cord. The *spinal cord* can be thought of as an extension of the brain. It enters the cervical spine from above through an opening called the foramen magnum and terminates below at the level of the first lumbar vertebra. Below the cord, the lumbar and sacral nerve roots continue within the arachnoid space and are called the cauda equina, or horse's tail (not to be confused with the other hindmost portion of a horse).

If you think of the spinal cord as a tree trunk, the nerve root is the first branch off the trunk. The anterior and posterior nerve roots emerge through an opening in the spinal canal called the intervertebral foramen and then unite almost immediately to form the spinal nerve. In all, there are 31 pairs of spinal nerves. These nerves are named and numbered according to the region of the vertebral spinal column with which they are associated. Shortly after the spinal nerves exit the spinal canal, they give off a branch called the *recurrent meningeal nerve,* also known as the recurrent nerve of von Luschka. This nerve innervates many pain-sensitive structures, including the meninges and their blood vessels, the dural sac of the nerve roots, the anterior and posterior longitudinal ligaments, and the outermost layer of the intervertebral disc. Then the spinal nerves divide into the anterior and posterior primary rami, which contain nerve fibers from both the anterior and posterior nerve roots as well as sympathetic fibers. The *anterior rami* supply the front and sides of the neck and trunk as well as the arms and legs. The *posterior rami,* on the other hand, supply the back of the neck and trunk. They divide into the cutaneous branch (to the skin), the muscular branch, and the articular branch. The latter supplies the facet joints.

Finally, there are unmyelinated sensory nerve endings within the supraspinous, interspinous, and longitudinal ligaments; the capsules of the facets; the lumbar fascia; and the erector spinae muscles. All of these tissues are potential sources of pain.

The Nervous System: The Transmitter of Pain

Imagine that you are a carpenter putting in a hard day's work building a house. You've swung that hammer a hundred thousand times before and hit the nail on the head with the precision of a surgeon. You are an expert tradesman and you know it. You hold that nail between your index finger and thumb as you raise the hammer one more time. Then you bring the hammer down with force. Tragically, you miss the mark. Instead of the crisp sound of the hammer on the head of the nail, you hear the dull thump of the hammer on your very own thumb. You let out a yelp but try to withhold the expletives that rapidly are coming to mind. The pain in your thumb is excruciating, and instinctively you begin to rub it. The diagram on the next page presents a schematic representation of what happens in the nervous system while this is going on.

Pain Receptors

Pain receptors, also known as *nociceptors,* are free nerve endings that detect tissue damage caused by injury, disease, or inflammation. The tissue damage results in the release of endogenous chemicals or pain-producing substances into the extracellular fluid around these pain receptors. These pain-producing substances include potassium and hydrogen ions, prostaglandins, bradykinin, histamine, serotonin, substance P, and many others. They all have a direct excitatory action on the membrane of the nociceptor, which converts mechanical, thermal, and chemical energy into electrical signals that are then transmitted to the spinal cord via nerve fibers.

There are basically three kinds of pain receptors. The first responds only to a great force, such as the hammer blow to your thumb. The second responds only to heat. The third responds to varying degrees of pressure, heat, and chemical changes and is called the "wide dynamic range" nociceptor.

The heat pain receptors and the wide-dynamic-range pain receptors can become sensitized, or irritated, following burns or nerve injuries, as the damaged nerve resprouts and regrows. As a result of sensitization, these receptors may send a pain signal in response to benign stimuli such as a light touch. This may play a significant role in the development of chronic pain.

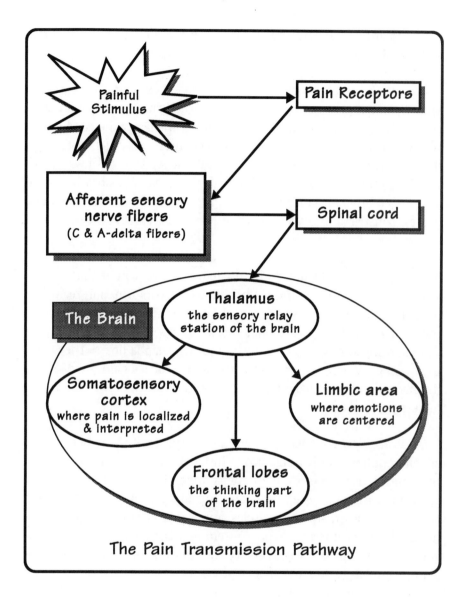

The Pain Transmission Pathway

Nerves

Nerves are bundles of nerve fibers that lie outside the central nervous system, that is, the brain and spinal cord. These nerves connect the various parts of the body with the central nervous system. Nerves are like two-lane highways. They carry information from the body parts to the brain and spinal cord and also transmit instructions from the brain and spinal cord back to those same body parts.

There are three categories of nerve fibers — *A, B,* and *C* — based on fiber diameter, presence or absence of a myelin sheath, and conduction velocity. In general, the larger the diameter, the faster the conduction. In addition, fibers that are myelinated carry messages much faster than those that are not. The myelin sheath is produced by the Schwann cell, which is found in close association with the nerve. The sheath is composed of a fatty substance that wraps around the nerve. In peripheral nerves, constrictions, called nodes of Ranvier, separate successive myelin segments.

A fibers are large diameter, myelinated, and fast conducting. Of the four subgroups, *A-alpha fibers* transmit sensory information regarding proprioception (joint position sense) and vibration at an approximate speed of 60 meters per second. *A-delta fibers* are relatively smaller diameter, myelinated fibers compared to the A-alpha fibers. They carry the message of temperature and sharp, well-localized pain — again like the hammer blow to your thumb — but at a much slower rate of 20 meters per second.

B fibers are slow conducting, myelinated, and small in diameter. They are efferent fibers, only transmitting instructions in one direction, from the central nervous system to the autonomic nervous system. The autonomic nervous system regulates involuntary bodily functions and controls the heart, smooth muscles, and glands. There are two components: the sympathetic nervous system and the parasympathetic nervous system. The B fibers regulate the preganglionic sympathetic fibers. Stimulation of these fibers produces vasoconstriction of blood vessels, a rise in blood pressure, an increase in heart rate, dilation of the pupils of the eyes, a slowing of the gastrointestinal tract, and erection of the hairs, commonly known as goose bumps. This may occur when an individual is frightened, stressed, or in pain.

Finally, *C fibers* are the smallest, unmyelinated, and slowest conducting of all the nerve fibers. Like the A-delta fibers, C fibers transmit information regarding temperature and pain. However, unlike the sharp, well-localized pain transmitted by the A-delta fibers, C fibers carry the message of aching, burning, poorly localized pain very slowly, at a rate of only two meters per second.

Both the A-delta and C fibers are nociceptive fibers. They carry the message of injury and pain from the pain receptor to the entry zone of the spinal cord, the dorsal horn. Here, they synapse, or connect, with interneurons of the substantia gelatinosa before ascending to the brain.

Central Nervous System: The Spinal Cord and Brain

The spinal cord and the brain are known as the central nervous system. The entry zone of the central nervous system is the dorsal horn of the spinal cord. Here, nerves carrying messages from various body parts synapse, or connect, with the next group of nerve fibers. This second set of nerve fibers, in turn, carries the signal up through the spinal cord to the brain. In effect, they pass the baton.

There are two main "roads" (or ascending pathways) within the spinal cord by which pain signals may travel to the brain: the *paleospino-thalamic tract* and the *neospinothalamic tract*. The prefix *paleo* means old, and the term *spinothalamic* indicates that the message is carried from the spine to the part of the brain called the thalamus. Sound logical? It is. Seem simple? Well, maybe not. The fibers that comprise this older pathway make many connections along the way and transmit messages relatively slowly. Like those conducted by C fibers, pain signals that travel along the paleospinothalamic tract are perceived as being deep, aching, burning, and poorly localized.

The other main "road" by which pain signals travel within the spinal cord is the *neo-* or *new spinothalamic tract*. In contrast to the paleo-spinothalamic tract, there are fewer connections made along the way, and pain messages are transmitted much faster and far more efficiently. Like the pain signals that are conducted by the A-delta fibers, pain signals that travel via the neospinothalamic tract are perceived as being sharp, intense, and well localized. Like the carpenter's injured thumb, you can pinpoint where it hurts.

About 80% of pain messages cross over from one side of the spinal cord to the other as they travel toward the brain. Many connections are made with various body parts all along the road. At the dorsal horn, for example, a message is sent to muscles causing them to contract, or tighten, in order to protect the individual from further injury. Other signals sent along the way cause the heart to beat faster, the blood pressure and respiratory rate to increase, stress hormones such as epinephrine to be released, and the blood glucose to rise. These are typical responses to painful stimuli and are automatic. We don't have to think about making any of this happen.

The pain signals carried by the spinal cord tracts arrive at a particular part of the brain called the *thalamus*. The thalamus is essentially the sensory relay station. From here, connections are made with various other parts of the brain, including:

- ♦ The *somatosensory cortex,* where pain signals are localized and interpreted

- ♦ The *frontal lobe,* where most of our thinking takes place

- ♦ The *limbic area,* where our emotions are centered

Thanks to the limbic system, pain signals have an emotional component in addition to the purely physical sensation of pain. This can significantly increase the degree of suffering an individual experiences. It is our limbic system that tells us that pain sucks. In response to this sensory input, the thalamus and brain stem send modulating signals back down the spinal cord to the dorsal horn, which suppress the input of pain signals emanating from the site of injury or irritation.

The Gate Control Theory of Pain

In 1965, Drs. Ronald Melzack and Patrick Wall introduced the *Gate Control Theory* of pain in an attempt to explain the mechanism by which a sensory-overloaded pathway to the brain will selectively eliminate or dampen the transmission of pain signals. This theory conceptualized a finite-sized sensory "gate" to the central nervous system located in the dorsal horn of the spinal cord. Theoretically, if this gate is flooded with other types of sensation, it will reach capacity and will be unable to accommodate additional sensory input. As a result, further pain input will be blocked.

The interneurons of the substantia gelatinosa, found within the dorsal horn, regulate the position of the gate. The degree to which the gate is open or closed is determined by the balance between large A-fiber input and the small A-delta and C-fiber input to the central nervous system. Supposedly, large fiber input inhibits or closes the gate, while the small fiber input facilitates or opens the gate for the spinal transmission of pain. The idea is that hyperstimulation of the nervous system can potentially drown out pain. For example, after the carpenter hit his thumb with the hammer, he rubbed it, thus applying pressure in the process. This rubbing action stimulates large-diameter, myelinated A-alpha fibers that travel at a speed of approximately 60 meters per second. In contrast, pain travels relatively slowly, at 2 to 20 meters per second. Therefore, the pressure sensation will arrive at the gate first and will preoccupy it. Massage and the application of an ace wrap also stimulate pressure receptors and block pain in a similar manner. The same concept applies when a chiropractor manipulates the spine. This activates receptors of proprioception (i.e., joint position sense), which also travels rapidly via A-alpha fibers, bombarding the gate; in effect, the gate will be kept so busy that the pain messages will not be able to get through as easily.

Pressure, vibration, and proprioception all travel rapidly via large-diameter, myelinated A-alpha fibers along the posterior columns of the spinal cord. Heat and cold, on the other hand, travel on the very same

Opening and Closing the Pain Gate

The balance between large- and small-fiber sensory input to the central nervous system can be tipped in favor of or to the detriment of the pain sufferer. Here's how:

Things that Open the Gate, Leading to More Pain

♦ Negative thoughts
♦ Anxiety
♦ Fear
♦ Depression
♦ Memory of pain
♦ Life situation crises
♦ Stress
♦ Cultural factors (which may also operate in favor of the pain sufferer; some studies show that the expression of pain varies with cultural background)

Things that Close the Gate, Leading to Less Pain

♦ **Cortical and thalamic methods of the brain:** Pain medications, tranquilizers, placebos, endorphins, antidepressants, relaxation techniques, biofeedback, meditation, euphoria, transcutaneous electrical nerve stimulation (TENS) and aerobic exercise (by increasing endorphins), TENS (by working both centrally and peripherally)
♦ **Spinal-cord-level blocking methods:** Dorsal column stimulator, endorphins, tractotomy
♦ **Peripheral blocking methods:** Acupuncture, electrical stimulation (TENS), heat, cold, massage, traction, manipulation, salves and ointments
♦ **Blocking or correcting the source of pain:** Spinal fusion, discectomy, chymopapain, facet neurectomy, nonsteroidal anti-inflammatory medications

pathways as pain, that is, via small, myelinated A-delta fibers and small unmyelinated C fibers along the spinothalamic tract of the spinal cord. Application of heat or cold interrupts transmission of pain along the same pathway.

The position of the gate is also affected by descending signals from the brain. Here's how it works. The injured body part sends a message to the brain via the spinal cord: "Ouch!" The brain registers the sensation, which is then altered by feelings, memories, and attitudes. It then sends signals back down the spinal cord to the gate that either increase or decrease the incoming pain messages. Thus, the factors that are frequently thought of as nonphysical (i.e., emotions, memories, life experiences, previous learning) can impact the amount of pain and suffering we experience. Indeed, mounting research shows that the strong link between our mind and body is indisputable.

If you have made it through this chapter, we congratulate you. You have gained not only a better understanding of the anatomy and physiology of pain, but our respect for your perseverance in learning about such a challenging subject. In the next chapter, we will address the medical work-up as it relates to chronic pain conditions. It is not always done properly, and we want to arm you with information that will protect you against an inadequate evaluation that can lead to erroneous conclusions and improper treatment. Stay tuned.

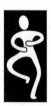

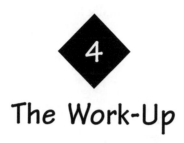

The Work-Up

Chronic Pain and the Evaluation Process

One of the most important precursors to effective chronic pain management is the establishment of an accurate diagnosis. Why is the person hurting? What's causing the pain? We see far too many individuals in our clinic who suffer from "pain of unknown etiology," unknown because someone — namely, the doctor — failed to do the necessary homework or to make the appropriate referral. Consequently, these people receive, at best, a generic treatment program, which can actually serve to make matters worse. We know that the longer a chronic pain syndrome exists, the more entrenched it becomes. Hence, the longer a pain sufferer goes without a proper diagnosis, the more difficult the problem is to treat — now and in the future.

An especially tragic example is the person who contracts shingles and is not diagnosed and treated properly within the first few weeks. A condition called postherpetic neuralgia can develop which carries with it a lifetime of excruciating, burning pain. Proper treatment, administered early on, has been shown to dramatically reduce the incidence of this disabling pain condition. But if the window of opportunity is missed by the doctor or the insurance company, which may balk at authorizing treatment, it is the patient who will potentially pay the high price of this transgression in terms of endless suffering.

We think patients deserve better. To maximize the chances of success, pain management should be tailored to address the individual's unique condition. A proper diagnosis requires a complete work-up. The initial step in this process is a thorough history and physical examination by a qualified physician. This is usually followed by appropriate testing to confirm the working diagnosis and to further elucidate the problem.

History

During the history-taking portion of the evaluation, the doctor listens to the patient's report of subjective symptoms. In the process, the doctor will ask many questions including, but not limited to, the following: Did the pain come on suddenly or gradually? Was the onset associated with trauma? What was the mechanism of injury? Did the patient slip and fall, for example, or was he or she injured while lifting? Where is the pain located? Is the nature of the pain burning, stabbing, numbness, tingling, sharp, shooting, dull, or aching? Does it feel like pins and needles? Does the pain travel down the arms or legs? How intense is the pain? Is it mild, moderate, or severe? Some doctors will ask patients to rate their pain on a scale from 0 (the absence of pain) to 10 (the most intense pain they have ever experienced).

The doctor will also ask how frequently the pain occurs. Is it constant or does it come and go? What makes the pain worse? What makes it better? Is there any weakness associated with the pain? Has the patient lost control of his or her bowel and bladder?

Is sexual function impaired in any way? Has the patient been experiencing any systemic signs of illness, such as fever, chills, sweats, or weight loss? Is there any personal or family history of cancer, especially cancer of the breast, thyroid, prostate, or kidney? Is there a previous history of injury? What tests have been done to evaluate the pain, and what were the results? When did the female patient last have a mammogram and PAP smear? What treatments, including medications, have been tried, and how effective were they?

In addition, the doctor will inquire about emotional and social factors that can be related to the pain experience. How is the patient's mood? Anxious? Depressed? Irritable? Has the patient been subjected to a lot of stressors lately, such as death or illness in the family, divorce, physical or emotional abuse, or financial hardship? How is the patient sleeping? Does the pain awaken him or her at night? Finally, and most important of all, the doctor will ask how the pain has impacted the person's lifestyle and ability to function.

Physical Examination

The doctor usually examines the patient shortly after taking a history. A detailed description of the physical examination is beyond the scope of this book. Briefly, however, the doctor will look, listen, and feel as he or she examines the individual for objective signs that are consistent with the subjective symptoms. Sensation, reflexes, muscle strength, bulk and tone, joint stability and range of motion, gait, and coordination will be assessed. In the case of the patient who comes in with a headache, the sinuses, temporomandibular joints, cranial nerves, and mental functions — such as concentration, memory, and judgment — will also be evaluated.

Lab Work

Analysis of blood and urine samples may render critically important information that can either nail down or rule out a diagnosis. The following table lists some of the more common laboratory tests that may be ordered by a physician to evaluate a patient with pain.

Lab Tests Used to Diagnose Pain Conditions

Test	Description
Alkaline phosphatase	Elevated in fractures, Paget's disease, bony metastasis, and osteomalacia.
Amylase	Elevated in pancreatitis, which can cause both abdominal and back pain.

Lab Tests Used to
Diagnose Pain Conditions (continued)

Test	Description
Antinuclear antibody	Abnormal in systemic lupus erythematosis and various other painful connective tissue diseases.
B12	May be low in peripheral neuropathy and myofascial pain.
Calcium	Elevated in some metabolic disorders such as parathyroidism and certain malignancies such as multiple myeloma. Normal in osteoporosis and osteoarthritis.
Erythrocyte sedimentation rate	Nonspecific lab value that is elevated in inflammation, malignancy, or temporal arteritis (a serious cause of headache associated with visual blurring which can lead to blindness). Normal in osteoarthritis and mechanical low-back pain.
Folate	May be low in peripheral neuropathy and myofascial pain.
Hemoglobin	May be low in malignancies such as multiple myeloma and in rheumatological diseases that cause chronic inflammation. Normal in mechanical back pain, including herniated disc, spinal stenosis, and muscle strain.
HLA-B27	Positive in ankylosing spondylitis.
Lipase	Elevated in pancreatitis, which can cause both abdominal and back pain.
Magnesium	May be low in myofascial pain.
Rheumatoid factor	Elevated in rheumatoid arthritis and a wide spectrum of autoimmune disorders and chronic infectious diseases.
Serum acid phosphatase	Elevated in cancer of the prostate, which can metastasize to the spine and pelvis.
Serum protein electrophoresis	Abnormal in multiple myeloma.

Lab Tests Used to
Diagnose Pain Conditions (continued)

Test	Description
Thyroid function studies	May be abnormal in muscular disorders that present with pain, weakness, and reflex changes.
Uric acid	Elevated in gouty arthritis.
Urinalysis	Used to rule out kidney infection.
White blood cell count	May be elevated in infection and malignancies. Normal in mechanical low-back pain.

X-rays

X-rays (roentgenograms) remain the initial step in the radiologic evaluation of the back. Conventional X-rays use radiation to penetrate body tissues and produce a photographic image. They provide good resolution of the bony structures and alignment but are ineffective in providing a clear image of soft tissues such as muscles, ligaments, and the intervertebral discs. In addition, they do not visualize the contents of the spinal canal, including the spinal cord.

The following diagnoses can be made by X-ray:

1. Fractures and dislocations

2. Arthritis

3. Abnormal curvatures of the spine, such as kyphosis (humpback), lordosis, (swayback), and scoliosis (lateral curvature)

4. Spondylosis (a defect of the facet joint of the vertebrae that can cause spinal instability)

5. Spondylolisthesis (when the defect of the facet joint actually results in the slippage of one vertebral body forward on another)

6. Degenerative disc disease (seen as abnormal narrowing of disc spaces between two vertebrae)

7. Abnormal straightening of the normal curvatures of the cervical (neck) and lumbar (lower back) spine due to muscle spasms such as occur with whiplash injuries

X-rays are relatively inexpensive compared with other imaging studies such as computerized axial tomography and magnetic resonance imaging (MRI) and are readily available in most areas. In addition, they are painless and fairly safe, as they expose patients to only low levels of radiation. However, they may pose risks to the unborn during pregnancy.

Computerized Axial Tomography

Computerized axial tomography (also known as a CAT scan or CT) is a special kind of X-ray that produces three-dimensional pictures of a cross-section of internal structures of the body. It is the method of choice for evaluating bony processes such as spinal stenosis (narrowing of the spinal canal). Unlike the X-ray, CT shows, in addition to bony structures, soft tissues such as ligaments, nerve roots, free fat, and the intervertebral disc. The spinal cord and disc fragments may also be visualized by this method.

While CT is a valuable tool for confirming a diagnosis that is based on a history and physical examination, it should never be used to make a primary diagnosis. Potential pitfalls of making clinical decisions on the basis of CT findings alone have been revealed in recent studies. In one such study, three neuroradiologists evaluated CT scans of 53 normal subjects and 6 with back pain. The physicians agreed in their interpretation only 11% of the time. Also, there was a 30% chance that a patient could undergo unnecessary surgery if the decision was based on the CT alone without consideration of the history and physical examination.

CT is also used to evaluate other body parts, such as the abdomen and the head. An abdominal aortic aneurysm, for example, is a potentially lethal cause of both back and abdominal pain that can be diagnosed by CT. Most patients with severe headaches require either a CT scan or an MRI to rule out structural lesions such as tumor, abscess (localized infection), hydrocephalus (water on the brain), stroke, hemorrhage (the escape of blood from the vessels), subdural hematoma (a localized collection of blood situated below the dura mater, which is the outermost membrane covering the brain and spinal cord), aneurysm (a sac formed by the dilatation of the wall of an artery, a vein, or the heart), and arteriovenous malformation (a tangle of dilated vessels which forms an abnormal communication between the arterial and venous system).

CT can be done on an outpatient basis. Although the patient is exposed to radiation, the test is considered to be relatively safe and painless. However, the patient must lie perfectly still for 30 to 45 minutes on a special table that passes through the center of a large scanning device. This may be difficult and uncomfortable for patients who suffer from back pain. CT scans, like MRIs, are sometimes done with contrast agents (which may sometimes be swallowed or injected, depending on the particular test) to enhance the images.

Magnetic Resonance Imaging

Magnetic resonance imaging (MRI) is the most significant advancement in medical imaging in many years. Unlike CT, MRI does not employ radiation to develop the image. Rather, it uses a magnetic force and a computer to do the job. While the strength of CT as a radiographic technique resides in its superb demonstration of bony detail and spatial relations of anatomic structures, the strength of MRI lies in its outstanding characterization of soft tissue abnormalities and contrast resolution.

MRI is an excellent technique for visualizing bones, nerves and nerve roots, muscles, ligaments, discs, and the brain and spinal cord. It is the procedure of choice for diagnosing joint problems, including meniscal and cruciate ligament injuries of the knee and rotator cuff abnormalities of the shoulder. In addition, bone tumors, bone metastasis (the spread of cancer from another part of the body to the bone), osteomyelitis (bone infection), arachnoiditis (inflammation of the arachnoidea, a delicate membrane covering the brain and spinal cord that is located between two other membranes, the dura mater, which is the outermost membrane, and the pia mater, which is the innermost membrane), and discitis (disc infection) are well demonstrated. Other applications include spinal imaging to rule out compressive radiculopathy, which in most cases is due to a herniated disc. Intravenous administration of a contrast medium (gadolinium triaminepentacetic acid) combined with MRI brings out detail that is helpful in distinguishing between recurrent disc herniation and scar tissue (epidural fibrosis).

An MRI of the head or neck may be ordered to evaluate individuals with headaches. While CT is better than MRI in ruling out hemorrhagic lesions of the brain, MRI is superior in identifying lesions of the pituitary gland, the brain stem, the occipital–cervical (head–neck) junction, and the cervical spine. Furthermore, it is the best test available for diagnosing multiple sclerosis.

There is no special preparation for undergoing MRI. The patient is placed on a scanning table which slides into a large cylindrical structure. About 20% of patients experience feelings of anxiety and claustrophobia while confined to this small space and may require a sedative. Open MRI machines, which are less claustrophobic, are available in some areas. However, they provide poorer resolution of the images obtained, thereby potentially compromising the quality of the study. Throughout the test, the patient will hear both loud humming and thumping sounds. Some facilities provide earphones so that the individual can listen to music in order to mask the noise. Generally, an MRI lasts about 45 to 60 minutes. Like CT, the patient must lie perfectly still during this time. For people who suffer from severe back pain, this is indeed the most difficult part of the procedure.

MRI is considered to be a very safe procedure. So far, minimal risks have been identified. However, it is not known whether it is entirely safe for women in the early stages of pregnancy. Patients who are on life-support systems (metallic machines), have metal clips on intracranial aneurysms, or have cardiac pacemakers are not suitable candidates for MRI. Metal clips may loosen or twist, and pacemakers may revert from a demand mode to a fixed mode of operation. Although nonmagnetic implants such as stainless steel are not attracted to the magnet, they do cause significant distortions in the MRI image obtained.

Myelography

Myelography is performed by first doing a lumbar puncture and then introducing a contrast medium such as Omnipague® into the subarachnoid space. By this means, the spinal cord and nerve roots can be visualized. CT is often done in conjunction with the myelogram to improve diagnostic accuracy.

Myelography may be ordered prior to surgery to localize the exact level of a lesion (e.g., a herniated disc). It is helpful in identifying irregular filling defects and is an important diagnostic tool in arachnoiditis, fusion of nerve roots, absent filling of nerve root sleeves, and constriction or obstruction of the thecal sac.

Possible side effects include headache, nausea, vomiting, and seizures, but it is uncertain whether these occur because of the contrast medium or as a result of the lumbar puncture itself. It is well known that lumbar punctures may cause bleeding in some cases and that bleeding may lead to the development of arachnoiditis. Thus, myelography may not only diagnose arachnoiditis but also actually induce it. The good news is that major complications are rare. Since the development of CT and MRI, myelography is ordered less frequently.

Electrodiagnostic Studies

Electrodiagnostic studies are well-established procedures in the diagnosis of neurological and muscular disorders. They are a direct extension of the neurologic portion of the physical examination.

Electromyography and Nerve Conduction Studies

The electromyography and nerve conduction study (EMG NCS) is performed to determine if there is nerve or muscle damage. It is usually ordered to evaluate patients with objective motor signs, such as weakness or atrophy, and/or subjective sensory symptoms, such as numbness, tingling, or radicular (shooting) pain. While CT and MRI are exceptional tests for identifying anatomic, structural lesions, only the EMG NCS directly assesses the physiological integrity of nerves and muscles.

Electromyogram

During the electromyogram, the physician inserts a small, sterile, disposable needle into selected muscles and records electrical activity. He or she can determine if the muscle is working normally by looking at the waveforms projected on an oscilloscope screen and by listening to the sounds the activity makes over a loudspeaker.

Nerve Conduction Studies

Nerve conduction studies test how well signals travel along a nerve. The test is performed by applying a brief electrical stimulus to one portion of a nerve while recording at another place along the same nerve. Both sensory and motor nerves are evaluated in this manner. The nerve's response to the stimulus is picked up by a recording instrument and is then measured and analyzed by the physician performing the test.

Evoked Potentials

Evoked potentials evaluate the function of nerve pathways that carry signals through the vision, hearing, and spinal cord pathways. Signals are produced in these nerves by applying pulses of light to the eyes, clicking sounds to the ears, or small, brief electrical stimuli to the nerves of the arms or legs. The nerve's response is recorded from surface electrodes placed over the head or the spinal cord.

These tests may be performed to evaluate headache associated with a number of neurological conditions including postconcussive syndrome (brain stem auditory evoked response), visual disturbances (visual evoked response), and sensory symptoms (somatosensory evoked response).

Electroencephalography

Electroencephalography, or EEG, is an electrophysiological test that evaluates the function of the cerebral cortex (the outer layer of the brain responsible for higher mental functions). The test measures electrical activity generated by the cortex and modified by the thalamus (the sensory relay station of the brain) and reticular activating system (the area of the brain stem responsible for level of alertness and consciousness).

The EEG is the key test for the diagnosis and management of seizure disorders. It is also frequently ordered to evaluate a patient who presents with headaches, in particular if they are associated with altered mental states such as confusion, memory impairment, or personality change.

Bone Densitometry

Bone densitometry is a safe, painless radiological technique that assesses the bone density of an individual and compares it to the average value for others of the same age, race, and gender. Osteoporosis is a common metabolic bone disease in which there is a loss of bone mass per unit volume. As a result, the bones become porous and brittle and may therefore fracture easily. This disease is best diagnosed by bone densitometry.

Bone Scan

A bone scan is a painless nuclear imaging study that is very sensitive for the early detection of a variety of bone lesions. A radioactive "tracer" is injected intravenously into the bloodstream. Bones that are undergoing rapid cell growth have increased uptake of this tracer substance, which shows up as a black area called a "hot spot."

Clinical indications for undergoing a bone scan include suspicion of the following:

1. A stress fracture that cannot be detected by plain X-ray

2. Bone metastases

3. Acute osteomyelitis (a bone infection which may not be detectable on plain X-ray for 7 to 10 days)

4. Arthritis

5. Paget's disease (a localized disorder of bone characterized by a remarkable degree of bone resorption and subsequent formation of disorganized and irregular new bone)

6. Osteoid osteoma (a benign skeletal tumor found predominantly in the lower extremities of young males)

7. Heterotopic ossification (bone formation in an abnormal place)

8. Reflex sympathetic dystrophy, or RSD (a syndrome of pain in an extremity that involves overactivity of the sympathetic nervous system and that does not involve a major nerve)

To diagnose some conditions, such as RSD, a three-phase bone scan should be ordered. During the initial phase, a radionuclide angiogram, or flow study, is obtained over the area of concern during the intravenous injection of the tracer. The "blood pool" image of the second phase is obtained immediately after the flow study and displays regional perfusion, including that of soft tissues. The delayed "static" image of the third phase is taken two to three hours after the injection. Active bony abnormality is reflected by increased uptake of the tracer.

The radiation dose given to the patient is relatively low, and because iodinated contrast material is not used, side effects and allergic reactions do not occur.

Discogram

The discogram is very helpful in resolving difficult cases. It is an invasive procedure in which a fine-gauge needle is placed into the disc space, followed by the injection of radiopaque dye. The normal disc accepts about one milliliter of dye, whereas an abnormal disc will accept three milliliters. In the case of an intact disc, no dye will escape and an oval will be seen on X-ray. If the disc is ruptured, however, the dye will be seen leaking out of the disc into the adjoining area.

One of the goals of the discogram is to accurately reproduce the pain experienced by the individual in order to identify the exact source of the problem. This aids the surgeon in deciding whether or not the patient needs surgery, and if so, at what level.

The major risk associated with the discogram is infection. The procedure is performed under sterile conditions to help prevent this complication. If, despite these precautions, an infection does develop, it can be treated with antibiotics.

Ultrasound

Ultrasound is a noninvasive test that evaluates tissues according to their echogenicity, that is, their ability to reflect sound waves. These sound waves are generated by a transducer, bounced off the tissue under study, and returned to a receiver, where an image is created. By this method, fluid can be easily distinguished from solid tissue in the thyroid gland, kidney, and liver, allowing for the differentiation of cysts from tumors. Gallbladder disease can also be evaluated by ultrasound. In addition, the uterus, fallopian tubes, and ovaries can be visualized using a full urinary bladder as a window. Doppler flow scanning in conjunction with ultrasound imaging of the vascular system is effective in the detection of partially or completely blocked veins and arteries, as may occur with blood clots or atherosclerosis.

Bone and air unfortunately do not adequately transmit sound. Therefore, ultrasound has limited use in the evaluation of the skeletal system, chest, and midabdomen. Structures in the pelvis and upper abdomen, however, may be visualized by ultrasound, as long as bowel gas does not interfere with the transmission of the sound waves.

Because no ionizing radiation or contrast material is used, ultrasound is exceptionally safe.

Thermography

Thermography is a noninvasive procedure that measures and images the infrared radiation (heat) emitted from the body surface. Because skin temperature is a reflection of autonomic nervous system activity, this test is most useful in diagnosing conditions such as RSD and Raynaud's disease.

As thermography is a noninvasive test that does not involve exposure to contrast dyes or ionizing radiation, it is therefore very safe.

Biopsy

A biopsy is an invasive procedure in which tissue is removed from the body and analyzed under a microscope using various staining techniques. Some lesions are accessible to needle biopsy and therefore do not require an operation. Others require an "open" biopsy.

A biopsy may be necessary in order to diagnose an infection, to culture and identify the responsible organism, and to determine which antibiotic will be effective in eradicating it. Evaluation of biopsy specimens is also extraordinarily helpful in identifying benign and malignant tumors.

Potential risks include bleeding, infection, and pain. Blood thinners, such as coumadin, heparin, and aspirin, are usually discontinued prior to the procedure. Bleeding is controlled by cryotherapy (cold), cauterization (heat), or the application of pressure. Chances of infection are minimized by performing the biopsy under sterile conditions. Pain due to the biopsy is generally managed with painkillers and the application of a cold compress.

Differential Neural Blockade

Differential neural blockade, or diagnostic nerve block, can be instrumental in identifying the cause of pain in a patient whose condition remains undiagnosed after the usual work-up. The aim is to determine the exact site, structures, nerves, pathway, or processes involved in pain generation. There are two basic approaches: a pharmacologic approach and an anatomic approach.

The pharmacological approach is based on the selective sensitivity of different types of sensory fibers to local anesthetics of varying concentrations. The sensitivity is related, in part, to the amount of myelin enveloping the fibers. The more myelin, the higher the concentration of local anesthetic needed to penetrate the nerve and block transmission. An example of this approach is the differential spinal block, which is very useful in certain circumstances but is limited to the evaluation of pain that involves the lower abdomen, pelvis, low back, and legs.

The anatomic approach bases the block site on the most likely origin of the pain. Direct injection of local anesthetic into superficial sites of pain (i.e., near the surface of the skin), for instance, can readily elicit the precise site and source of pain and offer a definitive diagnosis. Trigger points associated with myofascial pain and nerve entrapment in a postsurgical scar are good examples. Deep structures may also be evaluated by giving injections under radiologic guidance. Low-back pain may be defined more precisely by this method, and it is possible to distinguish whether pain is arising from nerve root damage, a facet joint, ligaments, or muscles. This is one of the most valuable applications of all the diagnostic block techniques.

Another application of neural diagnostic blocks is in the evaluation of arm pain. If the doctor suspects that arm pain is mediated by the sympathetic nervous system, for example, he or she will perform a stellate ganglion block. If this is unsuccessful, he or she may perform a brachial plexus or a peripheral nerve block. If no pain relief occurs with any of these blocks, the offending lesion may be located in the central nervous system (i.e., the brain or spinal cord).

A differential nerve block is an invasive procedure with the potential for complications. Although these rarely occur, they include allergic reactions, bleeding, increased pain, nerve damage, numbness, weakness, paralysis, infection, dizziness, and seizures. Contraindications include local skin infection at the injection site, bleeding disorder, and maintenance on blood thinners. In addition, the patient must have pain at the time of the procedure. If pain is absent, the procedure is postponed.

While nerve blocks are very helpful in identifying the precise site and mechanism of pain in many instances, they cannot offer a valid assessment about the presence or absence of psychological or behavioral factors contributing to the pain experience. Nor do they provide accurate forecasts for the duration of pain relief with "permanent" ablative procedures such as neurectomy.

Summary

Chronic pain may be due to one or more of a multitude of causes, including mechanical, infectious, vascular, neuropathic, autoimmune, and malignant conditions. An accurate diagnosis is essential in order to develop a specific treatment plan and to maximize the chances of successfully reducing pain and improving function. The process of establishing the diagnosis begins with a thorough history and physical examination by a qualified physician. Appropriate testing should then be ordered to confirm the suspected diagnosis. But beware! Countless pain patients — through no fault of their own — fail to undergo this vital process, to their own detriment. We do not want you to be among them. As an informed consumer, you have every right to demand a proper work-up.

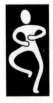

The Doctors Know
Best...Or Do They?

In essence, one orthopedic surgeon provided the following information:

Martha is a 36-year-old married mother of two with a history of a whiplash injury from a motor vehicle accident two years ago. She was at a stoplight, waiting to turn right, when a Ford Bronco rear-ended her at approximately five miles per hour. She complained of severe neck and back pain later that day and went to the emergency room, where X-rays were taken. They were normal. A diagnosis of neck strain was made, and she was given a five-day supply of Motrin. The pain got worse and, on the recommendation of a friend, she saw a chiropractor, Dr. Will Kracket, who gave her a series of cervical spine manipulations over the course of six weeks. The pain continued to worsen. Her internist put her on Percocet as needed for pain and referred her for physical therapy, where she received ultrasound, massage, and hot packs. She obtained only temporary relief from these measures, and she was subsequently referred to me for surgical consultation.

An MRI of the cervical spine showed disc bulges at C3–4 and C4–5. Because her symptoms had not improved with conservative treatment, she underwent cervical fusions at the above levels approximately one year ago. Her postoperative course was very difficult. She required excessive amounts of narcotic pain medication while in the hospital. She was noncompliant with my instructions to remain immobile after going home and began to complain of pain in the mid and lower back and of insomnia, irritability, and nervousness, for which her internist prescribed Valium. She resisted attempts to get her off narcotic pain medication and began to run out several days in advance of her scheduled refills.

I sent her back to physical therapy to address her pain complaints, but she refused to cooperate. The physical therapist reported that she complained of severe pain and was unwilling to exercise. She was highly emotional and complained that the exercise made her pain worse. She frequently missed her appointments and eventually was discharged from physical therapy due to poor motivation and nonresponsiveness to treatment.

Subsequent MRIs showed solid fusions and no other abnormalities in her thoracic and lumbar areas. Despite a successful surgery, she continued to complain of pain, even in areas unaffected by the cervical injury. She demanded that I run further tests, as she was sure that I had missed something. I sent her to anesthesiologist Dr. Ira Needleman for a series of epidural steroid injections, which, according to the patient, made her pain worse. As such injections block all pain signals, it was clear that there was no real reason for her pain. Yet she was using larger and larger doses of Percocet. As I soon found out, she was getting narcotic pain medication from another doctor. I told her that I would no longer treat her because of her dishonesty and discharged her back to her internist about four months ago.

—*Rod N. Plates, M.D.*
Orthopedic Surgeon

Martha's internist forwarded the following additional information:

I instructed Martha to take one Percocet every six hours as needed for pain. However, she consistently would run out a week or two before the end of the month. She called the office frequently for refills and was abusive to the staff while on the telephone. I found out that she, again, had obtained a prescription for narcotic pain medications from an urgent care doctor. At first she denied this, but then admitted that she had gotten the additional medication because she couldn't stand the pain. I informed her that I would no longer see her if this ever happened again. Although she resisted, I sent her to Dr. R.X. Pihl for psychiatric consultation. Given that there was no physical basis for her pain, he diagnosed a conversion (somatoform pain) disorder and recommended that she be placed on the tranquilizer Xanax three times daily to treat the anxiety and pain she was experiencing as a result of her psychological conflicts.

Martha became hysterical when I told her that Dr. Pihl had found that her pain was of psychological and not physical origin. I told her that she would simply have to learn to live with her pain. However, I did not carry out Dr. Pihl's recommendation to prescribe the tranquilizer Xanax, as I was increasingly concerned about her abuse of pain medications. She clearly had become addicted, and I wanted to avoid adding another addictive medication to her list. Although her pain symptoms were unfounded, she was using more than eight Percocet and four Valium tablets a day. Because of this, I referred her to the "12-step" chemical dependency treatment program at Johnny Walker Memorial Hospital. Unfortunately, she elected to leave against medical advice after she was detoxified (taken off all addicting medications). She was especially resistant to attending the required substance abuse support group meetings. The staff reported that Martha was in heavy denial as evidenced by her refusal to admit that she was an addict.

She now is back to taking pain medications, despite my repeated efforts to discontinue them. She has persistent complaints of severe neck and back pain and refuses to discuss further physical therapy. Quite frankly, I feel I have nothing else to offer her. Thank you for seeing this most difficult patient.

—*N.A. Rush, M.D.*

From this information, it seemed that Martha had failed miserably. She underwent the treatment prescribed by her chiropractor, her orthopedic surgeon, her physical therapists, and her internist. But it was clear from their descriptions that she was a "bad" patient. She bucked the system. She failed to comply with the prescribed exercise program. She questioned her surgeon's judgment and ability to correctly diagnose her problem. She rejected the doctors' opinion that her pain was not physical but rather psychological in origin. She "abused" her pain medications. She "abused" her doctor's office staff while demanding early refills. She refused to acknowledge the "fact" that she was an addict. She was angry and unpleasant. And she failed to get better despite the extra time invested in her case by her doctors and therapists. For her healthcare providers, Martha was simply no fun to work with.

In fact, our guess is that all of these providers actually *disliked* Martha! Forget the supposed objectivity of today's modern physician. Forget the Hippocratic oath. Forget the idealized sense of duty marching triumphant over personal views and reactions, "for the good of the patient." When it comes right down to it, doctors and therapists are human beings, albeit ones with particular kinds of training and experiences. While it is true that health professionals present themselves with varying degrees of openness, we all have personal reactions and feelings about our patients. Don't let anyone tell you otherwise. Some of us communicate these feelings, whether verbally or nonverbally, and some of us don't. In the end, however, we believe most patients have a pretty good idea as to whether or not their doctor or therapist likes them.

While we are not saying that being liked by your doctor will cure you of, say, pneumonia, the interpersonal relationship between you and your healthcare provider is an important contributing factor in determining your degree of progress, especially for such complex conditions as chronic pain. Skeptical? You are not alone — so are many physicians. After all, how can a good relationship with one's doctor influence pain intensity? How can it affect the biochemical action of pain medications? How can it impact one's use of medication? How can it yield better results from therapeutic exercise? All of these involve physical processes, whereas the doctor–patient relationship has to do with mental phenomena like thoughts and feelings.

The answers lie not only in our collective clinical experience but also in a virtual explosion of new scientific research that shows a powerful link between mind, body, and health. Suffice it to say, your relationship with your healthcare provider is an essential component of high-quality care, especially in the area of chronic pain management. In Martha's case, it was not difficult to discern that her doctors were more than upset with her. It was clear that they held Martha responsible for her own suffering and for alienating them. In their case descriptions, there was not even a hint that perhaps her "problematic" behavior was a not so illogical response to being misunderstood, mismanaged, and mistreated by the providers themselves. Yet, that is exactly what happened. Why?

The Doctor "Knows Best"

Our cultural tradition raises images of the all-knowing, all-caring physician whose education, intelligence, and wisdom were beyond reproach. He (and the physician was almost always a *he*) practiced a kind of *paternalistic* medicine in which the patient was informed of his or her condition only if the doctor felt that it was in the patient's best interest. Historically, the communication flowed from doctor to patient, usually concerning information about diagnosis and treatment. A patient who questioned either was decidedly out of step. He or she might expect a sharp rejoinder such as "Are you questioning my medical judgment?" or "What medical school did *you* go to?"

Sound archaic? Like the product of a 1950s "the doctor knows best" American culture? Guess again. Chances are, many readers have heard these very responses from at least one doctor in the past few years. We have actually witnessed other doctors utter these words to patients who ask "too many questions." When a patient does not agree with the diagnosis or chooses not to adhere to the treatment prescribed, he or she is assumed to either be ignorant or to have a "personality disorder." We cannot count the number of times we have been asked to see a "difficult" chronic pain patient with a "borderline" personality disorder (referring to a very serious psychiatric condition characterized by widely fluctuating emotions, intense though unstable relationships, and identity disturbances). In almost all cases, the individual, usually a female, did not have a borderline personality disorder, but did tend to assert herself emotionally and, therefore, posed a behavioral management challenge for the referring physician. Alternatively, the patient may be seen as suffering from a "knowledge deficit disorder" when disagreements arise. Most physicians certainly attempt to educate the patient so that he or she might be better informed and able to deal with his or her condition. However, disagreements often will arise not out of patient ignorance but out of the doctor's lack of appreciation for the patient's logic and personal perspective. When this happens, the patient's perspective is considered by the physician to be inadequate and unworthy of serious consideration. End of discussion! There simply is little or no effort put forth to understand the patient's perspective on his or her illness and treatment experiences.

Under such circumstances, the patient tends to be noncompliant with treatment, either because it does not make sense or because it is ineffective in his or her eyes. A common example is a therapeutic exercise program that is carried out too aggressively. When a physical therapist attempts to motivate a chronic pain patient with the adage "no pain, no gain," the therapist is unwittingly setting the patient up for failure. The patient's experience is that exercise causes more pain, despite the doctor's and the therapist's promises to the contrary. (Patients often are told that exercise will decrease their pain. This is not always true, despite the many other benefits of therapeutic exercise.) The patient's own experience tells him or her that it hurts more, especially when following instructions to "push past the pain." Thus, a credibility gap is created which logically leads to nonadherence to treatment recommendations. Unless the patient's experience is taken into account and fully appreciated by the therapist or doctor, the nonadherence can look a lot like poor motivation or overreacting to pain. It is through this lack of appreciation for the patient's perspective that doctors and therapists make the same errors again and again.

Although we have come a long way since the paternalistic era of medicine, the arrogance and lack of respect for the patient on the part of some physicians linger on. These attitudes and behaviors may cause serious harm to the patient with chronic pain. And while such an approach certainly is not medically necessary, *it is actually taught in medical schools today*!

The "Perils" of Medical Training

While you won't find "Medicine 101: The Practice of Arrogance in the Consultation Room" in any medical school curriculum, it *is* an inadvertent part of the educational experience, from day one. It starts with a sense of personal achievement for having been smart enough to get into medical school. It continues by being referred to as "Doctor," even before you are one. Professors are ascribed the status of ultimate authorities. There is no time to debate any point of interest, as there simply are too many facts to learn. There is a sense that, with the enormity of the knowledge base one has acquired and digested, there just can't be any part of the human body or human functioning that is not explainable by Western medical science. Such circumstances set the stage for the development of self-assuredness. But how does an adaptive sense of self-assuredness become transformed into arrogance or lack of respect for the patient by some?

Rounds

Typically starting in the third year of medical school, students begin to see patients on hospital wards and in medical clinics. Along with interns, residents, and attending physicians, they make "rounds," reviewing the course of each patient during his or her hospital stay. If you have never seen — or, indeed, experienced — doctors making rounds, it is really quite interesting. Typically, the resident or attending physician briefly discusses each case while standing outside the patient's door. Although unintended, the patient usually can hear this discussion from inside the room.

Then the group moves, en masse, into the patient's room, where they all huddle around the bed. The lead doctor will usually, though not always, greet the patient prior to making a few introductory remarks to the group. He or she will then proceed to examine the patient, perhaps with a stethoscope or other instrument. The others, especially the less senior participants, then repeat the procedure in turn while the patient lies passively. Everyone present participates in the discussion — everyone except the patient, that is. The discourse continues as if he or she were not there. When they are finished, the group exits the room while concluding remarks are made and/or questions are answered by the senior doctor, again usually within earshot of the patient.

Although there are many variations on this general theme, this type of interaction among doctors, doctors-in-training, and patients goes on in virtually every Western teaching hospital. There really is no other social situation like it. To be sure, it is a very effective way to teach medical students and interns about disease and its treatment. But, inadvertently, it also teaches that the owner of the body under scrutiny need not be part of the discourse. We have seen — indeed, participated in — this process countless times during our own training. When seen later, on a one-to-one basis, patients almost always relate how emotionally uncomfortable rounds make them. One of us (AC) made it a point to ask patients about their "rounding" experience. They often would describe feeling like a piece of meat to be inspected by all comers. In fact, every single patient, over the course of several years of conducting this informal survey, acknowledged that no one had ever before asked how they felt about it. The inescapable conclusion is that no one had been particularly interested in the impact of this strange social event on the person lying in the bed. Thus, it is not difficult to see why this part of the medical education process continues in its present form: It is an especially effective teaching method. But no one is asking if there is a downside. We believe that there is. Not only does it demean the patient's sense of dignity if not handled with sensitivity, but it also has the unintended effect of teaching our doctors-to-be that the patient's experience of his or her illness is not particularly important to healing and recovery. And, as we shall later see, this is far from the truth.

In this part of the medical education process, doctors-in-training are exposed to and participate in interactions wherein the patient — the human being in the bed — essentially is ancillary to the interchange between the doctor and the patient's body. Medical students learn, through modeling the behavior of others and through direct feedback from their superiors, that their primary interest should be the physical data (lab results, heart and lung sounds, radiological images, etc.) and that the patient need not be too involved in the treatment process. This lesson is reinforced day after day over the course of several years throughout medical training. Hence, we can see how treating the disease, *instead of the human being with the disease,* can become standard practice.

To be sure, there are many doctors who are sensitive to their patients' feelings and overall illness experience. Some include the patient in the discussion during rounds and attempt to make him or her feel at ease. Those who do are special indeed. For despite training practices that reinforce noninclusion of the patient's experience, there are some who never forget that there is a *real person* in the bed. But for those entering medical school who do not already exhibit healthy amounts of sensitivity, compassion, and humility toward their fellow human being, the training experience can lead not only to indifference toward the patient's experience of illness but to arrogance as well.

The "God Syndrome"

Webster's Unabridged Dictionary defines arrogance as an "offensive exhibition of assumed or real superiority." Most of us have encountered people who are so self-assured that their behavior crosses the line and becomes arrogance. After reading this paragraph, close your eyes and recall in detail an encounter you have had with such a person. Recall the circumstances and details of how this person presented himself or herself. Listen to the person's words and tone of voice. Watch his or her body language. After you get a pretty vivid picture, open your eyes and continue reading.

Notice how you felt emotionally and physically. If your ability to use imagery served you well, chances are you felt ill at ease or possibly downright angry. You also may have felt physically tense. Your heart and breathing rates may have quickened. If so, you have just experienced the mind–body connection. Now imagine that you have to turn to this same individual for help in relieving the suffering associated with chronic, unrelenting pain. What if your doctor were like this? We certainly have met more than a handful of such doctors who project an air of superiority. And in addition to being rather unpleasant to be around, we know that patients have been harmed by such arrogant behavior, which in the field of medicine is commonly referred to as the *"god syndrome."*

To understand how the "god syndrome" can develop and thrive within the medical community, consider how doctors are treated in our culture. Within the hospital environment, they are regarded with utmost deference. There is a special parking lot for physicians. They have their own dining room, often with free meals. Furthermore, doctors often can, and do, get away with treating others with disrespect. They can vent their anger or frustration unfairly upon others and there are rarely any consequences, in contrast to what would typically occur in almost any other social or occupational setting.

Indeed, we recently heard of a hospital department head physician who, during a case conference attended by other nonphysician professionals (physical therapists, speech pathologists, nurses, etc.), proceeded to scold one of the team members in the presence of case managers visiting from another institution. When told that his actions were inappropriate, he proceeded to announce that he was more than qualified to do each person's job and that he could criticize the performance of others whenever he cared to. The fact is that, in this example, the corrective feedback he received was a rare event. Such actions usually go unchallenged. But in this case, he had gone even further by asserting the false claim about his range of expertise. There were no further consequences. What do you think happened here? Could it be that this was the first time he exhibited such arrogant behavior? We think not. More than likely, he has acted this way many times in the past, not only with professional staff but with patients as well.

One of our patients, Gary, told us of his treatment course following a job-related back injury. Several months after the accident, he was referred to an orthopedic surgeon for evaluation. He had his X-rays and MRI scans with him and was hoping against hope for some kind of recommendation that would restore his quality of life. He waited for over two hours before he was escorted into the examination room. The doctor finally entered and, without introducing himself or otherwise greeting the patient, announced, "I'm going to tell you right up front that I will not prescribe you any pain medications." Gary experienced a flash of anger but managed to contain it. He responded by stating, "Doctor, I'm not here for medications. In fact, I want very badly to get off of them. I'm here simply to get your opinion about my condition and whether surgery would be a good idea or not." The doctor's demeanor changed and he became more respectful after Gary provided corrective feedback. But Gary is an assertive and cool-headed person. We wonder about the other patients treated by this doctor who may be less able to respond in such an effective manner. Nonetheless, Gary was wounded by this experience and thereafter became very cautious about trusting doctors. Thus, it was not only Gary who suffered from this misinformed and insensitive error but also the many well-informed and compassionate doctors he subsequently was to see.

Another patient, Diana, had undergone eight back surgeries. She was in excruciating pain, could not work, and had become very depressed over the years. She was referred to a neurosurgeon who, after examining her X-rays and MRI scans (he did not conduct a physical exam), told her that there were no remaining problems in her back and that she "shouldn't be hurting." He said that the pain was "all in your head" and implied that her real objective was to remain on disability so that she would not have to work for a living. This is a good example of the "god syndrome" at its worst. Diana was devastated and blamed herself for being disabled and in pain.

When we saw her a few weeks later, it was entirely clear that the doctor had missed the mark by a wide margin. Diana *was* in severe pain despite no obvious derangements on the films. There was absolutely no evidence that she was complaining of pain so as to remain on disability. In fact, she felt ashamed for not contributing to society. As it turned out, she had a clear case of chronic pain syndrome, complete with a major depressive illness stemming from her pain and debilitation. Unfortunately, she also was suffering from being abused by a doctor who was so sure of himself that he was unwilling to even consider that he might not hold a valid perspective. Had Diana not pursued an opinion from a specialized pain clinic, this encounter could have easily resulted in years of further pain, depression, and dependence upon the healthcare system. And Diana was not the only person who received this kind of treatment from this particular doctor. Almost without exception, we heard the same story over and over again despite many discussions with him regarding alternative interpretations of the data. He remained unconvinced. He also "happened" to be very popular with many of the worker's compensation insurance carriers, for obvious reasons.

On a positive note, Diana's life has improved significantly since undergoing her interdisciplinary pain management program over three years ago. Although she has good and bad days and remains on narcotic medication, she is now able to do some limited work and has begun to take an active role in her family life and social world again.

Our healthcare system, as well as our general cultural practices, can contribute to the development of insensitive and arrogant behavior on the part of doctors. They are treated with special consideration in many ways. They can misbehave interpersonally and there are typically no corrective consequences. Patients have told us of traumatic experiences with doctors, but then have gone on to provide excuses for the doctors' misconduct. They blame themselves for possibly provoking the doctor or explain away the unacceptable behavior by saying that perhaps the doctor was very busy that day. No. The fact is that there is *never* a good reason for patients to be treated with arrogance and disrespect. It merely constitutes a further injustice when the patient buys into this inexcusable aspect of chronic pain mismanagement. It is simply wrong.

While these examples represent some of the more blatant instances we have encountered, this type of patient mistreatment is all too common.

It typically occurs in a less obvious form, such as when patients are told that there is no reason for their pain or that they are "overreacting" to it. Such statements not only are misinformed on the part of the physician but also imply (falsely) that he or she fully understands all there is to know about how the human nervous system works. A quick glance at the scientific literature tells us that this is far from the truth. And it is sad to note just how much damage is done to patients when doctors lose their sense of humility in the face of the "state of nature" that is chronic pain.

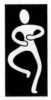

"It's All in Your Head" and Other Popular Fairy Tales

Individuals suffering from chronic pain conditions that have no clear *structural* or *organic* cause often have a very difficult challenge: to convince doctors (and others) that their pain is real. We cannot tell you how frequently this comes up when we ask people to tell us about their experiences in seeking relief.

Consider the following definitions of pain:

- ◆ "Bodily suffering or distress, as due to injury or illness" (*Random House College Dictionary*)

- ◆ "A primary condition of sensation or consciousness, the opposite of pleasure; the sensation which one feels when hurt (in body or mind); suffering, distress" (*Oxford English Dictionary*)

- ◆ "...an unpleasant sensory and emotional experience associated with actual or potential tissue damage, or described in terms of such damage" (International Association for the Study of Pain, Committee for Taxonomy, 1994)

On the surface, defining pain would seem to be no problem. Perhaps most of us would agree with Guildenberg and DeVaul (1985) when they said, "Pain is what hurts." All of us certainly know it when we feel it. But here's the problem: *Pain is a very personal experience that cannot be directly observed by anyone but the person within whom it resides.* Boom. That's it. That's the problem that underlies so much of the needless suffering we observe. It stems, in part, from the fact that there is no such thing as a pain meter. There is no test that measures the experience of pain without it first being *interpreted* by the observer. There is no way anyone can fully experience what it feels like to be inside another person's skin. The fact is that pain can only be *inferred* by another person from the experiencer's words, actions, or from observations of his or her body. And like the experience of love, only the person himself or herself can know its true reality.

But time and again, our patients, especially those with myofascial (or soft tissue) pain, have reported to us that they have been told by doctors, "There's nothing wrong. The pain is all in your head. I think you need to see a psychiatrist." If these doctors spoke more plainly, their statements could be summed up in the following series of propositions and conclusions:

Proposition 1: "My education and experience have provided me with a thorough understanding of chronic pain, even though I have never actually experienced it myself."

Proposition 2: "Your reported symptoms and the objective medical findings do not fit my model of (or way of understanding) pain."

Conclusion A: "Therefore, you are not experiencing *real* pain."

Proposition 3: "Since your pain is not *real,* you are either faking your symptoms (e.g., for narcotic medications, financial gain, attention, and/or to get out of working for a living) or you have a deep-seated psychological problem — about which I don't know very much — which only makes you think you are in pain."

Conclusion B: "Since your problem is outside my particular area of medical expertise, I will refer you to a psychiatrist who will be able to treat your psychological pain problem and/or addiction to pain medications."

Although you probably have never heard a doctor utter these exact words, chances are such thoughts (or some variant thereof) have crossed the mind of at least one doctor whom you have seen if you have had a myofascial-type chronic pain condition for a year or more. We know because we have heard doctors utter such beliefs to one another when the patient is not around. And these beliefs are often presented in a rather judgmental tone.

If you think about it, most of us would be at least somewhat judgmental if we *really* believed that someone was faking pain symptoms for financial gain or to obtain narcotic medications simply for the "high." Unfortunately, these *assumptions* are all too often regarded as *fact* by healthcare professionals who are not willing to entertain the possibility that they might have an incomplete understanding of the patient — that they might be *wrong*. The tragic result is that the victim ends up on trial and is often pronounced guilty.

The Emergency Room

A very common example of healthcare professionals serving as judge, jury, and executioner occurs every day in many emergency rooms. Ask anyone who suffers from severe, chronic migraine headaches, and there is a good chance he or she will tell you about having been mistreated in the emergency room. Like soft-tissue pain disorders, severe migraines are "hidden" from public view. No structural damage shows up on X-rays. No blood test reveals the problem. And all too often there is no compassion from healthcare providers who jump to the wrong conclusions: That the pain is not real and that the problem is either psychological or one of addiction or some other presumed psychological abnormality. The result? Frequently it is insult added to injury by way of accusations of "drug-seeking." One woman told us of visiting an emergency room for the first time. After describing her symptoms of severe pain, the screening nurse said to her, "I can tell you from the start that we're not giving you any pain medications." The woman, already suffering from excruciating pain, now felt accused of a crime of which she was not guilty. Our guess is that this nurse had never experienced the true reality of chronic, recurrent pain. And, like so many others, she jumped to a false conclusion regarding the motivation of the person before her: That she was "drug-seeking" and only claimed to be in pain in her quest to get "high." A miscarriage of justice, to be sure.

The Waddell Test

The physical examination of patients suffering from chronic pain often includes a series of five short procedures collectively known as the *Waddell test*. Arising from the growing sophistication in our understanding of chronic pain, Waddell and colleagues published a study in the journal *Spine* (1980) which showed that utilization of these five procedures could reliably identify patients in whom "nonorganic" factors were important in understanding their chronic low-back pain. These physical procedures were designed to test for pain responses in the (supposed) absence of any physiological pain mechanism. For example, pushing down on a patient's head while he or she is standing (the *axial loading* test) should not elicit low-back pain as a result of *anatomically based* organic mechanisms (e.g., ruptured vertebral discs). According to Waddell et al. (1980), one or two isolated findings should be ignored. But if the patient produced pain responses in three or more of the five tests (*nonanatomic tenderness, simulation, distraction, regional disturbances,* and *overreation*), it was considered to be significant. A more detailed behavioral evaluation should then be performed to assess the possibility that nonanatomic factors might be contributing to the pain condition.

The Waddell Test as a Weapon

But there is a dark side to the Waddell test as currently applied. It is frequently misused to harm people. This is accomplished through mis-

The Five Waddell Signs

1. **Nonanatomic tenderness.** Patient lies on stomach. Examiner presses on soft tissue around the spine. Positive sign = report of low-back pain. "Superficial" (i.e., surface) tenderness of the skin should be ignored in this test, but usually isn't in practice. Fails to take nonstructural modes of pain generation into account (e.g., muscle tension).

2. **Simulation** (axial loading). The examiner presses down on the standing patient's head. Positive sign = report of low-back pain. Fails to take nonstructural modes of pain generation into account.

3. **Distraction.** Examiner appears to be examining another body part while actually observing the effect on the painful area in question. Positive sign = pain only upon obvious manipulation of the painful area. Fails to take nonstructural modes of pain generation into account.

4. **Regional disturbances** (weakness, sensory). Positive sign = any painful response that is not consistent with accepted neuro-anatomy. Almost by definition, fibromyalgia sufferers will test positive on this one. Fails to take nonstructural modes of pain generation into account.

5. **Overreaction.** Positive sign = grimace, recoil, pain response to a mild physical stimulus. This requires a subjective judgment on the part of the examiner and is especially prone to bias. Fails to take nonstructural modes of pain generation into account.

application and misinterpretation of the test. To doctors without an adequate understanding of the link between mind and body, and/or to those with powerful financial incentives to invalidate the patient's pain condition, positive Waddell signs can be misconstrued to reflect out-right malingering. Using the tired old assumption that all back pain stems from problems in the spine, many doctors erroneously conclude that the patient is faking. We cannot tell you how often we see medical reports in which this false conclusion is drawn — especially in worker's compensation and personal injury cases. This practice not only reflects poorly on the examiner's command of the pain literature (or, more ominously, on the quality of his or her scruples), but it also happens to be extremely unfair to the patient. Yet, on a daily basis, it results in the inappropriate revocation of disability benefits and denial of court awards for legitimate and debilitating pain conditions. In short, the Waddell test was never designed — *nor should it be used* — as a test for malingering. In fact, Waddell et al. (1980) state:

> Selected physical signs that appeared to have a *predominantly* nonorganic basis were described early in this century, following the introduction of the Compensation Acts and the development of medicolegal practice. Initially these signs were interpreted as evidence of "malingering," although with increasing psychological knowledge this appeared to be an oversimplification... (p. 117).

There are four main problems with the Waddell test as commonly implemented:

1. Not all back pain is due to structural problems in the spine. Yet, the test assumes that (low-back) pain responses result from (a) structural pathology of the spine (thus the focus on signs consistent or inconsistent with anatomic nerve distribution) or (b) psychological pathology. However, there are large numbers of people suffering from back pain conditions that do not originate in either the spine or the mind. Fibromyalgia and myofascial pain syndromes are common examples. Although the precise physiological mechanism relating to these disorders is not yet fully understood, there is evidence that a lack of oxygenation to affected tissues may contribute to the pain. Nonanatomic tenderness, one of the Waddell tests, is almost universal in fibromyalgia. But to conclude that it therefore reflects psychological pathology would be to ignore other (less well-known) physiological pain mechanisms.

2. Almost all behavior can be viewed as occurring along a continuum. Yet many who use the Waddell test fail to take

the individual's unique learning history into account when interpreting positive signs. For example, a low-back pain response to the axial loading test (pushing down on the head) may simply reflect the patient's *anticipation* of physical pain due to prior experience with less than gentle examinations. (Indeed, many patients have reported undergoing very physically and emotionally stressful independent medical examinations.) Thus, a positive Waddell sign due to the anticipation of physical pain has absolutely nothing to do with psychological pathology. In addition, the unfortunate label *"overreaction"* (referring to one of the five Waddell test areas) fails to appreciate behavior as a state of nature — needing to be understood and not judged. The fact that an individual's response may happen to lie on one or the other end of the normal curve should not constitute grounds for condemnation of that individual.

3.   The Waddell test was developed and validated for use with low-back pain patients but is widely administered to individuals suffering from chronic pain in other areas of the body.

4.   It is often used to imply that a patient's pain is not physical and, therefore, not *"legitimate"* or *"real."* This is a clear misuse of the test and reflects either a gross misunderstanding of the chronic pain literature or a blatant misrepresentation for partisan purposes. "Anatomic" versus "nonanatomic" does *not* mean "legitimate" versus "illegitimate."

In medical settings, the application of scientific findings can be a matter of life and death, whereas in the insurance and legal arenas, it is more likely to be a matter of dollars and cents (and potentially lots of them). Attempts to save money routinely lead to the corruption of truth. And sadly, this is occurring every day with the misapplication of the Waddell test.

Bottom line: Examine your medical evaluation reports for references to Waddell signs. If they are present and used to raise questions about the

The Waddell Test in the Legal Arena: Potentially Useful Cross-Examination Questions

1. **"Doctor, you noted the presence of three (four or five) positive Waddell signs. What does that tell you?"**

Nonvalid Responses	*Valid Responses*
◆ "It tells me that there is no physical cause for the pain."	◆ "It tells me that nonspine-related sources of pain may be present."
◆ "...that there's really nothing wrong with the patient."	◆ "...that an evaluation by a behavioral pain specialist should have been performed."
◆ "...that the patient's problem is psychological."	

2. **"If there's really nothing wrong with the plaintiff, then how do you account for the positive Waddell signs?"**

Nonvalid Responses	*Valid Responses*
◆ "The patient just wanted me to think he/she was in pain when, in fact, there was no way that the Waddell procedures could have caused pain."	◆ "I don't know for sure. I can only hypothesize that there are nonspine-related physical sources and/or biobehavioral phenomena that contributed to his/her response."
◆ "He/she overreacted, indicating either hypochondriasis or malingering."	◆ "A behavioral pain specialist would be better able to answer that question."

3. **"Did you recommend a specialized behavioral pain evaluation to obtain clarification regarding the possible reasons for the positive Waddell signs?"**

Nonvalid Responses	*Valid Responses*
◆ "No."	◆ "Yes."
◆ "He/she saw a (nonpain) psychiatrist or psychologist who diagnosed somatoform pain disorder (or hypochondriasis)."	◆ "No, but that would have been appropriate given the positive Waddell signs."

The Waddell Test in the Legal Arena: Potentially Useful Cross-Examination Questions

4. **"Waddell et al. have developed the test as a means for determining the need for further specialized behavioral assessment, and yet, having found three (four or five) positive signs, you failed to recommend such an assessment. Can you tell me why?"**

Nonvalid Responses	*Valid Response*
◆ "I was able to definitively rule out any physical basis for the pain. Therefore, it was clear that the plaintiff had some other agenda." ◆ "The (nonpain specialist) psychiatrist diagnosed somatoform pain disorder (or hypochondriasis) after reviewing my findings."	◆ "I wasn't aware that the test was designed for that purpose. I apparently misunderstood it to be a test for whether there was a physical or psychological cause for the pain."

5. **"The Waddell test was developed and validated for use with individuals suffering from chronic low-back pain and yet the plaintiff has neck pain. Can you cite any literature that validates using the test on individuals with nonlow-back pain?"**

Nonvalid Response	*Valid Responses*
◆ "No, but I was able to determine that there was nothing physically wrong with him/her. Therefore, the patient doesn't really have pain."	◆ "No." ◆ "I wasn't aware that the test was designed for use only with chronic low-back pain patients …I apologize for my blatant ignorance. Please [now weeping] just disregard my entire testimony."

validity of your pain condition, let the red flags fly. This is especially true if your pain is work related or part of a personal injury situation. If you have an attorney, make sure that he or she is aware of these issues. We certainly don't want people who are faking an injury to be rewarded. Just like everyone else, we want to see fraud and abuse weeded out. But when ignorance and greed corrupt an otherwise legitimate medical test, a different kind of fraud and abuse is rewarded. Only this time it is the patient who gets swindled.

It's Really All in Your Head: The Sarno Hypothesis

In 1984, Dr. John E. Sarno, a specialist in physical medicine and rehabilitation, published a book entitled *Mind Over Back Pain,* which went on to become a best-seller. In it, and its sequels *Healing Back Pain* and *The Mind–Body Prescription,* Dr. Sarno proposed a radically new way of looking at chronic pain disorders and other maladies of the body, such as ulcers, arthritis, asthma, hay fever, migraine headaches, hiatal hernias, colitis, and even heartburn. Categorized under the general term *tension myositis syndrome,* he proposed that these physical conditions arise not from the usual structural or biological causes but from psychological conflict. In essence, Dr. Sarno proposed that the mind somehow tells the body to develop physical symptoms as a way to divert one's attention away from situations in life that have generated anger and anxiety. He notes that anger is deemed to be unacceptable in our culture and liberally borrows concepts from psychoanalytic thinkers like Sigmund Freud and Franz Alexander in making his case.

As you may know, Freud was a pioneer of the unconscious. It was he who theorized that emotions such as anger are so unacceptable that we repress them into our unconscious mind and "discharge" their energy by developing physical symptoms. One of Freud's students, Franz Alexander, picked up where his teacher left off. He proposed this...er...*interesting* theory that specific physical disorders are the result of corresponding emotional conflict. For example, your boss is so critical that it makes your blood boil: Boom. High blood pressure. Your perfectionism and rigidity become overwhelming: Bang. Rheumatoid arthritis. Your mother-in-law is such a pain in the butt: Ouch! Hemorrh…well, you get the picture. While it is not our aim to make fun of these early to mid-20th century theorists (much), we cannot refrain from reflecting on the fact that much has been learned about mind–body interactions since Freud and Alexander put pen to paper. But more about that later.

Dr. Sarno maintains that tension myositis syndrome disorders do not require medical intervention except for symptom relief during episodes of extreme exacerbation. In fact, he emphasizes that once tension myositis syndrome is diagnosed, medical tests, injections, medications, procedures, surgeries, and physical therapy should be avoided. He views these as merely feeding into the mind's attempt to divert attention away from the psychological conflict and to the supposed physical malady. As long as the charade continues, so will the pain. And modern biological medicine is playing right along.

Well, how does it sound so far? Pretty exotic, huh? But wait. There's more. According to Dr. Sarno, the cure comes by short-circuiting the mind's attempt to cover up the unacceptable emotions. Stop buying into the trickery, and the symptoms will vanish. The treatment? Read his books. That's right. Read his books, which expose the masquerade, and the mind will instantly know that you are on to its little game. The jig is up. You're not going to be fooled by its clever hoax. Period. End of story. Exclamation point.

And guess what. In some cases, it works! We have seen some pretty impressive reversals in chronic pain by basing our treatment on Dr. Sarno's hypothesis. In those cases, symptoms almost immediately diminished — or, more rarely, disappeared — when the patient was able to operate on the assumption that his or her mind was producing the symptoms in order to distract attention away from troubling emotional issues. We have seen lasting improvement result as these issues were identified and successfully addressed. Truly amazing.

The skeptic will justifiably question the reason for such improvement. After all, it absolutely flies in the face of our understanding of biomechanics and the way the body works.

♦ Could it be a placebo response? Maybe, but probably not. Placebo responses almost never last very long. In some cases, we have seen what appears to be permanent recovery.

♦ Could it be that, in challenging with skepticism the presumed physical cause of their pain, patients start on a more constructive coping path that eventually becomes self-reinforcing? Although this does happen in some cases, it does not explain the often immediate (e.g., within minutes) reversal of chronic pain conditions.

♦ Could it be that there was never any physical pain to begin with? Nope. Take our word for it.

None of these alternative hypotheses fit the data. Conventional, mainstream explanations work only when the facts are pushed, pulled, or otherwise contorted into place. They simply are not convincing when the data are approached with an open and objective mind.

So, does this mean that it really is all in your head? Dr. Sarno says yes. We say no, although our difference of opinion may be based more on semantics than substance. As we maintain throughout this book, the mind and body are so intimately intertwined that it is folly to force them into separate arenas (see Chapter 9: The Psychology of Chronic Pain and Illness). We suspect that Dr. Sarno, in putting forth a wholly unconventional hypothesis, is making his case in the simplest terms possible. Our culture is used to the mind–body distinction. Maintaining that it's all in your head helps the reader to get the point. Our preference is to treat the mind and body as inextricable parts of the same whole. For us, it is most definitely *not* all in your head.

Semantics aside, then, what's going on in cases where the Sarno approach seems to work? Our honest answer is we don't know. But we suspect that it has something to do with the brain regulating, from moment to moment, hormone release, muscle tension, and blood flow to the affected body parts. Thus far, there have been no scientific studies examining the validity of the hypothesis or treatment efficacy (does it work?), let alone mechanism of action (how does it work?). We can only go by Dr. Sarno's reported experience as well as our own. But we can say that, for some, the Sarno approach has a legitimate place in the treatment of chronic pain.

The Sarno Approach: Some Cautions

While we would agree that the mind–body connection does exist and that it plays a part in almost all chronic pain disorders, we would urge caution as to the extent of its application. While his hypothesis is appealing to many in that it diverts attention away from the prospect of *unappealing* treatment approaches (e.g., surgery), it has the potential to be dangerous if a proper work-up has not been done.

For example, we wonder what might happen if medically based or structural causes of pain were to go undiagnosed. What might result if surgically correctable, nerve-impinging deformities of the spine were missed due to the doctor ordering low-resolution X-rays instead of high-resolution MRI scans in an attempt to keep costs down? What if a person were then diagnosed with tension myositis syndrome and routed to a Sarno-oriented pain management program in which he or she was constantly admonished to ignore the pain — a program in which the person was put through a rigorous physical therapy regimen, only to meet with increased pain, suffering, and possibly damage to the spine? What if the appropriate MRI scans were taken two years later and, lo and behold, serious lesions were found and then surgically corrected? Could this kind of nightmare really happen? It can and it has. We have witnessed it.

The old real-estate adage says that the three most important elements are "location, location, location." In a similar vein, the three most important elements in healthcare are *"diagnosis, diagnosis, diagnosis."* While we agree with Dr. Sarno that mixing in physical treatments in true tension myositis cases can serve to strengthen the pain disorder (as though the mind sees that it is successfully deflecting attention away from the psychological issues from which it is "protecting" the patient), we urge caution. Biomechanical pathology occurs and needs to be treated appropriately. As is true with any serious condition, misdiagnosing tension myositis syndrome can lead to harm. As Groucho Marx once said, "Sometimes a cigar is just a cigar."

Fibromyalgia and Other "Soft Tissue" Disorders

Although we find fault with how the healthcare system treats individuals with chronic pain in general, we have found that those suffering from the "soft tissue" disorders have an especially difficult time in their search for adequate care. This is largely due to the fact that, to date, there exists no "objective" medical test, such as an X-ray or lab test, to confirm the presence of any physical abnormality. Given a lack of such findings, the sufferer's condition is often attributed to a psychological disorder. Doctors are trained to look primarily for structural abnormalities when investigating pain conditions. When no such abnormalities are found, it is easy to see how they can conclude that the pain is not "real" and that the problem is "all in the patient's head." Unfortunately, this stance on the doctor's part suffers from the lapse of logic we addressed earlier. That is, "If it doesn't show up on the tests, it doesn't exist." Wrong!

There are several disorders of the soft tissue, variously referred to as *myofascial pain syndrome, fibrositis,* or, more commonly, *fibromyalgia.* Individuals suffering from these conditions report symptoms ranging from sore, aching muscles to excess fatigue; mental confusion; sensitivity to light, sound, and odors; and sleep disturbances. Fibromyalgia syndrome is a particularly severe and debilitating form of myofascial disorder. Whereas myofascial pain syndrome typically involves fairly well-localized, regional pain and sensitivity, fibromyalgia syndrome is characterized by pain and tenderness throughout the body.

In hopes of reigning in the nature of this puzzling syndrome, the American College of Rheumatology established specific diagnostic criteria for fibromyalgia in 1990. In 1992, the World Health Organization adopted these criteria. These events allowed clinicians and researchers to more adequately specify the condition under clinical or scientific scrutiny. In general, the diagnosis of fibromyalgia syndrome requires the presence of widespread pain on both sides of the body as well as the identification of at least 11 of 18 predetermined "tender points." As these criteria have been put to use, researchers and clinicians have been better able to advance our understanding of this disorder.

In an editorial published in the *Journal of Rheumatology* (1995), Dr. Simon Carette asked, "What have we really accomplished" after 20 years of research in fibromyalgia? Although the research has documented physiological elements of the syndrome, such as disturbances of sleep, muscles, neurotransmitters, lack of aerobic fitness, and, more recently, elevations in substance P, it has not revealed much at all about the cause. Professor Carette concludes that "...we need to concentrate our efforts mainly on better understanding the *psychosocial* [emphasis added] factors predisposing the patients to develop this chronic pain syndrome as well as those that perpetuate the symptoms" (p. 592).

We couldn't agree more. Biomedical research has not brought us very far in terms of understanding this complex and potentially debilitating disorder. But a promising new line of research is examining the problem from a *biopsychosocial* perspective. This approach is often referred to as *behavioral medicine*: the application of psychological principles to problems in medicine. As individuals involved in this research, we can tell you that consistencies have developed across studies that may have powerful implications for the treatment of fibromyalgia.

At the 1993 meeting of the American Pain Society, we reported that individuals with fibromyalgia who were treated in an interdisciplinary chronic pain management program were significantly more likely than other chronic pain patients to have encountered emotional and sexual abuse. An expanded version of this study added childhood neglect as an additional contributory factor. Also, the more abuse factors an individual had encountered (e.g., alcoholic parent, physical mistreatment), the more likely a diagnosis of fibromyalgia or myofascial pain syndrome. Other studies are now reporting similar findings.

Do these findings prove that the skeptics were right all along? That fibromyalgia is "all in your head"? Absolutely not. The pain, fatigue, and debilitation experienced by individuals with fibromyalgia are as real as that suffered by individuals with, say, migraine headaches. We are convinced of that. But what it does suggest is that we have a lot of work to do in figuring out why exposure to such circumstances can heighten one's vulnerability to fibromyalgia. In this regard, we feel that there is an overlap between these variables and those implied by the Sarno hypothesis mentioned earlier. Although we are starting to develop some research strategies, our patients deserve credit for showing us where to look. Their response (and sometimes *nonresponse*) to treatment has guided our ideas about the possible cause and pathophysiology of the disorder, as well as our clinical approach. Are we talking about a miraculous cure? No. But we *are* talking about ways to manage this chronic condition that can significantly impact symptom severity and improve quality of life.

Behavioral Conditioning

Have you ever stopped to think about what causes you to act the way you do? Most of us do this all the time with regard to others, but what makes *us* tick? All of us work essentially the same way: Mother Nature has given us the capacity to learn from our experiences. In the larger scheme of things, this has led to a high degree of success for humans as a species. Now consider how long we would last if we did not learn from our experiences. Not very! (Take the spotted owl for example. Had it not, as a species, had the foresight to organize and finance expensive lobbying efforts against the logging of old-growth forests, it would be toast by now.) Not only has Mother Nature given the human species the capacity to adapt biologically to our world at large, but she has also provided a means by which we, as individuals, can adapt to our unique circumstances. The mechanism by which this occurs has gradually been uncovered by behavioral scientists over the past century. As part of a broader learning theory, *behavioral conditioning* refers to the ways in which we respond to changes in our environment.

In a nutshell, responses that are followed by positive consequences are strengthened, while those followed by unfavorable or neutral consequences are weakened. Behavior that is understood in this manner is called *operant* behavior. A large proportion of our actions constitute operant behavior. Examples range from simple behaviors such as choosing a favorite food from a menu at a fine restaurant ("Chef Ecoli's oysters Rockefeller is irresistible!") to more complex examples like preparing and sending in our taxes ("I think I'd like to avoid going to prison this year."). In each case, we encounter positive consequences and/or avoid negative ones as a result of our actions. Our behavior is thus strengthened.

Mind–Body Connections

The application of learning theory to problems in medicine such as fibromyalgia syndrome has started to yield significant benefits. Laboratory research has shown that behavioral conditioning can affect all kinds of functions in the body, such as heart rate, blood pressure, immune function, and even EEG (brain) waves. We also know that exposure to aversive or unpleasant stimuli can produce changes in *autonomic* nervous system activity. This is the part of the nervous system that takes care of all those automatic functions of the body. It is comprised of the *sympathetic* and *parasympathetic* systems. In general, the sympathetic nervous system speeds things up, while the parasympathetic slows them down. For example, recall how it physically feels to be accused of something of which you are not guilty. This is the sympathetic nervous system at work. Think about the course of events for a moment. For you male readers, suppose your wife accuses you of, say, being lost while driving around in circles trying to find the video store that has the one remaining copy of the original "Wrestlemania." What's worse, she actually suggests that you stop somewhere and ask for directions! Of course, you're not only insulted, incensed, and out- raged that she could even *think* you might be lost, but there's a little part of you that is absolutely terrified she might be right! Outrage coupled with fear. A stress response in the making.

In this case, however, it is not the threat of being the main course for a hungry saber-toothed tiger's dinner. No. It's far worse. It's the threat of looking like a complete idiot in front of the only woman you could get to marry you. Dining with the saber-toothed cat would be a plea- sure cruise in comparison. Thus, the mere thought of the anticipated consequences of one's behavior ("My behavior has led to the appear- ance of my getting us lost...Who am I kidding? We *are* lost!...And my wife is going to find out just what a complete moron I am.") can trigger a cascade of physical events in the sympathetic nervous system which we call a stress response. Get it? Thought...physical stress response. Mind...body. Husband...buffoon. Simple.

So, just what happens during a human stress response, whether in- duced by a physical or psychological threat? It's really an amazing process. The brain tells the pituitary gland to get ready for evasive action by flooding the bloodstream with stress hormones. This will divert energy from such routine activities as digestion and immune function to the large muscles of the legs, the lungs, and the heart. Simultaneously, the sympathetic nervous system tells the heart to beat more rapidly (get oxygen and energy to those leg muscles), the lungs to breathe faster (ditto), the peripheral blood vessels to constrict (you don't want to bleed too much when the wife — er...*the tiger* — gets hold of you), and the skin to perspire (the greased pig effect). Does "cold and clammy" ring a bell? This is your sympathetic nervous sys- tem responding to some kind of threat to your physical or emotional integrity. Whether a virus, a physical insult from an accident, or a personal insult from a co-worker — your nervous system doesn't know the difference. Boom. Stress response.

These are natural physical responses to stressful events. But what hap- pens to a person's long-term physiological functioning if he or she is repeatedly exposed to such events? Might prolonged exposure to an abusive environment actually bring about a conditioned response of the neuromuscular system, resulting in an increased vulnerability to developing fibromyalgia later in life? Is it possible that behaviors that were once associated with mistreatment (such as failing to take others' "needs" into account) could later trigger an increase in the body's tendency to release stress hormones in the blood or an exaggerated responsiveness of the sympathetic nervous system? Could a more thorough understanding of the ways in which the body's automatic functions respond to what happens to us emotionally illuminate the elusive link between mind and body? Could we get away with posing yet *another* complex question in this paragraph? Although our clinical experience suggests that all of the above are probably true, it will be up to formal scientific studies to provide more solid conclusions.

The Puzzle of Fibromyalgia: A Working Model

We have hypothesized that individuals exposed to emotional and sexual abuse are, in a sense, conditioned (or "taught") by their environment to ignore how they feel while simultaneously being conditioned to attend to the "needs" of others. If repeatedly exposed to these circumstances, behavior patterns emerge in which the individual ignores *internal stimuli* or his or her own emotional and physical feelings. He or she learns that the needs and desires of others take priority and that he or she must remain alert and attentive to them. Theoretically, these behavioral circumstances can create a conditioned state of readiness for action in the neuroendocrine, neuromuscular, and cardiovascular systems. In other words, the person is always on "alert." It is this conditioned state of the mind and body that may lead to a heightened vulnerability to myofascial pain syndrome and fibromyalgia.

In an informal survey taken at a Fibromyalgia/Chronic Fatigue Syndrome Support Group meeting in Las Vegas, 22 of 22 individuals (100%) who identified themselves as having fibromyalgia indicated that they have a marked tendency to "push" themselves. That is, they tend to subordinate their own internal stimuli (i.e., physical and emotional feelings) to the tasks that they perceive "need" to be accomplished.

Nineteen of 22 (86%) acknowledged being "perfectionistic." These percentages are very similar to those we obtained from a fibromyalgia support group in northern California a few years earlier and to patients we see in our respective practices. Although not scientifically obtained, these results suggest the possibility that current behavior patterns may be important in understanding fibromyalgia.

Our model would predict that, given a higher incidence of exposure to this conditioning pattern, fibromyalgia sufferers would show stronger tendencies to "push" themselves and to strive for perfection relative to other chronic pain patients. This would be so because the behaviors in question led to the avoidance of aversive events earlier in life (an example of behavior being strengthened via negative reinforcement). In other words, pushing hard in spite of how one feels and avoiding mistakes were adaptive behaviors in an environment geared toward pleasing others at the individual's expense.

At the same time, the neuromuscular, neuroendocrine, and cardiovascular systems, which must "support" these behavior patterns, have become conditioned to always be ready to take evasive action, even after the individual has moved away from the environment which produced the conditioned response. When encountering a subsequent trauma, either physical or emotional, we hypothesize that the sympathetic nervous system is primed to overrespond. As a result, the supply of oxygen delivered to the muscles is reduced, thus causing pain. Elevated muscle tension may then lead to a vicious cycle of muscle fatigue, pain from decreased oxygenation to the muscles, and further hyperreactivity of the sympathetic nervous system.

Personal Questions

Sandy came to us for consultation after hearing us speak at a local community meeting. At 50 years of age, she had a long history of severe pain in many areas of the body. She was disabled but continued to engage in volunteer work despite her pain. She was divorced, lived alone, and had a strained relationship with her grown daughter. She had been on countless medications for her pain and had undergone many physical procedures, all without lasting success. She had been diagnosed with various spine-related disorders, but a rheumatologist had recognized the symptoms of fibromyalgia a few years prior to her first visit with us. After a thorough physical exam and careful review of her medical history, MRIs, and lab tests, we agreed with the diagnosis.

At our first meeting, one thing was obvious. Sandy was extremely guarded and reluctant to reveal much about her personal life. She had seen her past medical and psychological reports which contained such terms as "conversion disorder," "psychosomatic," and (dare we say?) "hysteria." She was hurt and angry that previous doctors seemed to blame her for her pain, and she was not about to add us to the list. However, questions about one's psychosocial history and current circumstances are a standard — *and vitally important* — part of our interdisciplinary pain evaluation. For example, we ask people to tell us about their upbringing. Were the patient's parents relaxed, affectionate, and respectful of his or her feelings as a child? Or were the parents typically strict, rigid, and insistent that he or she conform to their expectations, regardless of how the patient felt? Was there ever a time when the patient was mistreated physically or sexually? Did either parent drink too much? If so, how could the patient tell? Was the patient well taken care of as a child? Was he or she ever left to fend for himself or herself? Was he or she responsible at an early age for managing the household or for raising younger siblings? Other questions posed to our patients pertain to their current circumstances. These include queries regarding the nature of the individual's marital relationship. Is it mutually supportive? Do others in the person's life seem to really care about his or her feelings? Does he or she tend to take responsibility for solving others' problems?

Now these are very personal questions. In most cases, no one has ever asked such sensitive and seemingly irrelevant questions of those we see. Just think. When was the last time you were in a social setting and someone asked, "So, ever been emotionally abused?" It is simply not proper to ask these types of questions. Similarly, most people probably have never been quizzed about such things from their medical doctor when seeking help for pain.

Recognizing that we run the risk of coming across as being excessively nosy, we have developed over the years ways of asking these questions with some precision and sensitivity. But Sandy was pretty sharp. She recognized "irrelevant" and potentially "incriminating" questions when she heard them. After all, what in the world did her *screwy mother* have to do with — Ah ha! *Now we're getting somewhere!* Sandy took a chance in trusting us with some very painful details of her personal history after we assured her that we would treat the information with the utmost respect and confidentiality. It turned out that her stepfather had sexually abused Sandy over the course of several years. When she finally found the courage to tell her mother, she was told not to tell such "lies" and that God would punish her if she did. Sandy felt guilty, hurt, angry, and betrayed by her mother, who was always critical and never affectionate with her. Her mother seemed to take every opportunity to condemn Sandy. A favorite opportunity for inducing guilt would be any instance in which Sandy did something good for herself, like developing a healthy adult relationship with a man. Through years of conditioning, Sandy had learned that anything that felt positive or made her happy reflected her "selfishness" and was "wrong." Try as she might, she could never gain her mother's approval. And she tried hard. Even to this day, she pushes herself — almost beyond belief — to help others through her volunteer work. Early on, however, she learned from her mother that no matter how much she does, it's *never* enough. So she pushes harder. Her mind is never idle, even when her body succumbs to fatigue and pain and she *has* to rest. No. In fact, things get worse. She feels that she is forever falling behind, that she should be busy instead of "selfishly" lying in bed in an attempt to recover from her pain and fatigue. She plans. She worries. She hurts. So even when her body is not active, her brain is working overtime. It is signaling the pituitary gland to stay alert by dumping large quantities of stress hormone into the bloodstream. It is prodding the sympathetic nervous system to speed things up in anticipation of getting things done — all while lying in bed "relaxing." When her body does start to recover, there is another burst of activity in an attempt to catch up. More physical stress, more worry, and more pain. Look up vicious cycle in the dictionary. Sandy's picture should be there.

Okay. So it sounds like we're blaming Sandy for her painful malady. Like she's doing it to herself by working so hard and worrying so much. Next thing you know we'll be telling her to just relax and take a vacation, right? Wrong. To illustrate our perspective on the matter, we invite you to take the following pop quiz.

Pop Quiz

Check the correct answer.

Sandy's vicious cycle...

☐ a. Is something she was born with.

☐ b. Is of her own making and she should just snap out of it. Shame on her!

☐ c. Involves thoughts and behaviors that once helped her to survive in a crazy environment but that are now difficult to unlearn.

If you answered *a* (it's something she was born with), cash in your "Get-Out-of-Jail-Free" card and proceed directly to "GO" (i.e., the beginning of this chapter).

If you answered *b* (it's of her own making and she should just snap out of it), you either think like Sandy's mother or you *are* Sandy's mother.

However, if you answered *c* (involves thoughts and behaviors that once helped her to survive in a crazy environment but that are now difficult to unlearn), congratulations. You have earned a perfect score! Recall our earlier discussion of reinforcement in which we explained that behaviors which help us to avoid unpleasant circumstances are strengthened. This is called *negative* reinforcement (not to be confused with punishment, which serves to *weaken* the behavior it follows). Look up negative reinforcement in the dictionary. You guessed it. Sandy's picture again. Indeed, her hard-driving, self-denying thoughts and behaviors were so successful in warding off the wrath of her mother (and occasionally her stepfather) that they were strengthened and honed to perfection. She carried them with her into adulthood, long after she left her mother's home. Unfortunately, contact with her critical, angry mother continued over the years, thus keeping the offending thoughts and behaviors alive and well. However, Sandy has made excellent progress in counterconditioning those old responses, with a little coaching from us. We are now starting to see a woman with the courage to challenge the old ways in favor of experimenting with more self-nurturing behaviors. And her fibromyalgia has eased up as well.

Sound like a bunch of hocus-pocus? Like your standard psychological gobbledygook? Not at all. In fact, it is *biobehavioral* gobbledygook. There is a big difference. In this analysis we are attempting to show the link between behavior and physical illness. Advances in our understanding of biology and behavior have allowed us to start filling in the blank space between mind and body. And courageous individuals like Sandy have helped us to bridge the gap.

Hardware versus Software

This proposed model of fibromyalgia and myofascial pain syndrome is still under investigation and must be treated as a work in progress rather than fact. Nevertheless, we have found it to be clinically useful in that it guides our behavioral treatment approach. We humans are like computers. We are comprised of "hardware" (the brain and body) which, depending on our components, runs at various speeds, operates at certain temperatures, and can malfunction if overworked. But it is the *software* that tells the hardware what to do. Got a piece of computer hardware that keeps crashing? Perhaps it is the software that is telling that component to operate in overdrive mode when it really doesn't need to. Don't keep repairing the chip. Modify the software! In a way, we seek to help people to revise their brain's "software" which was once successful in enabling them to cope with earlier, more stressful, circumstances but which now only produces excess stress and strain on the system.

Computer Repair 101

Essentially, the focus of our behavioral management approach to fibromyalgia and myofascial pain syndrome is to retrain the brain so that it realizes it no longer needs to prepare the body for evasive action (the fight-or-flight stress response). Unless this is done, we can massage or otherwise do things to the affected parts of the body all day long, but the computer residing between our ears will continue to send the tension (and other) signals that cause the symptoms to return. As both hardware and software engineers of the human computer, we seek to treat symptoms medically while counterconditioning the old nonvalidating behaviors. This is done by reinforcing responses that essentially show respect for one's physical and emotional feelings. In other words, we help people learn how to be good to themselves. Fine-tune the software and the hardware starts working more efficiently. It only makes sense.

When an individual is successful in doing this, we see significant improvement in his or her physical symptoms. This approach takes work. It is not a "passive" form of treatment. It takes considerable effort and a bit of courage to let go of behaviors that were once adaptive and "protective." But for those bold enough to experiment with giving themselves permission to put their own desires and needs at the top of the priority list, the positive consequences that naturally follow strengthen adaptation to the new, less dysfunctional environment.

It's All in Your Head — Not!

Whether your pain is related to migraines, fibromyalgia, or a ruptured disc in the spine, only you know how it really feels. In addition to the physical pain, there is also disappointment and frustration from having to limit your life activities. You have to deal with disrupted relationships and try to communicate the suffering produced by these factors to your loved ones and healthcare providers, who often do not adequately understand. Personally, we do not know a single person who has been helped by having been told that the pain is "all in your head." But we do know plenty of people who have been deeply harmed by this sentiment. And while we can forgive well-intentioned doctors for engaging in this transgression out of ignorance, we have a more difficult time with those who convey this message with an unhealthy dose of judgment and contempt. Not only is it unprofessional, unpardonable, and just plain unfair, it is also downright unhealthy to the extent that it contributes to an already overly active stress response brought on by that for which help is being sought: the experience of pain and suffering.

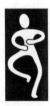

Narcotics and the Fear of Addiction: Or Much Ado about Almost Nothing

Jason was a handsome, 24-year-old athlete who was involved in a motorcycle accident that changed his life forever. He sustained a spinal cord injury that resulted in the paralysis of both legs. Shortly thereafter, Jason underwent major surgery to stabilize his spine. Following his recovery from the operation, he went through a physical rehabilitation program where he learned how to deal effectively with his disability.

Fortunately, Jason retained the full use of his upper extremities. With proper instruction and guidance, he was able to care for himself independently. But Jason, the athlete, was now permanently confined to a wheelchair and was even unable to control his urinary flow. He had to insert a catheter through his penis and into his bladder several times a day to empty it of urine. To compound his problems, he had constant, excruciating pain in his back and both legs.

Jason found that the pain was even more debilitating than his spinal cord injury. Because of his extreme discomfort, he was unable to work, and he became a financial burden to his family and society. The pain also interfered with his sleep. He would fall asleep but awaken several times during the night and have a hard time getting back to sleep. The hours between 1:00 A.M. and 6:00 A.M. were especially uncomfortable, lonely, and depressing. Jason began to experience feelings of hopelessness and despair.

Then it happened. Jason's rehabilitation doctor discovered that small doses of morphine, taken daily by mouth, obliterated his pain. The quality of Jason's life seemed to improve rapidly with the use of the pain medication. He was able to sleep better and return to the work force full time, and his depression became a thing of the past. Life looked a whole lot better.

Jason's interest in women was even renewed. Although it was an adjustment to pursue a relationship from wheelchair level, he was not deterred. He met Sarah, a schoolteacher, through a mutual friend. They began to date, and before long their relationship evolved into a serious commitment. In June of that year, they became engaged and made plans to be married the following September.

Then one day, several weeks before the wedding, Jason's doctor received a letter from the State Board of Medicine raising serious questions about his practice of prescribing narcotics. The board put him on notice that it would be watching his prescribing pattern very closely and that he could face disciplinary action — perhaps even lose his medical license — if he was found to be "irresponsible," as the board defined it. Fearful of losing his license, the physician stopped prescribing the medication. Jason's debilitating pain soon returned, and before long he was unable to work. The insomnia and depression he thought were behind him repaid him an unwelcome visit. His worst fears had come true. He had again become a burden to his family and society, and this time, there truly seemed to be no hope on the horizon.

As so often happens, Jason took his grief out on the person closest to him, Sarah. His irritability knew no bounds now that his pain was out of control and his life was crumbling around him. The final blow came when Sarah called off the wedding. Jason sank into a deeper depression and eventually pulled the trigger that ended his life.

Did justice prevail? Were the best interests of this courageous man served? We think not. This is just one of countless examples of the tragedy of needless pain.

Conventional Wisdom

According to conventional wisdom, the good and wise physician never prescribes narcotics for chronic, nonmalignant (noncancer) pain because of the possibility of *tolerance, physical dependence,* and *psychological dependence.* But is conventional wisdom based on fact or fiction? The field of pain medicine is a relatively new specialty that has come a long way in the last decade. Conventional wisdom, on the other hand, has come under much needed scrutiny, and it turns out to be erroneous. There is now solid research evidence that shows the fallacy of conventional wisdom. Let's look at this issue more closely.

Drug Tolerance, Physical Dependence, and Psychological Dependence

Drug tolerance is an involuntary physiological reaction whereby a given dosage of a drug becomes less effective and an increasing dose must be given to achieve the same effect.

Physical dependence is an involuntary physiological condition that occurs after repeated administration of a narcotic over at least several weeks. Abrupt discontinuation of the drug results in a syndrome characterized by agitation, tremors (shaking), an elevated heart rate, fever, sneezing, yawning, and tearing from the eyes.

Psychological dependence is synonymous with addiction. It is a pattern of compulsive drug use characterized by continuous craving for a narcotic and the need to use it for effects other than pain relief. The individual exhibits "drug-seeking" behavior, leading to overwhelming involvement with obtaining and using the drug.

Pseudoaddiction, A Key Concept

Pseudoaddiction is an iatrogenic (i.e., doctor-induced) syndrome caused by undermedication of pain. For example, patient Joseph Bloe comes to Dr. Miserlee with a severe back strain after lifting a heavy bag of cement at work. Dr. Miserlee prescribes a drug that is not strong enough to alleviate the pain and/or does not last long enough to provide relief during the entire time between doses. Joe experiences minimal pain relief after taking the medication, or he experiences significant pain relief but only for two hours. According to the prescription, he must wait another four hours before taking another pill. His pain is clearly undermedicated.

Since Joe does not want to be in pain (who would?), he responds in a logical manner. He asks for stronger medication and/or more frequent doses of the drugs, a seemingly reasonable request. But Joe meets resistance. He watches Dr. Miserlee cross his arms in front of his chest. He sees the skeptical look on the doctor's face. Joe knows he is in for a battle.

If Joe wants to win the battle, he must first convince Dr. Miserlee that the pain is real and of sufficient severity to warrant additional medication. So Joe decides to put on an Academy Award-winning performance. He moans and groans rather loudly. He grimaces and holds the affected body part in a protective manner. He also unknowingly produces a pain response during a physical exam mistakenly used by physicians to differentiate "real" from "imagined" pain (the Waddell test; see Chapter 6).

As a result, Dr. Miserlee perceives Joe to be a behavioral problem, one of those "nut cases." The doctor responds by avoiding contact with him. Joe, in turn, feels angry and abandoned. He concludes that perhaps he did not effectively convey the extent of his suffering. A vicious cycle is set up, leading to distrust on the part of both the patient and the doctor. At some point, Joe is mislabeled as an addict and his pain complaints are no longer taken seriously by Dr. Miserlee, who withholds needed pain medication for fear that he may be contributing to Joe's "addiction."

This syndrome is called *pseudo*addiction because of the striking resemblance of the behavior pattern to that of truly addicted individuals, especially the all-consuming, compulsive drive to acquire and use narcotics. The difference is that, in the case of pseudoaddiction, the person is driven by a need and desire for genuine pain relief. And in the case of true addiction (involving psychological dependence), the person is driven by the desire for the mood-altering effects — the "high" — and the avoidance of unpleasant physical withdrawal symptoms. In essence, addiction stems from a person's choice to experience a "high," whereas pseudoaddiction results from undertreatment of a medical condition.

Unfortunately, we see real-life examples of pseudoaddiction all too frequently. Patients like Joe suffer from severe pain and *no one believes them*! They are treated like third-class citizens. They are condemned by their families, the medical establishment, our "watchdog" state and federal agencies, and society at large. They are unfairly mislabeled as addicts.

Beware of the "12 Steps"

Another tragic result we often see occurs when "pseudoaddicted" patients are referred by their doctors to programs that specialize in the treatment of substance abuse. Such programs usually embrace the principles and methods of Alcoholics Anonymous and other so-called "*12-step*" approaches to addiction. These programs are not geared toward, nor are they equipped to handle, individuals with chronic pain. While we applaud their success with those who seek help for true addiction, many a chronic pain patient has been harmed emotionally and physically by the inappropriate use of "12-step" techniques for the treatment of pseudoaddiction. If pseudoaddiction is considered as stemming from the inadequate medical treatment of chronic pain, it becomes apparent that the "cure" lies not in changing the patient's behavior but rather in changing the *doctor's* behavior. If the doctor had treated the pain appropriately in the first place, the problem would cease to exist. Yet, it is the patient who is held responsible for the doctor's inadequacies; it is the patient who "must be fixed." The injustice deepens as the patient is then referred to a 12-step program for treatment of "addiction." Let's take a look at what happened to Joe.

He reluctantly agreed to enter a 14-day in-hospital chemical dependency program as prescribed by Dr. Miserlee. Upon arrival, most of his personal belongings were confiscated, he was instructed to don a hospital gown, and he was given a physical exam by one of the program physicians. He was told that he could "earn" telephone and other "privileges" by adhering to the program rules. For the next 48 hours, he was medically "detoxified" of all addictive substances. This means that he was medically monitored through the withdrawal process and was given other medications to minimize the potentially harmful effects that the body undergoes. As withdrawal progressed, Joe reported some of the greatest discomfort he had ever experienced. On top of the unpleasantness of withdrawal itself, there was the now unmedicated nociception, or physical pain, and the sense of powerlessness over it. Joe's requests for effective pain-relieving medication were met with denial and seen as typical of addictive behavior. He contemplated checking out of the hospital against medical advice, but decided to stick it out, despite his increased suffering.

After a few days, Joe's withdrawal symptoms eased, but his pain roared back to life. He was now getting only ibuprofen and was expected to get out of bed and attend the support group meetings on the ward. With great effort, he did. As Joe looked around the room, he saw one participant after another stand up and say, "Hi. I'm [so and so] and I'm an addict." The group, in unison, responded, "Hi [so and so]." Joe instantly started wondering why he was required to attend this meeting. After all, he was taking the medications prescribed by Dr. Miserlee, and they were his only "lifeline" in a sea of unrelenting pain. He wasn't seeking a "high," just pain relief so that he could function. As he saw it, he had nothing in common with these people. When his turn came, Joe simply introduced himself and stated that he was there — at his doctor's insistence — to get off of pain pills. He became terribly ill-at-ease as he could sense that the others expected him to announce that he, too, was an addict.

Later that day, Joe met with his program counselor, Stuart Stepman, and told him of his reservations about being identified as an addict. He also made it known that his pain was worse and that he would need something stronger than ibuprofen if he were to spend much time out of bed.

But Stuart had heard it all before. According to his way of thinking, addicts were, by their very nature, "manipulative and deceitful." The problem was the "disease," the addiction. It was then that Joe's "education" began. He was told that he was, in fact, an addict and that his "denial" explained his misgivings about the group, his nonidentification with the other addicts, and his requests for pain medications. In fact, Stuart himself had been an addict at one time and was still in "recovery": "Once an addict, always an addict." Stuart knew all the "tricks." Unfortunately for Joe (but fortunately for Stuart), Stuart had never had chronic pain and therefore had no experience base from which to interpret Joe's statements. After all, Joe's behavior was just like that of an addict. Why waste time even considering that there might be another, more valid, explanation for his behavior? The doctors, the staff, and the other "recovering" addicts all saw Joe as an addict. There was no question about that. In Stuart's mind, Joe's first task was to work on the first step: admitting that he was an "addict."

Over the next few days, no attention was paid to helping Joe cope with his pain and the accompanying debilitation. There was no discussion with the counselors, the doctor, or the support group members about how to deal with this very real problem. In their view, the problem was Joe's supposed refusal to own up to his "disease." After all, he hadn't even reached step one yet. Yet, despite his almost overwhelming sense of demoralization and hopelessness, Joe remained unconvinced and eventually left the hospital against medical advice. To make matters even worse, he was now without medical support, as Dr. Miserlee refused to take him back as a patient due to his "noncompliance" with the chemical dependency program.

An isolated example? Not at all. Over the years, we have worked with dozens of chronic pain sufferers who have lived to tell this story. It is painful to hear, especially since the vast majority of these people, after undergoing a coordinated interdisciplinary pain program, went on to achieve good pain control, improved functioning, decreased depression and anxiety, and *reduced reliance on pain medication.* Their successes essentially contradict the *hypothesis* that the "real" problem was addiction. No. The *real* problem was misguided treatment and an inflexible group of healthcare providers that had little capacity, or desire, to question whether or not they were on the right track. Through ignorance, indifference, and inertia, the system failed these individuals in a most unjust way. And the same thing is happening to others at this very moment.

As chronic pain specialists, we take what may be considered by many to be a radical position regarding the prescribing of narcotics (although it appears to be getting less radical all the time). We believe that treatment with narcotics should be considered in cases of chronic nonmalignant pain that is not relieved by other, more conservative, methods (such as physical therapy, chiropractic manipulation, nonnarcotic pain medications, nerve blocks, and even bona fide interdisciplinary pain programs — the very Cadillac of pain management). In our view, the physician has a moral and ethical obligation to distinguish between addiction and pseudoaddiction and to treat pain conscientiously. As professionals, we should not be timid about prescribing narcotics when they are effective. They should be used in as high a dose as is required to control the pain, for as long as the pain persists, according to the patient's report rather than the doctor's estimate of how much the patient "should" need. The critical qualifier is that the individual's ability to function should not be compromised by untoward side effects such as oversedation.

Our position is supported by the California Medical Board and is strongly reinforced by the knowledge that the risk of tolerance or addiction is actually very low, whereas the potential benefit in terms of an individual's quality of life can be very high. For example, an individual may be able to work while taking pain medication, but without it, he or she may be home- or even bed-bound. Gainful employment is an excellent benefit and far outweighs the risks of taking the medication, if handled appropriately by the physician. But the ability to go out to dinner with a loved one or to tolerate sitting through a two-hour movie is just as important. Forget conventional wisdom. The issue is quality of life.

A Look at the Evidence

Drs. Russell Portenoy and Kathleen Foley of the world-renowned Sloan-Kettering Medical Center studied the effects of narcotic administration in 38 patients with severe nonmalignant pain. Half of the patients received opioids (another term for narcotics) for four or more years, while six were treated for more than seven years. Sixty percent reported that their pain was either eliminated or significantly reduced. Only 2 of the 38 patients had difficulty managing their pain medications, both of whom had a history of drug abuse prior to the onset of chronic pain. Portenoy and Foley concluded that narcotic administration can be a safe and humane alternative to no treatment or to surgical intervention in patients with chronic, intractable, noncancer pain.

An isolated study with an isolated finding? Not at all. This conclusion is supported by numerous other studies.

Zenz, Strumpf, and Tryba studied 100 patients who were chronically given narcotics for pain that was nonresponsive to other treatments. Fifty-one reported good pain relief and 28 had only partial relief. Only 21 reported no benefit from the medication. Pain relief was associated with improved performance and functioning. The most common side effects were nausea and constipation. Of the 100 chronic pain sufferers in the study, there were no cases of addiction to narcotics! The researchers concluded that opioids can be safe and effective in the management of chronic nonmalignant pain.

Taub described 313 patients with intractable (unrelieved) pain who were maintained on opioids for up to six years. Only 13 of the 313 experienced serious problems in managing their medications. Of the 13, all had a prior history of substance abuse. No incidences of tolerance or toxicity (significant side effects) occurred, and all patients appeared to benefit from the narcotic medications.

Tennant and Uelman studied the experience of 22 patients who were maintained on narcotics after failing to benefit from treatment at pain clinics. Two-thirds returned to work, and all had fewer subsequent medical visits for pain, including trips to the emergency room.

France described 16 chronic pain patients who were maintained on narcotics as part of a comprehensive pain management program. No clinically significant physical tolerance or side effects developed, and each patient's ability to function improved.

"Well," you may say, "that's nice, but those are not the biggest studies in the world. I mean, 16, 22, 38, 100, and 313 patients? There are *millions* of chronic pain sufferers. Can't you do any better than that?" The answer is *yes* (so glad you asked). There are now two studies with over 10,000 subjects — and the conclusions are the same!

Porter and Jick of the Boston University Medical Center followed up on 11,882 patients who were given narcotics to relieve pain stemming from a variety of medical problems while they were hospitalized. None had a prior history of substance abuse. Of the 11,882 patients, only 4 subsequently had a problem in managing their narcotic medications, and in only one case was the problem considered major.

Perry and Heidrich presented equally impressive results from a survey of more than 10,000 burn victims. While hospitalized, these patients underwent multiple debridements, an extremely painful procedure in which dead tissue is removed from the wound. Most received narcotics for weeks to months. Not a single case of later addiction could be attributed to the opioids given for pain relief during the hospitalization. Of the 10,000 patients, only 22 abused the narcotic pain medications after discharge, all of whom had a history of substance abuse prior to the onset of chronic pain.

The results of these studies stand in sharp contrast to the emphatic cultural prohibition against opioid use in chronic pain patients. It is time that the medical community revise its medieval attitudes about — *and miserly practice of* — prescribing narcotics. But our society at large must also undergo an attitude adjustment regarding opioids. Too many members of our society equate taking narcotics for pain relief with the abuse of street drugs. In actuality, they are comparing apples and oranges.

So, as you can see, the barriers between the sufferer and the solution are many. They include the erroneous beliefs and purposeful actions (and inactions) of uninformed physicians and federal and state bureaucracies such as the Drug Enforcement Administration (DEA). Other barriers include the dilemma encountered by more informed physicians whose hands are tied by the "watchdog" agencies responsible for policing the prescription of controlled substances. The sad result is that the individual suffering from chronic pain pays the price for an overzealous agency that cares little for the consequences of curbing the legitimate use of pain medication.

Beware of the Medication Trap

While we advocate the appropriate use of narcotic medications for chronic nonmalignant pain, we also must emphasize that this approach should be used as *part of a coordinated effort between doctor and patient*. Narcotic pain medications are rarely the answer in and of themselves. Too often, we treat individuals for whom pain medications have been the only approach used. Their doctors never considered the multifaceted nature of chronic pain — that is, the psychosocial as well as physical aspects — and that the goal of improving function frequently involves taking the time and effort to address the person's social, emotional, occupational, and familial circumstances. The sole focus is treating the physical pain component by way of narcotics.

Unfortunately, this "medication trap" can lead to increased lethargy, withdrawal, and further loss of function. In fact, many of these individuals absolutely insist that they need more medication despite the fact that what they are taking is not working very well for them. Yet they spend most of the day in bed or being otherwise inactive. We believe that this is because they have not been given appropriate alternatives. In almost all such cases, the individual has never undergone an interdisciplinary chronic pain evaluation from which a coordinated treatment plan would emerge. If you take narcotic pain medication as your only real way of coping with chronic pain but find that it does not result in improved functioning, it is time to have a talk with your doctor about a specialized chronic pain treatment program. As we shall see, this coordinated approach can be our most powerful weapon in combating chronic pain and the debilitation that stems therefrom.

The California Board of Medicine Sets Precedent

On July 29, 1994, California became the first state to openly acknowledge that patients are enduring pain needlessly. Minorities, women, children, the elderly, and persons with AIDS were found to be at the greatest risk for undertreatment. The board issued a formal statement, the first of its kind from a state medical authority, regarding the use of narcotic medication for both acute and chronic pain conditions. In this statement, doctors were strongly urged to prescribe narcotics to relieve suffering in those individuals afflicted with pain, whether due to trauma, surgery, cancer, or a nonmalignant cause such as back pain that persists after surgery (the so-called "failed back syndrome").

The catalyst for this historic action was the *Governor's Summit on Effective Pain Management*. This body of 120 healthcare professionals, after studying the research evidence, concluded that patients with pain are undertreated for a number of reasons. Among these are the following:

- ♦ Pain management traditionally has been a low priority in our healthcare system. Unlike cancer, there never has been a "War on Pain."

- ♦ Insurance reimbursement for specialized pain management treatment has been limited.

- ♦ Misdiagnosis frequently occurs.

- ♦ Physicians fear state and federal regulators because of archaic prescription laws.

- ♦ Physicians and others have exaggerated fears of causing "addiction."

This list certainly shows that the barriers to the appropriate medical use of narcotic medications are many and extend into the very fabric of our culture.

The summit recommended revising the laws that impede appropriate access to pain medication and passing laws that create a positive legal duty on the part of the physician to effectively treat pain. Patients, according to the summit report, should be told that they have a right to quality pain management. In addition, it was recommended that education in pain management be made a requirement for medical licensure.

Marijuana

Personal testimonies about the benefits of marijuana abound in some pain centers. "It's great!...It's the best!...It helped ease the pain when nothing else would!...I was finally able to eat and sleep normally again." Because it is an illicit drug in most parts of the world, pain sufferers usually learn of the alleged effectiveness of this substance in relieving pain by word of mouth and behind closed doors. But controlled studies are sorely lacking — in large part because of the extremely restrictive criteria imposed by the DEA for authorizing marijuana research.

Tetrahydrocannabinol (THC; brand name Marinol®) is a synthetic agent that is the major psychoactive component of the marijuana plant, hemp. The drug may be administered orally, intravenously, or by inhalation. Two reliable clinical signs of cannabis effect are red eyes (conjunctival injection) and increased heart rate.

THC is prescribed for a number of clinical conditions. First and foremost, it is used to alleviate severe nausea and vomiting associated with cancer chemotherapy. It is also prescribed as an appetite stimulant in the treatment of AIDS-related anorexia and weight loss. In addition, the drug is used to treat asthma and glaucoma, as well as the spasticity, tremor, and unsteadiness associated with multiple sclerosis. Finally, it has also been used for analgesic purposes.

To date, studies that have been carried out to evaluate the potential pain-alleviating properties of the drug have shown it to have questionable efficacy. Pain is a subjective experience that is strongly influenced by a multitude of factors, including mood, anxiety, personality, personal expectations, and the power of suggestion. The improvement in pain reported by individuals receiving the drug may be influenced by both physiological and psychological factors. For example, reports of pain reduction may, in fact, reflect decreased worry, anxiety, muscle tension, and overall suffering. These studies have generally overlooked these potentially contributory factors. But we might add that even if these factors do constitute the primary mechanisms of action, they are valid therapeutic effects in and of themselves.

True double-blind controlled studies are difficult to carry out, especially when some research participants may be familiar with the subjective effects, such as euphoria. Many of these studies administer such high doses that the side effects become intolerable. Untoward side effects may include drowsiness, hallucinations, muddled thinking, visual changes, weakness, dry mouth, anxiety, loss of coordination, mood changes, tachycardia (heart rate over 100 beats per minute), palpitations, and a drop in blood pressure. In addition, the medication may cause psychological addiction in predisposed individuals. To date, some of the evidence suggests that the risks of taking THC in doses high enough to potentially alleviate pain may outweigh the benefits. On the other hand, the mass of credible anecdotal reports of its merits in alleviating suffering cannot be discounted.

"Medical" Marijuana

In recent years, several states have, by popular vote, passed "medical marijuana" laws that essentially allow licensed physicians to prescribe marijuana for the treatment of medical conditions. Such proposed legislation has led to some of the most contentious campaigns in recent years due to the strong feelings among anti-drug and pro-patient rights advocates. In general, the anti-drug folks hung their hats on the following assertions:

1. Making marijuana available for ("ostensible") medical uses would also make it more available to addicts.

2. The "medical" part of the proposed law is merely a ruse by recreational users to weaken the prohibition against marijuana.

In monitoring this debate, it seemed to us that the anti-drug activists displayed a remarkable lack of acknowledgment of the testimony of patients with maladies such as glaucoma and chronic pain who told of their own first-hand experience of reduced suffering and improved quality of life. It was glossed over, discounted, and, in more extreme cases, ridiculed as amounting to a veiled excuse to get high. We heard some with a specialty in addictionology (or addiction medicine) arrogantly condescend to chronically ill patients that getting off all "addictive" medications was in their best interest. Besides, they said, detoxification from addictive substances was the "accepted" first step in treating chronic pain (wrong). It appeared that the addictionologists simply did not believe these patients. Why?

Specialists in addictionology spend their professional time, day in and day out, dealing with people whose lives are adversely affected by the use of addictive drugs. These patients are in trouble and seek help because they cannot control their addictive behavior. In the addictionologist's training and clinical experience, the same pattern emerges over and over. And like the rest of us, they begin to think and operate in the world according to their own (experientially constructed) view of reality. The only chronic pain patients addictionologists see are either those who also have problems with addiction (as contrasted to physical dependence) or those who are sent by physicians who mistakenly think they are addicted (because they are considered to be taking "too much" pain medication). Even in cases where pain medications are truly effective in treating the pain, addictionologists are prone to see only the drug-seeking, pill-taking, and physical dependency aspects — which they mistakenly label "addiction." To most of them, it reflects a "disease" that should be "treated." Hence, when one is primed to see the world through addiction-colored glasses, it can be quite difficult to consider that the alternative reality of chronic pain truly exists when "addictive" substances such as marijuana are part of the landscape.

Most of us use our cars safely for legitimate purposes. But if we had little or no personal experience with them and our primary source of information about using them came from accident investigation experts (whose mandate involves reducing the accident rate), it would be easy to conclude that automobiles are an unacceptable danger to society and should be outlawed. And it would be easy to discount the testimony of those who drive carefully and responsibly. ("It's just a smokescreen so that they can go out joyriding.") Ridiculous! And just as not all drivers are reckless, not all consumers of marijuana are addicts. The only real difference between the two issues is that the vast majority of us do have personal experience using automobiles safely and for worthy purposes. On the other hand, relatively few in our society have personal experience with chronic pain and the things that alleviate it.

The moral of the story is that we should all look outside our own realm of life experience and consider that it may not always apply to every issue affecting others. And while we are not necessarily medical mari-juana advocates, we *are* patient rights advocates who believe in taking an empirical — *and compassionate* — approach to treating pain and human suffering.

Oregon Passes Assisted Suicide Law

In 1995, the state of Oregon passed the Death with Dignity Act. This legislation legalized physician-assisted suicide within that jurisdiction. It is limited by the geographic boundaries of the state and by restric-tions on the type of circumstances that qualify a physician to assist in the death of a patient. Essentially, there are three criteria: A patient must be terminally ill, mentally competent, and physically able to take medications on his or her own.

This legislation represented a fundamental shift in focus relative to medical tradition and generated enormous controversy both within and outside the healthcare field. Because we routinely work with chronic pain patients who, by definition, are experiencing ongoing suffering, our concern is that many of those who may elect to discontinue their lives in this manner would not be in such a state of despair if their pain and overall suffering were adequately treated. Several studies show that there are close connections between pain — physical and emotional — and the "existential" suffering that drives people to want to end their lives.

We have grave concerns about requests for assisted suicide because we have methods at our disposal for effectively treating pain and emotional problems stemming therefrom. We believe that these methods should be employed before thoughts of assisted suicide are seriously consid-ered. It is a fact that many of those suffering from such extreme physi-cal and emotional circumstances are never given access to the kinds of treatment that will help — that will make life worth living again. In terms of so-called "rational" suicide, *you don't know if it's rational if you don't know the alternatives*. And, as addressed earlier, the barriers to reaching more people in need of such treatment are substantial.

Suicide is the eighth leading cause of death in the United States and accounts for over 30,000 deaths annually. At greatest risk are elderly white men, among whom the suicide rate is five times the national average. Recent studies indicate that about 90 percent of suicide victims have a diagnosable psychiatric condition at the time of death. In one study, 75 percent of the elderly who took their own lives had seen a primary care physician within a month of death. Yet, their emotional pain apparently went undetected and/or inadequately treated.

In a study of public attitudes in the United States, 69 percent of people queried indicated that they would consider suicide if their pain were not adequately controlled. In the Netherlands, previously the only Western country where active voluntary euthanasia is permitted by law, 46 percent of the patients who requested and obtained physician assistance in suicide reported pain as one of the symptoms leading to their decision to die.

Several vulnerability factors that contribute to increased suicide risk in chronically ill patients have been identified. They include pain, depression, hopelessness, delirium due to metabolic imbalances, disinhibition (nonawareness of socially appropriate behavior), loss of control, feelings of helplessness, exhaustion and fatigue, prior suicide history or a family history of suicide, advanced illness and poor prognosis, and a preexisting psychiatric illness. Of these, the perception that one has lost personal control over one's life is the most pervasive and the most frightening. It is this fear that has led many to support the legalization of assisted suicide. Yet, as we shall later see, fear of suffering can be eased with understanding, compassion, and the right clinical measures.

"Doctor Death"

In June 1990, Dr. Jack Kevorkian, a pathologist from Michigan, made national headlines when he performed the first publicly acknowledged physician-assisted suicide in the United States, which he called "medicide." The "patient" was Janet Adkins, a mentally competent woman with rapidly progressive Alzheimer's disease. Her death was brought about by a device Dr. Kevorkian dubbed the "Mercitron," a "suicide machine" that delivers a lethal injection to the individual.

Mrs. Adkins and her husband, Ron, lived in Portland, Oregon. They first contacted Dr. Kevorkian in November of 1989 after reading about his campaign in an article in *Newsweek*. Janet, a wife, mother, grand-mother, teacher, musician, and outdoorsperson, had been diagnosed with Alzheimer's disease four months earlier, after undergoing evalu-ation for a progressive impairment of her memory. At that time, she had made a "rational" decision to end her life prematurely rather than endure to the end, the natural course of the disease.

Her husband and their three sons argued against such a plan and persuaded her to participate in an experimental trial of a new drug, Tacrine (tacrine hydrochloride), at the University of Washington in Seattle. Dr. Kevorkian offered his support for the plan, as, by his cri-teria, any candidate for physician-assisted suicide must have exhausted all other potentially beneficial medical interventions. Janet reluctantly agreed to enroll in the program in January 1990. Unfortunately, in her case, the drug was ineffective. In fact, Janet's condition grew steadily worse. Subsequently, she became even more determined to end her life and to control the events leading to her death while her mental facul-ties would still allow her to do so. Time was of the essence.

Dr. Kevorkian reviewed Janet's medical record, which corroborated her story. Then he spoke with her personal physician, who did not support the proposed plan of action or the concept of assisted suicide. He be-lieved that Mrs. Adkins would remain mentally competent for at least another year. Dr. Kevorkian then spoke with Janet's husband and con-cluded, on the basis of that discussion regarding the progression of symptoms, that her personal physician was mistaken. The time to act was now.

Dr. Kevorkian encountered a series of roadblocks when he attempted to find a suitable place to carry out the act. This had posed no problem for a Michigan resident, but was quite another matter for an out-of-state subject. Because of lease restrictions, he could not use his own or his sister's apartment. He inquired at countless motels, office buildings, churches, clinics, and funeral homes, all without success. While many of the owners, proprietors, and landlords expressed sympathy for the endeavor, most were concerned about the potential impact on their business enterprises. They felt it would be bad for public relations. After exhausting all other possibilities, Dr. Kevorkian finally settled on his now infamous 1968 rusted-out van and a public campground.

On July 2, 1990, Dr. Kevorkian and his two sisters met Janet, her husband, and a close friend at the motel at which they were staying. Janet signed a statement of informed consent indicating that she understood the process and the implications, that she had freedom of choice, and that she was determined to proceed with the plan. Then Dr. Kevorkian's sister videotaped his interview with Janet and Ron, thus documenting her resolve to proceed with the plan. That night, they all had dinner together at a well-known local restaurant. Two days later, on June 4, Dr. Kevorkian drove his old van to a park in Oakland County. Meanwhile, his sisters drove to the motel to pick up Janet, who chose to say her parting good-byes to her husband and friend at the motel. Ron and the friend were inconsolable. Janet had written a brief note, again expressing her desire to die and to exonerate all those who were involved in aiding this effort. Then she left with Dr. Kevorkian's sisters for the campground. They arrived at 9:30 A.M.

Dr. Kevorkian had already set up the Mercitron, but unfortunately there was an accidental spill of some of the thiopental, a fast-acting barbiturate (sleep medication), necessitating a two-and-a-half-hour round trip to fetch more of the drug. Therefore, the actual event did not take place until the afternoon. Janet entered the van alone. She laid down fully clothed, resting her head on a clean pillow. Dr. Kevorkian placed electrodes on her wrists and ankles to monitor her cardiac (heart) status. With some difficulty, he started an intravenous line that infused normal saline. The Lord's Prayer was read. Then Janet hit the Mercitron switch that released a lethal injection of the thiopental, followed by potassium chloride, into her veins. The latter substance stopped Janet's heart. She became unconscious within seconds. Death occurred at 2:30 P.M.

Dr. Kevorkian, a brilliant eccentric, was prosecuted for his deeds in Wade County in 1990. Apparently to make a statement of defiance as he sat in court, he studied Japanese verbs and practiced mirror writing in full view of the jury. He was acquitted.

Since then, many more men and women, longing for death and relief from suffering, have perished with his help. About half of these people had a history of cancer. The rest were afflicted with a variety of medical illnesses, including Alzheimer's disease, multiple sclerosis, fibromyalgia, chronic fatigue syndrome, lung disease, and amyotrophic lateral sclerosis (Lou Gehrig's disease). In earlier cases, the individuals died by the Mercitron method. Later (after the authorities suspended Dr. Kevorkian's medical license and he could no longer prescribe or purchase prescription drugs), they died by carbon monoxide poisoning, administered by face mask, after the subjects removed a clamp from the gas hose.

Dr. Kevorkian came to be a familiar face in the courts. The judges knew him well. He was prosecuted repeatedly and acquitted as many times. It seemed that there was growing sympathy and support for his cause among the general populace. This changing tide of opinion regarding the deeply entrenched taboo against "mercy killing" or euthanasia was powerfully reinforced by the personal testimony of family members expressing their gratitude to Dr. Kevorkian for "helping" their loved ones.

In May 1995, a state court of appeals handed down a decision upholding a five-year-old injunction against Dr. Kevorkian. This decision tightened the legal noose created by the Michigan Supreme Court in December 1994, when it ruled that the act of assisting suicide was a crime based on common law. This was despite the fact that, in most states, suicide itself is not a crime. The U.S. Supreme Court refused to hear Dr. Kevorkian's appeal. Despite the obstacles, he made it eminently clear that he would not be deterred by the legislature or the judiciary. He would stay the course of his convictions.

But in April 1999, Dr. Kevorkian was convicted of second-degree murder after having videotaped himself injecting a man with lethal drugs.

Prior to this, the "patients" themselves were the ones who brought about their own demise by throwing a switch on the suicide machine. The videotape ran until the man was dead. The story, and the videotape, were aired on CBS's "60 Minutes," causing quite a stir. Prosecutors finally had hard evidence — evidence intentionally produced by Kevorkian himself — of murder. He was sentenced to prison, much to the dismay of the deceased's family and other supporters.

But Is Death the Only Alternative?

In his writings, Dr. Kevorkian stated that his highest ethical standard is individual self-determination. He further asserted that he has dedicated his life to a war against suffering. In a one-man crusade, he took on the legal community as well as the political, theological, and medical establishments. It is evident, based upon his actions, that he played by his own rules, since, in his view, those of society are clearly wanting. In the process, this energetic, single-minded man was dubbed "Doctor Death."

We believe that his goal, though possibly misguided, is a noble one: to relieve suffering in terminally ill and severely incapacitated, pain-ridden individuals who have made a "rational" decision to end their lives. But what constitutes a rational decision? Were these individuals mentally competent? If so, according to whom and by what criteria? Were they advised of all possible therapeutic approaches before proceeding with the plan to extinguish their earthly existence? These questions remain unanswered.

Our concern is that at least some of these people had treatable pain conditions. We know. A few years ago we evaluated a woman who suffered from fibromyalgia syndrome. Formerly a very active person, she became despondent over her loss of function due to pain and fatigue. Her condition was well known to us, as it was really no different from many others we had treated successfully. Our evaluation led to a coordinated treatment plan that was designed to reduce symptoms and improve her physical and emotional states. We found the prognosis to be good. She was pleased and agreed to start the treatment program in a few weeks. Tragically, she never did.

I (AC) remember well the day she called to announce that, contrary to our previous discussion, she would *not* be entering treatment. Despite my reasoned optimism that we could help her, she assertively held to her belief that our approach was not for her. She never really gave a reason. I vividly recall being haunted the rest of the day with a feeling of personal failure. I can still see myself driving home down I-15 while thinking, *"Why couldn't I reach her?"* This was strange because, on occasion, others had chosen not to pursue treatment, and it had never really bothered me too much. Why was this case different?

Several weeks later, we were stunned to learn that she had traveled to Michigan for a meeting with Dr. Kevorkian. She died that very day. Our guess is that he had agreed to "help" her at some point between our feedback session and the phone call. Her sudden — *and drastic* — change of heart now made sense. We wonder if Dr. Kevorkian would have intervened had he known about our successful experience with similar cases in general and our positive prognosis for her in particular.

The nagging question that looms large in our minds is: *How many assisted suicides could have been averted had the individual's pain, debilitation, and suffering been adequately treated?* At present, we don't know. We can merely speculate. But it is a very real possibility that if doctors had done more to alleviate physical and emotional suffering, we could run Dr. Kevorkian — as well intentioned as he may be — out of business, without his having to go to jail.

Let's Move that Mountain

You, the patient and owner of your own body, can help move that mountain of medical ignorance. You have a vested interest. But to do so, you must first educate yourself about the truth regarding the risks and benefits of taking narcotics for chronic pain. Armed with the facts, we believe that you will be able to advocate more effectively on your own behalf.

In our opinion, your primary care physician is one of the best people to help you, if there is no pain specialist in your area. The vast majority of primary care doctors chose their specialty because they like people. They usually will take more time to get to know you and your concerns. Most are, by nature, compassionate, good communicators, and may be far less burdened with ego problems compared with other specialists.

Have a heart-to-heart talk with your doctor. Approach him or her with the same respect that you would want. Offer to provide some relevant reading material. Consider using a highlighter or a written list to underscore key points. But remember that your doctor is busy. It takes time for new research findings to find their way into his or her hands. The primary care physician, unlike other specialists who are responsible for only one or two of the body's systems, must stay informed about new developments regarding all eight of the body's systems. And given the finite number of hours in a day, it is a mathematical impossibility to keep abreast of the latest in all areas. A person would have to read ten hours a day, every day. Yet we believe that most primary care physicians will be open to new information, that they genuinely want to help their patients, and that they are your strong potential allies. Do your part to make this important relationship work for you.

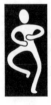

Pain Medications

In Chapter 7, we addressed the use of narcotics for chronic nonmalignant pain. In this chapter, we discuss other important classes of medications that may be helpful in alleviating the signs and symptoms of chronic pain syndrome. These include acetaminophen (Tylenol®), aspirin (acetylsalicylic acid), nonsteroidal anti-inflammatory drugs, steroids, antidepressants, muscle relaxants, antiseizure medications, blood pressure medications, and many others.

All drugs have a risk–benefit profile of which the patient and physician should be aware in order to make wise choices. The PDR (*Physicians' Desk Reference*) can be a very helpful source of information, but a word to the wise. At times, it can also be considered a public nuisance, since it lists every conceivable side effect. Talk about intimidating! Some patients overreact to this information and believe that they will fall victim to each and every one. A few patients may even blame the doctor for side effects they would never have experienced in the first place. "I thought you cared about me!" they exclaim. Countless hours are spent fretting about the risks, forgetting about the benefits. These individuals may even refuse to try medication that may truly help them, all because of a book called the PDR. Remember: every individual is unique, and it is important that you and your physician tailor your medication regimen according to your response to a given drug, and not according to some abstract, theoretical possibility.

Adjuvant Pain Medications

- Acetaminophen (Tylenol®)
- Aspirin (acetylsalicylic acid)
- Nonsteroidal anti-inflammatory drugs (NSAIDs)
- Steroids
- Local anesthetics (e.g., lidocaine, mexiletine)
- Antidepressants
- Muscle relaxants
- Botulinum toxin
- Anticonvulsants
- Benzodiazepines
- Buspirone (BuSpar®)
- Neuroleptics (antipsychotics)
- Antihistamines
- Sleep medication
- Barbiturates/sedatives
- Amphetamines
- Tramadol (Ultram®)
- NMDA-receptor blockers (e.g., ketamine, amantadine, dextro-methorphan)
- Triptans (Imitrex®, Amerge®, Zomig®)
- Ergotamine derivatives
- Isometheptene mucate/dichloralphenazone/acetaminophen (Midrin®)
- Caffeine
- Lithium carbonate (lithium)
- Oxygen
- *Tanacetum parthenium* (feverfew)
- Clonidine hydrochloride (Catapres®), an alpha-2-adrenergic agonist
- Propranolol (Inderal®; beta blocker)
- Calcium channel blockers
- Topical analgesics
- Capsaicin (Zostrix®)
- Glucosamine sulfate and chondroitin sulfate
- Calcitonin
- ABT-594

Acetaminophen (Tylenol®)

Acetaminophen is an analgesic that is effective in relieving mild to moderate pain. Unlike aspirin and nonsteroidal anti-inflammatory drugs, it has minimal effect on inflammation but rather works centrally. Acetaminophen is metabolized chiefly by the liver. While traditionally considered a remarkably safe drug when taken as prescribed, there is growing concern regarding potential side effects. Prolonged or high daily doses of acetaminophen can cause both serious kidney and liver damage and death. Overuse of acetaminophen may be responsible for as many as 5,000 cases of kidney failure in the United States each year. An alarming study reported in the *New England Journal of Medicine* found that taking just one Tylenol® or other acetaminophen-containing medication per day may double the risk of kidney failure. Fasting and alcohol ingestion may increase the risk of acetaminophen hepatotoxicity (liver damage). The maximum daily dose of acetaminophen for short-term use is 4,000 milligrams (mg). There are over 44 different trade names of acetaminophen-containing products (see sidebar: How Much Acetaminophen Is in Your Pain Medication?). Chronic use should be avoided.

Aspirin

"Take two aspirin and call me in the morning," replies the concerned doctor. While this may be good advice for many medical problems, aspirin is not a panacea. Nevertheless, this drug has been around since time immemorial, and it is still on the market and going strong. What staying power! Why? Because it is relatively safe and effective. And the price is right — just pennies a pill. You don't even need a prescription. So forget about going to the doctor, a time-consuming project to say the least. Just jump in your automobile and head to the nearest drug store.

Aspirin has three key properties:

◆ Analgesic (relieves mild to moderate pain)

How Much Acetaminophen Is in Your Pain Medication?

Medication	Contents
Darvocet-N® 100	acetaminophen 650 mg propoxyphene napsylate 100 mg
Esgic®	acetaminophen 500 mg butalbital 50 mg caffeine 65 mg
Excedrin® ES	acetaminophen 250 mg aspirin 250 mg caffeine 65 mg
Fioricet®	acetaminophen 325 mg butalbital 50 mg caffeine 40 mg
Lorcet® 10/650	acetaminophen 650 mg hydrocodone 10 mg
Lortab® 7.5/500	acetaminophen 500 mg hydrocodone bitartrate 7.5 mg
Lortab® 5/500	acetaminophen 500 mg hydrocodone bitartrate 5 mg
Vicodin®	acetaminophen 500 mg hydrocodone bitartrate 5 mg
Vicodin ES®	acetaminophen 750 mg hydrocodone bitartrate 7.5 mg
Percocet®	acetaminophen 325 mg oxycodone hydrochloride 5 mg
Tylox®	acetaminophen 500 mg oxycodone hydrochloride 5 mg
Tylenol® RS	acetaminophen 325 mg
Tylenol® ES	acetaminophen 500 mg
Tylenol® #3	acetaminophen 300 mg codeine 30 mg
Tylenol® #4	acetaminophen 300 mg codeine 60 mg

♦ Antipyretic (reduces fever)

♦ Anti-inflammatory (reduces inflammation)

Aspirin acts through both central and peripheral inhibition of prostaglandin production. It has a ceiling effect in that dosages above three tablets every four hours provide no additional benefit. In fact, higher doses increase the likelihood of undesirable side effects.

Like all drugs, this over-the-counter medication has a downside. Aspirin impairs platelet function, which in turn impairs the ability of the blood to coagulate. Hence, there may be prolonged bleeding in the event of an injury as minor as a nosebleed or as major as a laceration. Aspirin may also cause tinnitus (ringing in the ears) that may not resolve with discontinuation of the drug. In addition, it can cause stomach ulcers, gastritis, and esophagitis and may exacerbate asthma. Furthermore, aspirin may cause fluid retention and kidney and liver abnormalities. In the worst-case scenario, overdosing on aspirin can cause coma. Thus, even this relatively safe drug can be dangerous if not used appropriately.

Enteric-coated aspirin (Ecotrin®) is now available to prevent irritation of the stomach. Other aspirin products such as Bufferin® and Ascriptin® contain antacids such as Maalox® to reduce acidity and to protect the lining of the stomach.

Contraindications include allergy to the medication, asthma, peptic ulcer disease, diabetes, renal insufficiency, pregnancy, and viral infection in children. In addition, aspirin should not be taken if you are on a prescription drug to thin your blood, such as heparin or coumadin.

Nonsteroidal Anti-Inflammatory Drugs

Like aspirin, nonsteroidal anti-inflammatory drugs, or NSAIDs (pronounced EN-sayds), are effective in relieving mild to moderate pain. They, too, suppress inflammation, for example arthritis, by inhibiting

Nonsteroidal Anti-Inflammatory Drugs

♦ Celecoxib (Celebrex®, a COX-2 inhibitor)
♦ Choline magnesium trisalicylate (Trilisate®)
♦ Diclofenac (Voltaren®)
♦ Diclofenac sodium/misoprostal (Arthrotec®)
♦ Diflunisal (Dolobid®)
♦ Ibuprofen (Motrin®, Advil®)
♦ Indomethacin (Indocin®)
♦ Ketoprofen (Orudis®)
♦ Ketorolac tromethamine (Toradol®, available in injectable form)
♦ Naproxen (Naprosyn®)
♦ Naproxen sodium (Anaprox® DS, Alleve®, Naprelan®)
♦ Piroxicam (Feldene®)
♦ Sulindac (Clinoril®)
♦ Tolmentin (Tolectin®)

the enzyme cyclooxygenase. This, in turn, decreases the production of prostaglandins and other pain-intensifying substances activated by tissue damage.

While NSAIDs are extremely useful drugs for many pain conditions, each year more than 100,000 people are hospitalized for gastrointestinal complications resulting from their use. Over 16,000 people die. These medications are not as benign as many people, including doc-

Potential Side Effects of Aspirin and NSAIDs

♦ Gastritis, esophagitis, ulcers
♦ Renal (kidney) insufficiency
♦ Liver abnormalities
♦ Fluid retention
♦ Platelet inhibition (and therefore possible prolonged bleeding)
♦ Tinnitus (ringing in the ears)
♦ Exacerbation of asthma

Medications to Counter Gastric Distress Due to Aspirin and NSAIDs

♦ Aluminum sucrose sulfate (Sucralfate®)
♦ Cimetidine (Tagamet®)
♦ Famotidine (Pepcid®)
♦ Lansoprazole (Prevacid®)
♦ Maalox®
♦ Misoprostol (Cytotec®)
♦ Omeprazole (Prilosec®)
♦ Ranatidine (Zantac®)
♦ Cimetidine (300 mg four times per day has been found to be effective in relieving neuropathic pain due to postherpetic neuralgia)

---

tors, think and should not be taken long term for the management of chronic pain conditions unless a definite inflammatory component, such as rheumatoid arthritis, is involved. Such patients should be closely monitored for signs or symptoms of peptic ulcer disease and renal insufficiency. Lab work should be checked routinely as well.

Overall, NSAIDs share the same side effects as aspirin. The main differences are in their half-lives (the time required for the disintegration of half the medication), frequency of dosing, and cost. Aspirin requires frequent dosing, every four hours, while some NSAIDs require the same every four-hour regimen and some require only once-a-day dosing. Aspirin is cheap, whereas NSAIDs are potentially costly. Some NSAIDs are available over the counter, and others require a prescription. NSAIDs can enhance the efficacy of opioids in patients with inflammatory-based pain.

Choline Magnesium Trisalicylate (Trilisate®)

Trilisate® is an NSAID that is a nonacetylated salicylate. Unlike most NSAIDs, this drug does not interfere with platelet function, which therefore minimizes the risk of bleeding.

Ketorolac (Toradol®)

Ketorolac is the first injectable NSAID introduced in the United States. Like other NSAIDs, it decreases inflammation by inhibiting prostaglandin synthesis. In addition, it inhibits production of the by-products of inflammation and the chemical messengers of pain. Ketorolac is a potent analgesic. At doses of 30 to 90 mg, it is at least as effective as 12 mg of morphine. At a dose of 10 mg, it is equianalgesic to 30 mg of pentazocine (Talwin®).

Side effects include platelet inhibition and prolonged bleeding time, injection site pain, liver impairment, somnolence, sweating, nausea, and other gastrointestinal complaints. Ketorolac can also precipitate acute renal insufficiency in patients with preexisting renal dysfunction. It should not be used in combination with other NSAIDs, but may be used in conjunction with opioids.

Ketorolac-induced gastrointestinal damage has been well documented in the literature. Clinically life-threatening gastrointestinal bleeding occurs in 1.8% of ketorolac patients. Because of this, new dosing guidelines have been established. Current guidelines in the United States limit treatment to five days. In Europe, the maximum daily dose is 90 mg in the nonelderly and 60 mg in the elderly.

Celebrex® (Celecoxib)

An exciting new development among NSAIDs is celecoxib (Celebrex®), a COX-2 inhibitor. Like all NSAIDs, celecoxib relieves arthritic pain by blocking the production of the enzyme cyclooxygenase (COX for short). This, in turn, inhibits the production of prostaglandins, the substances responsible for the pain and inflammation of arthritis. In the 1980s, two enzymes were identified that make prostaglandins, COX-1 and COX-2. While COX-2 was identified as the driver of the disease symptoms, COX-1 was actually found to protect the digestive system from its own erosive acids. The drug celecoxib was developed to block COX-2 but without interfering with COX-1, thereby reducing the risks of serious side effects such as bleeding ulcers.

Unlike most NSAIDs, celecoxib does not impair platelet count or function and therefore does not prolong bleeding. However, renal effects are similar to other NSAIDs. While borderline elevations of liver enzymes may occur in up to 15% of patients taking NSAIDs, the incidence of such elevations is significantly less, 6%, in patients taking celecoxib. The rate of notable elevations of liver enzymes is 1% in patients taking other NSAIDs compared to only 0.2% of patients taking celecoxib. While celecoxib has been tested in more than 14,000 people, no patient has taken it for more than a year. Long-term effects are unknown.

Corticosteroids

The mere mention of the word "steroid" frequently evokes fear and perhaps repulsion in the hearts of many. It conjures up visions of bodybuilders with massive, rippling muscles who couldn't possibly be earthlings. These individuals have abused the medication for personal gain. Their bodies testify to this. And so do their health records, which in some cases document liver disease that has occurred as a result of their unrestrained enthusiasm for muscle bulk. And we've all heard about the dreaded condition osteoporosis, which occurs as a complication of legitimate treatment for medical conditions such as rheumatoid arthritis and lung disease. And that's only the beginning of an endless list of potential complications that may occur as a result of steroid use (see sidebar: Potential Complications of Steroid Use). "No," you say, "this definitely is not the drug for me." But wait!

Don't be too quick to judge a drug by its reputation. There is an upside to steroid therapy. A plethora of painful medical conditions exists for which steroid therapy is effective. For a multitude of reasons, corticosteroids should be considered legitimate drugs in the armamentarium of the pain specialist. The steroids most often used to treat pain are synthetic analogues of cortisol, a glucocorticoid that is normally pro-

Potential Complications of Steroid Use

- Growth retardation in children
- Cataracts
- Osteoporosis
- Aseptic necrosis of the femoral head
- Proximal myopathy
- Delayed wound healing
- Decreased resistance to bacterial and yeast infections
- Buffalo hump
- Skin striae
- Mood disturbances
- Psychosis
- Adrenal suppression
- Cushing's syndrome
- Increased blood pressure
- Glucose intolerance
- Restlessness, nervousness, insomnia
- Increased appetite
- Weight gain
- Hirsutism (increased body hair)
- Gastrointestinal bleeding

duced by the adrenal cortex. The advantage of the analogues — which include prednisone and its derivatives — is that they cause less sodium retention compared with cortisol.

How do steroids alleviate pain? They do so by reducing swelling and inflammation. Steroids can be given by injection or by mouth. They may be administered by injection into the joints (intra-articular) to treat arthritis. This may include the facet joints or the sacroiliac joints, among others. Steroids may also be injected into bursa to treat bursitis or into the tendon sheath to treat tendonitis. In addition, they may be injected around the site of peripheral nerves, such as the occipital nerves, in order to treat a painful headache known as occipital neuralgia. Injections into the epidural space of the spine may be helpful in the treatment of nerve root compression (radiculopathy) in order to delay or avoid more invasive procedures such as surgery. They may also be effective when administered subcutaneously for the treatment of acute herpes zoster (shingles). Finally, they may be administered into trigger points of the muscle in individuals suffering from myofascial pain syndrome. Talk about versatile!

The literature regarding the use of intrathecal steroids is extensive and clearly conflicting. According to some reports, intrathecal steroid injections are fraught with serious complications, including adhesive arachnoiditis and cryptococcal and tuberculous meningitis, and should, therefore, not be used. However, other reports indicate that they are beneficial and safe for the treatment of various low-back problems, especially failed back surgery syndrome. Many of these papers implicate the propylene glycol rather than the methylprednisolone as being potentially harmful. So far the jury is still out.

Steroids may also be administered orally. Currently, there is no research evidence to indicate that high-dose oral steroids administered in "bursts" of 7 to 10 days produce significant side effects as long as the patient does not have significant medical problems, especially diabetes, peptic ulcer disease, or an infection. Short, tapering courses given in initially high doses are advised to optimize benefits and minimize long-term adverse side effects.

Oral steroids are helpful in the management of acute exacerbations of vascular headaches, including migraines, temporal arteritis, and cluster headaches. Steroids may also be very effective in the treatment of herpes zoster. With oral, intravenous, or intradermal administration, dramatic relief of pain has been reported within $3\frac{1}{2}$ days, compared to an average of $3\frac{1}{2}$ weeks without steroid therapy. The best results are obtained when treatment is started early in the course of the disease. Of critical importance is the fact that systemic corticosteroid treatment decreases the number of patients who develop a painful chronic condition known as postherpetic neuralgia, which can occur as an aftermath of the acute herpes zoster infection. This is one of the greatest challenges with which the pain specialist must deal (not to mention the patient).

Steroids offer the advantages of mild euphoria and a sense of well-being, a definite plus for a patient population that is usually depressed. Caution should be exercised if oral thrush (candidiasis), fluid retention, psychiatric disturbance, or diabetes is present. Contraindications include peptic ulcer disease, active infection, and bleeding disorders.

Local Anesthetics

Lidocaine is a short-acting anesthetic that has dual action. It works primarily by blocking the sodium channels of the neurons, thereby disrupting the flow of signals to the spinal cord. In addition, it is a weak NMDA receptor antagonist. Lidocaine in injectable form is frequently given in conjunction with steroid injections. It can also be administered nasally in a 4% gel or solution for migraine headaches. Controlled studies of EMLA®, a topical mixture of 2.5% lidocaine and 2.5% prilocaine, have shown it to be effective in reducing pain associated with venipuncture, lumbar puncture, and arterial puncture. The cream should be applied liberally over the site for one hour prior to the procedure and covered with an occlusive dressing. EMLA® can also be applied to painful skin lesions related to peripheral nerve disease such as postherpetic neuralgia. Finally, viscous lidocaine is frequently used to treat oropharyngeal ulceration.

Mexitil® is a derivative of lidocaine that is available in pill form. Its membrane-stabilizing effect dampens the impulses from rapidly firing, damaged nerves, thereby alleviating neuropathic pain. Individuals suffering from cardiac or liver disease or seizure disorder generally should not take these medications for pain relief.

Antidepressants

The biogenic amine theory suggests that depression is caused by a deficiency of the neurotransmitter serotonin or norepinephrine. Coincidentally, the levels of these neurotransmitters are also low in chronic pain syndrome. Imagine that! These substances are actively secreted into the synapses (the interconnection between nerve cells) by presynaptic neurons (nerve cells) and then taken back up by receptors at the postsynaptic neuron. Subsequently, they are either catabolized (broken down) by the enzyme monoamine oxidase, or they are stored. Antidepressant medications increase the levels of serotonin and/or norepinephrine in one or more of three ways:

♦ By increasing the production of serotonin and/or norepinephrine

♦ By inhibiting the reuptake of serotonin and/or norepinephrine by the postsynaptic neuron

♦ By decreasing the breakdown (catabolism) of serotonin and/ or norepinephrine by inhibiting the enzyme monoamine oxidase

Antidepressants are helpful in the management of chronic pain syndrome in several key ways. They improve mood and sleep, and they alleviate pain directly.

Tricyclic Antidepressants

Tricyclic antidepressants (TCAs) are used as the first-line adjuvant therapy for neuropathic pain. They are also helpful in the management of headaches. Additional benefits include the amelioration of depression and insomnia associated with chronic pain syndrome. Amitriptyline (Elavil®) is the most widely used drug of this type, but it has dose-limiting anticholinergic side effects (dry mouth and eyes, impotence, constipation, and urinary retention). Can't poop! Can't pee! All for a little pain relief. Talk about robbing Peter to pay Paul. Other side effects include sedation and daytime drowsiness.

Nortriptyline (Pamelor®) and desipramine hydrochloride (Desipramine®) cause fewer of these side effects. Low doses of these drugs (10 to 25 mg) should be administered at nighttime and then titrated up every few days to the maximum dose tolerated. Nightly doses of 100 to 150 mg of nortriptyline and 150 to 300 mg of desipramine may be needed for effective pain relief.

Warning: TCAs can lower seizure threshold and should be used cautiously if at all in patients with epilepsy.

Selective Serotonin Reuptake Inhibitors

Selective serotonin reuptake inhibitors, or SSRIs, constitute a relatively new class of antidepressants. Studies show that these drugs have a much improved side-effect profile compared with TCAs. They are well tolerated and have a markedly reduced risk of toxicity in overdose. Patient compliance with SSRIs is much greater than with TCAs for a number of reasons:

♦ Fewer side effects

♦ Decreased need for dose titration

♦ Once-daily dosing

Fluoxetine hydrochloride (Prozac®) is the most widely prescribed brand-name antidepressant in the world. For many individuals, this medication is truly a miracle drug. Like other SSRIs, it requires only once-a-day dosing. It is well tolerated by most individuals. However, some individuals who suffer from an anxiety disorder may not be able to tolerate fluoxetine as it is associated with anxiety, nervousness, and insomnia in 10 to 15% of patients. It is the only antidepressant that is

---

Selective Serotonin Reuptake Inhibitors

♦ Fluoxetine hydrochloride (Prozac®)
♦ Paroxetine (Paxil®)
♦ Sertraline (Zoloft®)
♦ Citalopram hydrobromide (Celexa®)

associated with weight loss. For millions of American women, this is an endearing selling point. However, for a minority, such as those suffering from weight loss associated with cancer, fluoxetine is not recommended.

On occasion, we see patients that are horrified at the suggestion of taking Prozac®. They have heard through the media that it causes people to do all sorts of terrible things (axe murders, etc.). But our consistent experience is that it is an exceptionally effective antidepressant medication with an exceptionally favorable side-effect profile. (And to date, we have yet to be involved in a homicide investigation. Not even close.)

Monoamine Oxidase Inhibitors

Monoamine oxidase inhibitors (MAOIs) have been around for years. Call them dinosaurs if you like. They are prescribed primarily for the treatment of depression. With the introduction of tricyclics, their use has significantly decreased. Thank God!

Even though they have also been reported to be effective for chronic pain, especially atypical facial pain, they have never been widely prescribed by physicians other than psychiatrists. This is primarily because of their horrendous safety profile. Although they are relatively free of anticholinergic side effects, they may cause hypertensive crises, orthostatic hypotension, hepatotoxicity, urinary retention, insomnia, and significant drug and dietary interactions. Tyramine-containing foods and beverages, including cheeses, pickled herring, sardines, chicken livers, figs, and red wine, must be studiously avoided.

Monoamine Oxidase Inhibitors

♦ Tranylpromine sulfate (Parnate®)
♦ Phenelzine sulfate (Nardil®)

Patients on MAOIs must also avoid numerous medications. The list is staggering. It is also imperative that pain patients on MAOIs avoid narcotics, in particular meperidine (Demerol®) because the combination can be fatal. That means it can kill you! Our advice? Avoid these drugs. There are better antidepressants on the market. Don't take the risk, if at all possible.

St. John's Wort

St. John's wort (*Hypercum perforatum*) is an herb that comes from a perennial flowering plant. It has been used for medicinal purposes for thousands of years. Most recently, it has been identified as an effective and safe agent for the treatment of mild to moderate depression. The standard dose is 300 mg three times a day. For severe depression, a higher dose (e.g., 600 mg three times a day) of this botanical is needed. Studies have also demonstrated its efficacy in treating seasonal affective disorder. Some investigations indicate that it may have antiviral activity. This medication enhances wound healing and has anti-inflammatory and analgesic activity.

St. John's wort is unique in that it seems to impact all known neurotransmitters directly or indirectly through receptor sensitivity and regulation. It also seems to have a beneficial impact on cortisol and melatonin levels, which are factors in some individuals who suffer from depression. Because it is natural, this herb is especially popular among those individuals who embrace a holistic philosophy regarding medical care. In addition, studies comparing St. John's wort to numerous other antidepressants have shown equivalent results regarding effectiveness and a much more favorable side-effect profile. The downside is the inconvenience of frequent dosing with St. John's wort (three times a day) compared with once-a-day dosing for most antidepressants.

Muscle Relaxants

Got a spasm? Take an antispasmodic. Also known as muscle relaxants, these drugs act centrally to reduce muscle tone and excitability. The

Very Sedating Antidepressants

♦ Amitriptyline (Elavil®; TCA). Primarily increases serotonin. Severe anticholinergic side effects.
♦ Doxepin hydrochloride (Sinequan®; TCA). Also an H2 blocker, helpful in treating allergies, gastritis, and ulcers.
♦ Trazadone (Desyrel®)

Moderately Sedating Antidepressants

♦ Nortriptyline (Pamelor®). TCA, a metabolite of amitriptyline. Acts mainly on serotonin. Fewer cardiac side effects compared with other TCAs.
♦ Imipramine (Tofranil®; TCA). Acts on both serotonin and norepinephrine.
♦ Maprotiline hydrochloride (Ludiomil®; Tetracyclic). Acts primarily on norepinephrine. It is the antidepressant that is most likely to cause seizures.

Nonsedating Antidepressants

♦ Fluoxetine (Prozac®; SSRI).
♦ Desipramine hydrochloride (Desipramine®; TCA). Acts primarily on norepinephrine.
♦ Protriptyline (Vivactil®; TCA). Acts primarily on norepinephrine. It is considered to be the least sedating and the most activating.

only exception to this rule is dantrolene sodium (*Dantrium®*), a calcium antagonist that acts peripherally on the skeletal muscle by interfering with the intracellular release of calcium. This drug has the potential for hepatotoxicity. Therefore, liver enzymes should be closely monitored.

All of the centrally acting muscle relaxants cause sedation. Their exact mechanism of action is unknown. Lioresal (*Baclofen®*) is unique in that it has analgesic properties above and beyond its muscle relaxant effect. It has been found to be effective for neuropathic pain such as trigeminal neuralgia and facial postherpetic neuralgia but ineffective for diabetic neuropathy and limb postherpetic neuralgia. Baclofen® in-

Muscle Relaxants

♦ Carisoprodol (Soma®)
♦ Cyclobenzamine (Flexeril®)
♦ Dantrolene sodium (Dantrium®)
♦ Diazepam (Valium®, a benzodiazepine)
♦ Lioresal (Baclofen®)
♦ Metaxalone (Skelaxin®)
♦ Methocarbamol (Robaxin®)
♦ Orphenadrine (Norflex®)
♦ Botulinum toxin type A (Botox®)

hibits the excitatory inputs to the spinal cord and may also reduce substance P, a key mediator of pain. This medication can be administered intrathecally for the treatment of spasm-related pain and burning and lancinating dysesthesias (allodynia and hyperalgesias) associated with central pain syndromes including spinal cord lesions and multiple sclerosis. This includes the relief of allodynia, the sensation of pain in response to nonnoxious stimuli such as a light breeze, and hyperalgesia, which is a heightened sense of pain in response to nociceptive stimulation. These are among the most difficult chronic pain conditions to treat. However, nociceptive pain as elicited by stimulation of the C and A-delta fibers by pinch stimulus is not relieved by intrathecal Baclofen®.

Cyclobenzamine (*Flexeril*®) is structurally related to the tricyclic antidepressants. As such, it shares many of the same contraindications, including heart disease and narrow angle glaucoma. This muscle relaxant is a useful adjunct in the management of fibromyalgia. Carisoprodal (*Soma*®) is structurally and pharmacologically related to meprobamate, an anxiolytic (antianxiety). It therefore has the added benefit of a tranquilizing effect in addition to its muscle-relaxing effect. Diazepam (*Valium*®) is not only an effective muscle relaxant but also an anxiolytic agent and an anticonvulsant. It is a benzodiazepine and can be habit forming.

Botox® (Botulinum Toxin Type A)

Botulinum toxin, or *Botox®*, is a potent neurotoxin that is produced by the bacterium *Clostridium botulinum*. It blocks neuromuscular conduction by binding to receptor sites on motor nerve terminals, entering the nerve terminals, and inhibiting the release of acetylcholine. This medication has been shown to be effective in the management of a wide range of painful conditions associated with muscle spasm. Currently, botulinum toxin serotype A has been approved by the FDA only for the treatment of strabismus, blepharospasm, and seventh-nerve disorders in patients 12 years of age and older. However, current research suggests a potential role for Botox® in the treatment of the following:

♦ Myofascial pain disorders

♦ Dystonias

♦ Headaches

♦ Spasmodic torticollis

♦ Craniofacial pain caused by bruxism and spasm of the muscles of mastication

♦ Chronic low-back pain associated with spasm

Botox® should be injected directly into the involved muscle by a clinician who is thoroughly knowledgeable about the physiologic and clinical effects of the toxin as well as the local anatomy. The safe and effective use of Botox® depends on proper storage of the product, selection of the correct dose, and proper reconstitution and administration techniques. The duration of therapeutic effect typically varies from one to three months and is dependent on the dose administered and the clinical problem under treatment. Because frequent repeat injections may induce antibody formation and cause clinical resistance to further treatment, Botox® generally should not be given more than once every three months. Transient side effects can include dysphagia (difficulty swallowing), ptosis (drooping eyelid), diploplia (double vision), weakness, fatigue, malaise, local pain at the site of the injection, weakness of the voice, and skin rash.

Anticonvulsants

Developed for the medical management of seizures, anticonvulsants have also been shown to be effective in a number of pain disorders. These drugs provide analgesia for headaches, including migraine headaches. In addition, they alleviate the brief, lancinating pain associated with radiculopathies and neuropathies, such as trigeminal neuralgia and postherpetic neuralgias. Finally, they have been reported to ameliorate the symptoms of reflex sympathetic dystrophy (RSD) and arachnoiditis.

Anticonvulsants alter the perception of pain centrally and block the rapid, repetitive firing of damaged nerves that have grown new sprouts in response to injury. This, in turn, hinders the aberrant spread of excitation to normal neurons. Carbamazepine (Tegretol®), valproic acid (Depakote®), and phenytoin (Dilantin®) achieve this by enhancing sodium channel activation. Clonazepam (Klonopin®) and diazepam (Valium®) do so by increasing GABA-A receptor inhibition. While it has been established that gabapentin (Neurontin®) is an analogue of GABA, its exact mechanism of action is unknown.

The use of anticonvulsants in the treatment of neuropathic and other pain states is often limited by the high incidence of adverse side effects. Carbamazepine is known for its propensity to cause blood abnormalities. Ataxia (gait disturbance), nausea, sedation, and diploplia (double vision) may also occur. Phenytoin is associated with hirsutism (aberrant hair growth), ataxia, diploplia, confusion, epigastric pain, nausea, vomiting, and gingival (gum) hyperplasia. Clonazepam and diazepam may cause transient drowsiness, ataxia, and disinhibition, such as hostility or emotional lability. Lethargy may occur early in a course of treatment, but tends to subside with chronic use. Valproic acid is associated with nausea, vomiting, anorexia, diarrhea, sedation, tremor, rashes, transient alopecia (hair loss), altered liver functions, and weight

---

Anticonvulsants Used for Neuropathic Pain

- ♦ Valproic acid (Depakote®)
- ♦ Phenytoin (Dilantin®)
- ♦ Clonazepam (Klonopin®)
- ♦ Gabapentin (Neurontin®)
- ♦ Carbamazepine (Tegretol®)
- ♦ Diazepam (Valium®)

---

gain. All of the anticonvulsants can cause cognitive and behavioral effects and alterations in memory, mental processing, and motor response time. Abrupt discontinuation of these medications can induce a seizure even in patients without a history of seizures. For that reason, they should be tapered gradually over time.

Gabapentin has a lower incidence of untoward side effects compared to the other drugs in this class. It is exceptionally well tolerated and seems to have a benign efficacy-to-toxicity ratio. Even so, approximately 3% of individuals taking gabapentin develop adverse effects such as sedation, nausea, dizziness, ataxia, fatigue, nystagmus, rhinitis, diploplia, amblyopia, and tremor. Nevertheless, in terms of both safety and efficacy, gabapentin is the best anticonvulsant, followed by carbamazepine and valproic acid, which are superior to phenytoin.

Carbamazepine (Tegretol®) has proven to be beneficial in reducing pain associated with arachnoiditis, radicular pain, acute herpes zoster, and postherpetic neuralgia. In addition, it is the drug of choice in treating trigeminal neuralgia (neuralgia of the sensory nerve to the face). Approximately 70% of patients who suffer from this condition will respond to pharmacologic treatment alone. In fact, a therapeutic response to carbamazepine is virtually pathognomonic for trigeminal neuralgia and can be considered a "diagnostic" test with high reliability. Rarely will carbamazepine depress the white blood cell count (you know, those little guys that fight infection). Therefore, a white blood cell count should be obtained prior to the initiation of therapy, next after two and four weeks, and then three to four months thereafter. An initial leukocyte count of less than 4,000 is a contraindication to treatment. A decline in white blood cell count to less than 3,000 or an absolute neutrophil count of less than 1,500 should result in prompt discontinuation of therapy.

In 1994, gabapentin (Neurontin®) was approved for use in the United States. Since then, a growing body of literature has indicated that gabapentin is effective for a wide spectrum of pain problems ranging from migraine headaches to neuropathic conditions. The amelioration of symptoms of RSD with gabapentin was first reported in 1995. RSD is an extremely painful and debilitating disorder that is characterized by burning pain, allodynia, hyperpathia, vasomotor and sudomotor disturbances, edema, and bone, skin, and soft tissue changes. This syndrome frequently follows trauma, surgery, stroke, myocardial infarction, infection, and endocrine disease. It represents one of our greatest challenges. In a small study of nine patients with refractory RSD, all had previously undergone multiple treatments that included physical therapy, occupational therapy, stellate ganglion blocks, and lumbar sympathetic blocks. Trials of gabapentin were then instituted, resulting in dramatic relief of pain in the majority of patients. In addition, early evidence of disease reversal was noted in most of the patients.

In another small study, 10 patients out of a total of 15 to 20 patients with a variety of neuropathic pain states refractory to multiple other treatments showed responses that ranged from "great" pain relief to "cured." The duration of pain was 4 months to 16 years. The response rate appears to be 50 to 66%. Three of the patients were able to return to work, and others reported a significant improvement in their lifestyles. Gabapentin was discontinued by half of the patients and the pain promptly returned. Good pain control returned with resumption of the medicine. These results are very encouraging.

Gabapentin is currently being prescribed in doses up to 3,600 mg per day in divided doses.

Benzodiazepines

The first benzodiazepine released for use in the U.S. market was an anxiolytic, chlordiazepoxide (*Librium*®), in 1961. Diazepam (*Valium*®), the prototypical benzodiazepine, soon followed in 1964. Since then, at least 16 other "benzos" have become available for clinical use. The prescribing of benzodiazepines has been viewed with mixed feelings in the field of pain medicine. Because they may cause both physical and psychological dependence, all benzodiazepines are subject to control under the Federal Controlled Substance Act of 1970. However, many investigators have recently stated that the dependence and abuse potential of this class of drugs has been overemphasized. They cite the incredibly high number of doses taken and the relatively low incidence of dependency and abusive use.

Benzodiazepines are prescribed for anxiety, insomnia, muscle spasms, and neuropathic pain associated with chronic pain. When used for short periods of time, these drugs improve sleep and reduce anxiety. However, with extended use, a number of adverse side effects may occur. Normal sleep patterns are interrupted, including a reduction in the amount of time spent in stages 3, 4, and REM (rapid eye movement) sleep. This, in turn, may actually increase anxiety. Benzodiazepines facilitate GABA, a neurotransmitter that inhibits serotonin. As seroto-

---

Benzodiazepines

- Lorazepam (Ativan®)
- Flurazepam (Dalman®)
- Triazolam (Halcion®)
- Clonazepam (Klonopin®)
- Chlordiazepoxide (Librium®)
- Temazepam (Restoril®)
- Oxazepam (Serax®)
- Diazepam (Valium®)
- Alprazolam (Xanax®)

nin is believed to alleviate pain and depression, benzodiazepines may actually increase the perception of both.

At least 40 to 60% of patients admitted to chronic pain programs are on one or more benzodiazepines. Many have been taking them on a chronic basis for years. This pattern of prescribing and using benzodiazepine drugs is contrary to the accepted guidelines of the American Psychiatric Association Task Force on Benzodiazepine Dependency. Despite the widespread use of benzodiazepines in this patient population, it has been suggested that, in addition to being helpful, benzodiazepines may actually be harmful. Some have gone so far as to say that prescribing this medication on a chronic basis constitutes abuse.

One wonders why referring physicians, frequently primary care physicians who have known their patients for years, would continue to prescribe this medication, often for extended periods of time, and why on earth these poor suffering patients would continue to take these awful, awful drugs. Could it be that they actually helped more than they hurt?

Clonazepam (*Klonopin*®) is the benzodiazepine most widely used for seizure disorders. It has also been found to be effective in the treatment of neuropathic pain. Clonazepam relieves the lancinating, burning, or pins-and-needles sensation associated with neuropathy and phantom limb syndrome. Some patients report that it improves sleep. Fibromyalgia patients indicate that it is invaluable in the management of restless leg syndrome. Contrary to expectation, clonazepam has been shown to increase the synthesis of our friend serotonin and to increase its concentration at synaptic receptor sites. The risk of tolerance is low and is outweighed by the potential benefits.

Alprazolam (*Xanax*®) is another excellent benzodiazepine that has not only anxiolytic effects but also analgesic, antidepressant, anticonvulsant, and antispasmodic effects. Talk about a wonder drug! In one study, the average pain score over the course of a 12-week trial decreased significantly for both males and females. Alprazolam is the only benzodiazepine shown to be as effective in the treatment of depression as heterocyclic antidepressant medications. Compared with diazepam

Potential Adverse Side Effects of Benzodiazepines

♦ Anterograde amnesia
♦ Cognitive impairment
♦ Confusion
♦ Disinhibition in bipolar patients during the manic phase
♦ Dizziness
♦ Drowsiness
♦ Fatigue
♦ Gastrointestinal symptoms such as nausea
♦ Psychomotor dysfunction
♦ Rare serious behavioral changes such as agitation, hallucinations, bizarre behavior, paranoia
♦ Rare paradoxical central nervous system excitation
♦ Syncope
♦ Vertigo

(Valium®), alprazolam (Xanax®) is a more potent muscle relaxant and anticonvulsant. In addition, it is well documented that alprazolam is more effective than other benzodiazepines in the treatment of panic disorders. Anxiety increases when pain is in poor control. This heightened anxiety in turn increases muscle tension, which further increases pain, which in turn increases anxiety. It's a vicious cycle. The best way to interrupt this cycle is to *directly* reduce the pain by one means or another. If this is unsuccessful, the next best approach is to *indirectly* reduce the pain and suffering by decreasing anxiety pharmacologically. That's where alprazolam comes in. Does it help? Ask the patient.

While many "experts" do not recommend the routine use of benzodiazepines for the treatment of chronic pain syndrome, the patients themselves adamantly state that these medications relieve suffering.

♦ *They* — the patients — loudly proclaim their benefits from the rooftop. (Should the actual sufferers have a vote?) *They* say it helps.

- *We* — the medical establishment — say it doesn't.

- *They* say they sleep better, not well perhaps, but far better than without the medication.

- *We* say that studies indicate that prolonged use of this medication interrupts normal sleep patterns.

- *They* say that, in their case, they are sleeping better.

- *We* say that they'll become more anxious with prolonged use because of sleep cycle disturbance.

- *They* say, to the contrary, that they feel less anxious and more relaxed. Furthermore, they are better able to cope with the pain and disability. And they are more active.

- *We* say that research suggests that serotonin alleviates pain and that prolonged use of benzodiazepines *theoretically* depletes serotonin and increases pain perception.

- *They* say that, nevertheless, their pain is reduced. Furthermore, they don't care what the studies show or how they are "supposed to" respond theoretically.

- *We* say *we* went to medical school — *you* didn't.

- *They* say they live with the pain every day — *you* don't. (Who is the *real* expert?)

- *We* say you'll get addicted if you keep taking the benzos for a long period of time. In good conscience, we can't keep prescribing these drugs. The literature doesn't support this practice, nor does the DEA.

- *They* say we don't care if we get "addicted." With the medication, we have a life. Without it, we can't even get out of bed, much less the house.

The tug-of-war goes on...

Buspirone (BuSpar®)

Clinical anxiety disorders are common in the United States today, with a prevalence of 4 to 8%. Anxiety is often seen in association with chronic pain syndrome. For decades, the benzodiazepine anxiolytics were the mainstay of treatment. Although they are extremely effective, they possess a number of adverse side effects, including drowsiness, impaired cognition and motor function, the potentiation of the effects of alcohol, and for some patients possible depression. They also have the potential for dependence, addiction, and withdrawal syndrome. Nevertheless, in the opinions of those who matter the most (you know, the guys and gals suffering from chronic pain), the benefits of benzodiazepines far outweigh the risks. But it's nice to have alternatives.

In 1986, buspirone, a new anxiolytic, was introduced into the United States. This drug differs pharmacologically from the benzodiazepines. It does not cause tolerance, addiction, or physical dependence. Therefore, it is not a controlled substance, unlike the benzodiazepines. Buspirone also differs from the benzodiazepines in that it does not exert anticonvulsant or muscle relaxant effects.

Although the mechanism of action is not well understood, it has been established that buspirone does not interact with the benzodiazepine GABA receptors and that it is a serotonin (5-HT1a) receptor agonist. In addition, it has moderate affinity for brain D2 dopamine receptors.

Buspirone is well tolerated by most individuals. Potential side effects include dizziness, drowsiness, nervousness, nausea, and headaches. A major plus is that it does not impair cognition. The downside is that buspirone cannot be given on an "as-needed" basis. So if you're stressed about a public speaking engagement or a job interview, taking buspirone 30 minutes prior to the event will not help you. (Better reach for the benzos.) The onset of antianxiety effects with buspirone usually does not become apparent for one to two weeks.

Neuroleptics (Antipsychotics)

"Antipsychotics." Sounds scary. But wait! Their use in pain management has nothing to do with treating psychiatric illness. The phenothiazine fluphenazine (*Prolixin®*) and the butyrophenone compound haloperidol (*Haldol®*) are the neuroleptics most often used to treat pain. Although these drugs are frequently used alone, they may also be used in combination with antidepressants. Antipsychotic dosages are rarely indicated to treat chronic pain. Instead, very low doses (1 to 4 mg of Haldol® or Prolixin®) are usually prescribed. While it is known that neuroleptics block the neurotransmitter dopamine, their mechanism of action in alleviating pain is unknown. They may potentiate the effect of analgesics or they may have a direct analgesic effect. Both theories are as yet unproven.

Side effects include sedation, anticholinergic effects (dry eyes and mouth, urinary retention, constipation, impotence), orthostatic hypotension, multiple cardiac effects, extrapyramidal signs (drooling, difficulty swallowing, tremors, and cogwheel rigidity), and other movement disorders such as tardive dyskinesia. Because of the potential seriousness of the side-effect profile, prolonged treatment with neuroleptics for longer than six months is not advisable

Antihistamines

Hydroxyzine (Vistaril®, Atarax®) has analgesic, antiemetic, and sedative effects in addition to its antihistamine effects. It potentiates the effect of opioids, producing greater and more prolonged pain relief.

Sleep Medication

Many individuals who suffer from chronic pain syndrome would give their right arm if they could get a good night's sleep on a regular basis. It stands to reason that if you can sleep better, you'll be able to tolerate the pain better. But sleep remains an elusive friend for many. If a person cannot sleep, the question is why. If the answer is "because pain awakens him or her," then sleep medication is not the solution to the problem. Better try a long-acting painkiller instead. If such a medication is taken and still the patient can't sleep, then it's time to try something else. Believe it or not, hydroxyzine (Vistaril®), an antihistamine, is a very good next choice. This medication is helpful as a soporific and an anxiolytic should "brain overload" be the reason for difficulty sleeping. In addition, it potentiates the effect of the narcotic and prolongs its activity, should pain be the primary reason for unsatisfactory sleep. If hydroxyzine is ineffective, another good alternative is an antidepressant such as amitriptyline (Elavil®) or trazodone (Desyrel®). Antidepressants not only are helpful for sleep deprivation, but they also improve mood and alleviate pain. What a deal! All that in one little pill. For you holistic folks, melatonin is the drug of choice for sleep. It is "el naturel." Melatonin is a hormone that is produced from either tryptophan or serotonin in the pineal gland at the base of the brain. You can buy it at your local health store. Finally, if none of these measures do the trick, it's time for a trial of a bona fide sleep medication.

Chloral hydrate, an oldie but goody, has been around forever. Unfortunately, it is no longer available in pill form. You have to drink the potion. Avoid the barbiturate secobarbital sodium (Seconal®). It's nasty stuff. In fact, it is *the* medication recommended by the Hemlock Society should a pain patient decide to prematurely leave this world. (Could Hell be an actual place? We're afraid so, folks. You think it's tough here? Hell is a *really* bad eternal address. If you visit, you won't want to stay. The problem is there are no return flights.)

Several benzodiazepines are sleep medications. These include triazolam (*Halcion*®), temazepam (*Restoril*®), and flurazepam (*Dalmane*®). Benzodiazepines are reported to interrupt normal sleep cycles. In particular, they reduce the amount of time spent in REM sleep. The worst choice among the benzos is flurazepam (Dalmane®) because its half-life is several days. It hangs around forever.

Finally, there is zolpidem (*Ambien*®), the best sleep medication on the market today, in our opinion. Unlike the benzos, Ambien® generally preserves the stages of normal sleep. The onset of sleep usually occurs within 15 to 30 minutes of taking the pill. The half-life of Ambien® is 2½ hours, long enough for a good night's sleep and short enough to be alert in the morning. Now, the trick is to get your insurer to pay for it. Good luck!

It is recommended by "those who know best" that one should take sleep medication for limited periods of time only. Try telling that to a chronic pain patient who has had an hour or two of sleep per night for the last 10 days. "Hello…Earth to doctor. Earth to doctor."

Barbiturates/Sedatives

Barbiturates are sedative–hypnotic drugs that do not have analgesic properties. In fact, some studies indicate that even small amounts of barbiturates can actually increase pain perception. On the other hand, there are significant numbers of patients who report that Fiorinal®, a compound that includes the barbiturate butalbital, is effective in the treatment of severe headaches. In our opinion, the good clinician does not discount the view of the patient who suffers with a given pain problem because a research study contradicts it. Nevertheless, these drugs should generally be avoided in the management of pain and must be prescribed with caution.

Amphetamines

Amphetamines are sympathomimetic amines with central nervous system stimulant activity. Central nervous system effects are mediated by the release of norepinephrine and dopamine. Amphetamines may produce additive analgesia when given with narcotics. In addition, these drugs may reduce the sedative effects of narcotics and counter severe fatigue that often accompanies chronic pain syndrome. Unfortunately,

---

Statistical Research Studies and the "Nonaverage" Patient

Most medical research studies are statistical in nature and therefore measure effects for the average patient. The experience of the nonaverage patient is generally considered to be incidental to the "main effect" (as well as an irritating source of "error variance" to the researcher).

Yet, the nonaverage patient's experience is just as important — if not more so. This is because atypical cases teach us about principles that underlie exceptions to the rule. By definition, not everyone is average. Therefore, practitioners who attempt to shoehorn their square patients into round therapeutic holes — and then blame them for the terrible fit — are committing a pretty big boo-boo.

---

amphetamines have a high potential for abuse and are therefore not recommended for the management of these conditions.

Tramadol (Ultram®)

Tramadol (*Ultram®*) is a centrally acting analgesic with dual actions. First, although it is not a controlled substance, it binds with mu-opioid receptors and possesses weak opioid agonist activity. Second, it inhibits the reuptake of norepinephrine and serotonin, two important neurotransmitters that suppress pain. In this regard, its action is similar to that of tricyclic antidepressants.

Ultram® is a synthetic analgesic that is used primarily for chronic rather than acute pain. It is effective in the treatment of moderate to moderately severe pain. The analgesic equivalency of 50 mg of Ultram® is 30 mg of codeine in combination with 650 mg of acetaminophen (Tylenol®) or 60 mg of codeine. Adverse side effects include dizziness, drowsiness, seizures, nausea, constipation, headache, and sweating.

NMDA-Receptor Antagonists

N-Methyl-D-aspartate (NMDA)-receptor antagonists represent a new class of analgesic drugs that is currently undergoing research. NMDA receptors are present in the nerve cells of the brain and spinal cord. They play a critical role in modulating the body's response to pain. By blocking these receptors, NMDA-receptor antagonists alleviate neuropathic pain, enhance opioid analgesia, and reduce central sensitization to pain. Included in this class are ketamine, amantadine, and dextromethorphan.

Ketamine is an NMDA-receptor antagonist that has been used as a dissociative anesthetic for decades. Because of its low cost and high efficiency, it is still widely used in developing countries. Recently, ketamine has been found to be effective in relieving pain associated with neuropathy, reflex sympathetic dystrophy, multiple sclerosis, and cancer. It decreases the amplification of pain by the spinal neurons. Ketamine can be administered orally, topically, subcutaneously, epidurally, and intrathecally. Bioavailability by oral administration is only about 17%.

Amantadine is an antiviral medication that has been used for over two decades to treat intractable chronic pain. It was originally used in 1973 to treat acute herpetic neuralgia. At the time, its mechanism of action was unknown and its benefit was attributed to its antiviral capability. Not until 1995 was it recognized to be an NMDA-receptor antagonist.

Dextromethorphan is a weak NMDA-receptor antagonist that reduces the sensitization of pain-related spinal neurons, thereby decreasing both nociceptive and nonnociceptive inputs to the central nervous system. Dextromethorphan is not yet available on the market, but it is currently being evaluated in a drug trial.

5-Hydroxytryptophan Agonists: The Triptans

Migraine headaches have been identified as a distinct clinical entity for over a millennium. Typically, they are unilateral, episodic headaches that are pounding in nature and associated with nausea, vomiting, photophobia (light sensitivity), and sonophobia (sound sensitivity). They occur more commonly in females. It is well established that dilatation of the cranial blood vessels, including the carotid system and the vessels of the dura mater, produces intense pain. Such dilatation associated with migraine headaches activates the somatic nervous system and initiates an inflammatory response mediated by the release of substance P and the potent vasodilator calcitonin gene-related peptide. Pain transmission via the trigeminal nerve also activates this pain-modulating system.

Recent advances in knowledge of the role that the neurotransmitter 5-hydroxytryptamine (5-HT) plays in migraine headaches has led to the development of a new class of drugs, the triptans. These drugs are effective in relieving not only the pain associated with migraine headaches but also the associated symptoms, such as nausea and photophobia. Therefore, concomitant administration of antiemetics is usually not necessary. This simple truth puts triptans a step above other migraine headache remedies, which include:

♦ Sumatriptan (Imitrex®)

♦ Naratriptan (Amerge®)

♦ Zolmitriptan (Zomig®)

Sumatriptan (*Imitrex®*) is a highly specific 5-HT1B/1D agonist that relieves migraine headaches with or without aura. It is the most frequently prescribed drug in the United States for acute migraine headache. Sumatriptan reduces pain by constricting blood vessels. This vasoconstriction appears to be limited primarily to the large cranial vessels. Fortunately, sumatriptan does not seem to decrease cerebral blood flow and exerts only a weak effect on the coronary vessels, with vasoconstriction only 25% as great as that of the cranial vessels. Sumatriptan may also inhibit the release of substance P and calcitonin gene-related peptide from the nerve endings of the trigeminal nerve located in the dura mater. Sumatriptan lacks intrinsic analgesic properties and crosses the blood–brain barrier minimally. Therefore, it is unlikely that a central mechanism explains its efficacy in alleviating the pain associated with migraine headaches. The fact that it is nonsedating also suggests that it does not work centrally.

Sumatriptan (Imitrex®) is available as a tablet, an injectable, and a nasal spray. The advantage of the latter two forms of administration is that up to 90% of migraine sufferers report nausea and 50% vomiting. In addition, gastrointestinal motility is diminished during migraines, resulting in slower absorption of the oral medication and delayed onset of relief. The nasal spray and the injectable form are an enormous advantage in this scenario. Up to 70% of female migraine sufferers experience attacks associated with the menstrual cycle. Sumatriptan has been found to be effective for menstrual migraine. Like most abortive therapies, sumatriptan must be given early on at the first indication of aura or headache.

Naratriptan hydrochloride (*Amerge®*) provides a single-dose, nonsedating alternative to repeated dosing with short-acting drugs. It is longer acting and provides a full day of migraine relief for many. Up to 66% of patients achieve relief from the headache within four hours. Of these initial responders, up to 81% experience no recurrence within 24 hours. A rebound headache occurs, by definition, when the trigger of the migraine is a withdrawal from the agent taken to treat it. In contrast, a recurrence is defined as a migraine that outlasts the life span of the drug used to treat it. Migraines can persist for 4 to 72 hours. Because the duration of effect of many drugs is shorter than the duration of the headache, repeat doses are often necessary. This problem is at least partially alleviated by Amerge®.

Zomig® is a selective 5-HT1 agonist with high affinity for both 5-HT1B and 5-HT1D receptors. It acts both centrally and peripherally to produce cranial vessel constriction and inhibition of neuropeptide release. Zomig® crosses the blood–brain barrier and acts on the trigeminal nerve system. The advantage of this drug is that it is effective even when given later in the course of a migraine, when the headache is at a peak. Like the other triptans, it alleviates the nausea, photophobia (light sensitivity), and phonophobia (sound sensitivity) associated with attacks. Zomig® is effective in 66% of patients at two hours and 78% at four hours.

Triptans should be prescribed only when a clear diagnosis of migraine has been established. They should never be administered to patients with hemiplegic or basilar migraines. In addition, triptans are contraindicated for patients with uncontrolled blood pressure, severe renal or hepatic impairment, or cerebrovascular or peripheral vascular disease. Because all 5-HT1 agonists can cause coronary artery vasospasm, they are also contraindicated for patients with a history of ischemic heart disease, myocardial infarction, or other cardiac disease. Even patients who have risk factors for cardiovascular disease without a diagnosis should not take this medication until a cardiovascular evaluation has been performed. It is strongly recommended that these individuals receive their first dose in the doctor's office. It should not be given within 24 hours of other 5-HT1 agonists or an ergotamine-containing drug or ergot-type medication such as dihydroergotamine or methysergide.

Ergotamine Derivatives

Ergotamine is prescribed to abort or prevent vascular headaches such as migraines and cluster headaches. This drug has partial agonist and partial antagonist activity of alpha-adrenergic, dopaminergic, and tryptaminergic receptors, depending on the site. It is also a highly active uterine stimulant. Ergotamine constricts both cranial and peripheral vessels. It does not, however, reduce cerebral hemispheric blood flow.

Ergot derivatives are associated with a fairly high incidence of side effects, including nausea, vomiting, numbness, tingling, muscle cramping, weakness, chest pain, tachycardia, and bradycardia. Coadministration with antiemetics (antinausea medication) is frequently necessary. Ergotamine is contraindicated in pregnancy and peripheral vascular disease. To avoid the occurrence of rebound headaches, ergots should be limited to less than two days a week and should not be given for extended periods of time.

DHE-45 (dihydroergotamine) is a hydrogenated derivative of ergotamine that differs mainly in the degree of activity. DHE stimulates the uterus much less and has markedly reduced vasoactive action. Finally, it is $1/12$ as nauseating. DHE is given in injectable form, either intramuscularly or intravenously.

Sansert® (methysergide maleate) is prescribed for the prevention of vascular headaches, not for the management of acute attacks. It is a semisynthetic ergot derivative that blocks the effects of serotonin but has no intrinsic vasoconstrictor properties. Its mechanism of action is unknown. Sansert® is reserved for patients whose headaches are severe, frequent, debilitating, and unresponsive to other treatment. In fact, it is the drug of choice in the treatment of episodic cluster headaches in individuals under the age of 30. The success rate is 65%.

With long-term, uninterrupted administration, serious complications may occur, including retroperitoneal fibrosis, pleuropulmonary fibrosis, and fibrotic thickening of the heart valves. Therefore, patients should be under close medical supervision, and continuous therapy should not exceed six months.

Isometheptene/Dichloralphenazone/ Acetaminophen (Midrin®)

Midrin® is a combination product that is prescribed for both tension and migraine headaches. Among the ingredients is isometheptene, a sympathomimetic, which constricts both dilated cranial and cerebral blood vessels. The second component is dichloralphenazone, a mild sedative that reduces the patient's emotional reaction to the pain. Finally, acetaminophen (Tylenol®) relieves mild to moderate pain for all types of headaches.

According to the FDA, Midrin® is classified as only "possibly effective" for the treatment of migraine headaches. Because of concerns regarding dependency and rebound headaches, it is recommended that combination drugs such as Midrin® be used only after simple analgesics have been tried on a scheduled basis. Combination products should be utilized only for short periods of time and on an intermittent basis.

Caffeine

Caffeine, one of the most widely used drugs in the world, is a central nervous system stimulant. This methylxanthine is found in coffee, tea, cola drinks, chocolate, and many over-the-counter medications. It is an analgesic adjuvant and has some analgesic action in itself for acute pain. Caffeine in combination with aspirin and acetaminophen (in Excedrin®) and butalbital (the barbiturate in Fiorinal®) is much more effective in alleviating pain than the individual ingredients used alone.

Caffeine modulates the perception of pain in a variety of acute pain states. Doses of at least 65 mg of caffeine have been shown to relieve pain when given with aspirin-like or opioid drugs for tension headaches, migraines, dental pain, uterine cramping, and other acute pain syndromes. It causes vasoconstriction of cerebral blood vessels, which may account for its effectiveness in relieving headaches.

So far, there is limited research available regarding the effect of caffeine in chronic pain conditions. Theoretically, caffeine may actually increase pain and suffering associated with chronic pain conditions. This is because caffeine is known to increase striated muscle tension, raise arousal levels, potentiate anxiety responses, and disturb sleep. However, one recent study of caffeine and chronic low-back pain found no evidence to support this concern. Specifically, patients who consumed higher than average amounts of caffeine did not differ appreciably from moderate and low caffeine consumers on standard measures of pain severity, pain-related disability, mood, and sleep. The results provided little support for the clinical recommendation that chronic pain patients should restrict caffeine consumption in order to reduce pain and suffering.

Caffeine in doses of 64 to 100 mg produces analgesic effects. This is less than or equal to one cup of coffee. A fatal dose is 10 grams, which is equal to 100 cups of coffee. (Hold the cream and sugar, please.)

Oxygen

Oxygen inhalation is one of the safest and most effective ways to abort an acute cluster headache. In addition, it has been used to relieve pain associated with migraine headaches. Oxygen is delivered at 10 liters per minute via a close-fitting mask for 10 to 15 minutes. Home use is indicated for some patients. It may also help prevent high-altitude-induced headaches during travel. Patients must not smoke while using this treatment modality. Oh, and entering a burning building should also be avoided.

Tanacetum parthenium (Feverfew)

Feverfew is an herb that, like aspirin, impedes platelet aggregation and prostaglandin synthesis. It acts as an antihistamine by inhibiting the release of histamines. Additionally, feverfew reduces the release of se-rotonin from thrombocytes (cells that produce platelets) and polymor-phonuclear leukocytes.

Feverfew is used primarily for migraine, allergies, arthritis, and rheu-matic diseases. No side effects are known in conjunction with the proper administration of feverfew in designated therapeutic dosages.

Clonidine Hydrochloride (Catapres®), An Alpha-2-Adrenergic Agonist

Descending noradrenergic pathways originating in the brain stem con-tribute to pain control at the level of the spinal cord. Stimulation of the locus coeruleus releases norepinephrine at the level of the dorsal column of the spinal cord. Norepinephrine, in turn, stimulates alpha-2 receptors, especially those located in the substantia gelatinosa of the dorsal horn. This discovery has led to further research regarding the potential analgesic effect of alpha-2-adrenergic agonists such as clonidine. Numerous laboratory studies have shown that these drugs inhibit the wide-dynamic-range neurons evoked by A-delta and C-fiber stimulation and by doing so relieve pain.

Clonidine appears to work synergistically with both opioids and local anesthetics. For example, it potentiates the inhibitory effect of morphine on the activity of wide-dynamic-range neurons of the spinal cord. The combination provides a significant prolongation of analgesia. Clonidine together with local anesthetics also prolongs the duration of pain relief.

Clonidine has proven to be helpful in the management of diverse pain disorders. Approximately 50% of chronic pain patients report some pain relief when given clonidine. Of these, 44% admit to an improvement in quality of life. Clonidine is beneficial in the prophylaxis of migraine headaches and for the alleviation of pain associated with RSD, diabetic neuropathy, postherpetic neuralgia, and the ischemic pain of vascular insufficiency. In sympathetically maintained pain, clonidine may act by blocking the release of norepinephrine by activating the alpha-2 receptors on the sympathetic nerve terminals. Clonidine has also been used successfully in combination with methadone for opiate detoxification. It prevents or reverses the hyperalgesia and behavioral symptoms associated with opioid withdrawal.

Clonidine may be administered parenterally by injection either intramuscularly or intravenously. It may also be administered topically by a transdermal patch (Catapres-TTS®) or gel. Finally, it can be given intrathecally or epidurally. Side effects include hypotension, bradycardia, cardiac arrhythmias, dry mouth, constipation, impotence, sedation, and transient abnormalities in liver function tests. The sedation is easily reversed but precludes the simultaneous use of benzodiazepines.

Propranolol (Inderal®): A Beta Blocker

Propranolol (*Inderal®*) is a nonselective beta blocker that competes for both beta 1 and beta 2 receptors. Beta 1 receptors are found mostly on cells in the heart and the intestines. Beta 2 receptors are found in the smooth muscles of the blood vessels and bronchi. Propranolol is commonly used for migraine prophylaxis. It is often prescribed for headaches that are not responsive to acute therapy or that occur in a predictable pattern, such as those associated with the menstrual cycle. They are helpful in reducing both the frequency and severity of these headaches. In addition, propranolol is effective in the management of anxiety that is associated not only with chronic pain syndrome but also with mitral valve prolapse.

Side effects include somnolence or insomnia, nightmares, decreased libido, fatigue, and depression. Beta blockers should be avoided in patients taking monoamine oxidase inhibitors or who have asthma, chronic obstructive pulmonary disease, peripheral vascular disease, congestive heart failure, bradycardia, cardiac arrhythmias, heart block, diabetes, or a history of depression. Abrupt withdrawal of a beta blocker can result in unstable angina, ventricular tachycardia, fatal myocardial infarction (heart attack), and sudden death. Milder reactions to abrupt discontinuation of the medication include an increased heart rate, palpitations, tremor, diaphoresis, and anxiety. To avoid withdrawal syndrome, it is recommended that beta blockers be slowly tapered.

Calcium Channel Blockers

Calcium-channel-blocking drugs have been used for the prevention of migraine and cluster headaches for over 10 years. They inhibit arterial vasospasm and block platelet serotonin release. In addition, they affect cerebral blood flow and neurotransmission. Unlike the beta blockers, calcium channel blockers are made up of chemically unrelated compounds that comprise five different classes. They vary widely in efficacy and side effects because of their differing pharmacologic action at the cellular level. Calcium channel blockers include nifedipine, nimodipine, verapamil, diltiazem, prenylamine, and flunarizine.

In one study comparing nifedipine, nimodipine, and verapamil, the most effective drug in the treatment of migraine with aura but the least well tolerated was nifedipine. Postural hypotension, edema, flushing, and gastrointestinal complaints were common side effects. Verapamil was the most effective in treating mixed headaches and was the drug of choice for treating chronic cluster headache. The major side effect of verapamil is constipation, which occurs frequently and may be severe enough to warrant discontinuing the medication.

Lithium Carbonate

Lithium carbonate is widely used in psychiatry to treat bipolar affective disorders. It is also used to treat certain pain conditions. This drug has complex actions on the neurotransmitter serotonin and on the catecholamine system. Unfortunately, it has a very narrow margin of safety. Hazards of lithium treatment include thyroid, renal, dermatologic, neurotoxic, and cardiac abnormalities, not to mention nausea, vomiting, headaches, lethargy, and tremors. Despite the potential complications, lithium is the treatment of choice for chronic cluster and episodic cluster headaches in individuals over the age of 45. This is because of the typical severity and disability of cluster headaches and their unresponsiveness to other forms of therapy. The success rate of lithium carbonate prophylaxis in chronic cluster headache has been reported to exceed 80%.

The recommended dose is 300 mg twice a day. Because the lithium ion competes with intracellular sodium, concomitant use of diuretics or a sodium-restricted diet is contraindicated. Blood levels should be closely monitored.

Topical Analgesics (Liniments)

Topical analgesics such as Bengay®, Mineral Ice®, and Icy Hot® are generally applied to the skin overlying an area of pain such as an arthritic joint or a muscle spasm. The sensation of heat or cold produced by the liniment does not actually permeate the skin to reach the joint or muscle. Rather, it blocks the transmission of pain signals along the spinothalamic tract to the central nervous system, thereby reducing the perception of pain. This is not voodoo medicine, folks. Topical analgesics actually work in many cases, although the analgesic effect is transient.

Capsaicin (Zostrix®)

Capsaicin (Zostrix®) is a natural substance found in hot red chili peppers. This unusual agent both induces and relieves pain. Capsaicin acts on the capsaicin receptor, a specific marker for the nociceptor C fibers. This topical medication causes an initial short-term activation followed by a long-term desensitization of these fibers. The initial depolarization of the C fibers corresponds to the burning sensation experienced when the preparation is first applied. This burning sensation is attributed to the release of substance P, a pain-messenger neuropeptide, from the C fibers. With chronic application of capsaicin, there is a reduction in burning pain as a result of desensitization due to the depletion of substance P. The higher the dose, the faster the onset of analgesia. Theoretically, capsaicin can alleviate pain associated with postherpetic neuralgia, arthritis, cluster headaches, diabetic neuropathy, mastectomy, RSD, phantom limb pain, and postsurgical neuroma. However, the currently available ointments and creams have limited clinical value secondary to poor patient compliance, which requires multiple daily applications for weeks.

Glucosamine Sulfate and Chondroitin Sulfate

Glucosamine sulfate is derived from the chitin of crab shells, whereas the source of chondroitin sulfate is usually bovine trachea. The primary therapeutic indication for these two substances is in the treatment of degenerative diseases of the joints. Glucosamine plays a critical role in the formation of tendons, ligaments, skin, nails, heart valves, blood vessels, bones, and articular surfaces of joints. Glucosamine sulfate halts the progression of joint degeneration and promotes the regeneration of cartilage by stimulating the production of proteoglycans. The mechanism of action of chondroitin sulfate is similar in that it provides substrates for proteoglycan production and the formation of healthy joint matrix.

Unlike the NSAIDs, glucosamine does not inhibit the enzyme cyclooxygenase or the synthesis of prostaglandins. It is ineffective in suppressing the enzymes involved in inflammation. In studies comparing glucosamine sulfate to NSAIDs, long-term reduction of pain was more substantial for patients receiving glucosamine sulfate.

There are minimal mild side effects due to glucosamine sulfate, and all are reversible with discontinuation of the medicine. Chondroitin sulfate is also well tolerated. About 3% of individuals report slight dyspepsia and nausea following oral administration of chondroitin sulfate. Courses of both medications result in improvements that last only 6 to 12 weeks following cessation of a six-week period of treatment. Most individuals will benefit from repetitive courses or continuous administration. Although glucosamine sulfate and chondroitin sulfate are frequently administered together, currently there is no information available to suggest that the combination is more effective than glucosamine sulfate alone. The typical dosage regimen for glucosamine sulfate is 500 mg three times a day for a minimum of six weeks.

Calcitonin

Calcitonin is a polypeptide hormone that inhibits the activity of osteoclasts. Although the precise mechanism of action is unknown, it is reported to have analgesic properties. In particular, this medication decreases bone pain due to osteoporosis and compression fractures or metastasis. It also alleviates phantom limb pain.

ABT-594: Hope on the Horizon

In 1974, Dr. John Daly of the National Institutes of Health isolated a compound from a small, colorful frog called *Epipedobates tricolor* that was found within the rain forests of Ecuador. Dr. Daly named the compound epibatidine, in honor of the frog. Epibatidine is a potent analgesic that is 200 times more effective than morphine. As its effect is not blocked by naloxone, an opioid antagonist, it is believed that its mechanism of action is nonopioid. Through research efforts, it was discovered that it interacts with nicotinic acetylcholine receptors. The finding that the analgesic effects of epibatidine are blocked by mecamylamine, a nicotinic antagonist, in combination with previous research illustrating beneficial effects of nicotine, ignited intense interest in the chemistry of nicotine and nicotinic analogues. Unfortunately, because of its toxicity, epibatidine is not fit for human consumption. However, new analogues being synthesized hold promise. One of these analogues is ABT-594. The chemical structure is similar to that of drugs tested for the treatment of Alzheimer's disease, which also work on the nicotinic receptors of nerve cells. ABT-594 also closely resembles epibatidine but lacks the toxic elements. It does not cause constipation, a common side effect of narcotics, and it does not suppress respiration. Like epibatidine, it is 200 times stronger than morphine. The drug is now in the early stages of testing for human safety in Europe. Hope is on the horizon.

A Word about Polypharmacy

It stands to reason that the more drugs you take, the more interactions are possible in ways that no one can predict. Not even the most elite of pharmacologists knows what happens with multiple pills on board. So you would think that ideally the fewer pills taken to achieve the desired effect, the better. Simple is best. We agree — but not completely.

As we have seen, pain medications work in different ways on different receptors in different parts of the body. Some work peripherally, some centrally. Some are agonists, some antagonists for a multitude of receptors that potentially affect the pain experience. Many of these drugs work synergistically. That means the potential effect of two medications, for example, is not additive but multiplicative for the greater good. The downside is an increase in the potential for untoward side effects. You can't always have your cake and eat it, too.

For this reason, polypharmacy begrudgingly has its place in the management of chronic pain. But you must proceed cautiously, introducing one new medication at a time, usually at the lowest dose available, and then evaluate the clinical response before making adjustments. Nowhere is this more important than in the over-60 crowd. The liver and kidneys work less efficiently as we travel along the merry road of life. Therefore, medications do not clear as well from the body.

If you start five new medications at a time and feel better, you won't know which pill to thank. Maybe they all made a contribution. Maybe only one did. So you go to all the trouble of swallowing four additional pills a day, perhaps multiple times — all for naught. By the same token, if you start the same five pills simultaneously and develop one of the nasty side effects we've been talking about, you won't know which pill to flush down the toilet.

The moral of this story is that it is best to introduce one new pill at a time. Take a wait-and-see attitude. It may take weeks to months under the care of a pain specialist before the best medication regimen is established to your satisfaction. But if you hang in there, it will be worth it in the end.

Summary

Most individuals seen in pain clinics have pain that was not alleviated by therapy. The good news is that there is a plethora of medications available to treat chronic pain conditions. The options range from plain acetaminophen (Tylenol®) to narcotics and include aspirin, NSAIDs, steroids, antidepressants, muscle relaxants, anticonvulsants, tranquilizers, sleep preparations, and blood pressure medications, among a host of others. Only by tailoring the medication regimen to your particular pain condition can you find the optimal customized program. Remember: One size *does not* fit all. While these medications rarely cure the problem, they frequently help to make life with the unwelcome "friend" called pain more tolerable. Finding the appropriate medication regimen can improve the quality of your existence not only as a result of lessening pain but also by improving your sleep, mood, and ability to function. For most individuals, the proper combination of medications is a critical component in meeting the challenge of chronic pain.

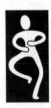

The Psychology of Chronic Pain and Illness

Bill Dearborn struggled to the receptionist's window, cane in hand and carrying his latest prescription. Handing it to Audrey, the receptionist, he said, "I'm supposed to see Dr. Chino at two o'clock. Is he going to be on time? Because if he's late, I'm not waiting." As was his usual practice, Bill was half an hour early. He had always prided himself on being punctual, even if others didn't show him the same consideration. He was aware that he was being less than cordial to Audrey, but he really didn't care. Of *course* he was irritable. He hurt like the dickens, and he wasn't about to wait one, two, or perhaps three hours to see a doctor who would spend only 15 minutes with him and who would provide him with no useful answers. After all, he had been through this routine on many occasions in the past, each time vowing never to subject himself to it again. "My time's just as valuable as any doctor's," he muttered under his breath. Like a character he had seen in a movie years ago, he was mad as hell and he wasn't going to take it anymore.

"There shouldn't be a wait, Mr. Dearborn," Audrey replied with a friendly smile. "Dr. Chino usually runs pretty much on time. Why don't you have a seat and fill out these forms. He should be with you shortly."

"Oh, here we go again," Bill muttered to himself as he hobbled over to a chair. "More useless forms asking the same stupid questions that I've answered a hundred times before: Where does it hurt? How long have

I been hurting? What medications do I take? Have I ever had the chicken pox? And, most importantly, who's going to pay the bill?" Upon settling into that sorry-excuse-for-a-waiting-room-chair, he was pleasantly surprised to see that there was no tortuous questionnaire, no request for what medications had been prescribed and by whom, and no queries asking about painful menstruation. There was only a short description of the services provided, their cost, and the billing policy. "This is different," Bill said to himself with relief. "But it's a waste of time nevertheless. What the heck am I even doing here? This Dr. Chino's a *psychologist,* for cryin' out loud, and my pain is *real*! The MRI proved that. And why would they have operated on my back if there weren't something wrong? A *psychologist*. I can't believe it."

Bill's mind flashed back to that terrible day two years ago when, while riding in his white Ford Bronco with an ex-football buddy, they were rear-ended by that *idiot* who was trying to drive while holding a cup of hot coffee between his legs. There was the impact, the trip to the emergency room, the constant unrelenting pain, the countless medical evaluations, the failed back surgery, the prescriptions, the physical therapy, the insurance hassles, the time off work, watching "The Jerry Springer Show" in the absence of anything better to do, the inability to concentrate, the inundation of weeds in the yard, the sleepless nights spent worrying about the inundation of weeds in the yard, the "problems" in the bedroom, the arguments at home with Janine and the kids, and — most aggravating of all — the never-ending indignity of being a chronic pain patient. To add insult to injury, now they wanted him to see a *shrink*!

"There's nothing wrong with my mind," Bill fumed inaudibly. "My pain is real, not imagined. And I'm dealing with it as well as anybody could. It's the pain that's causing all the problems, not me. What I need is for someone to fix the pain, not to tell me that I'm maladjusted. My pain is *real*! Doesn't anybody believe me?"

At 2:03 P.M., Bill checked his watch again just as a man in a shirt and tie walked up to him in the waiting room. Extending his hand, the man said, "Mr. Dearborn? Hi, I'm Dr. Chino. Sorry to keep you waiting. Would you like to come on back to my office?"

Bill shook the man's hand as he wondered if this *really* was Dr. Chino. After all, he was used to being summoned an hour or two (sometimes three) after his scheduled appointment time by a nurse and escorted to an examination room while being told that the doctor would be "right in." Thirty to 45 minutes later, while dressed only in a flimsy paper gown with bare legs and black socks exposed, the door would fly open. The doctor — attired in long pants, a dress shirt, and white lab coat made out of *real* cloth — would rush in while leafing through a thick file. Without looking up, he (and it almost always was a he) would say, "Hello, Mr. Dearborn. How are you?"

Bill found it odd that almost none of the doctors he had seen introduced themselves or seemed to make eye contact. This made him feel uncomfortable. (In fact, he wondered if the addition of reflector sunglasses would be the next trend in contemporary doctor apparel.) It was as if they knew *everything* about him, but he knew *nothing* about them. Even though he had been through the routine many times, it always left him feeling vulnerable and intimidated. It didn't seem fair. Bare legs, black socks, and flimsy paper versus pressed slacks, dress shirt — and *cloth*! Hardly a level playing field. But on one occasion, he even got up the nerve to look the doctor straight in the eye and ask, "And you are...?" This got the doctor's attention. And, thankfully, it seemed to yield Bill a modicum of respect.

Dr. Chino escorted Bill into his office and offered him a choice of chairs in which to sit. Looking around, Bill expected to see *the dreaded couch*. Yes, *the couch*. It brought to mind images of a sniveling, wretched, wreck of a man, lying back and whimpering about how he has always been misunderstood and mistreated while the psychotherapist sat impassively, scribbling notes on a yellow pad, saying not a word except to announce that their time was up and that they would continue next week. *The couch*. Where he — Bill — would soon be spilling all the gory details about his toilet training. But the closest thing to a couch in Dr. Chino's office was a recliner. Perhaps the good doctor's couch was in the shop for its scheduled 10,000-patient tune-up.

"We see a lot of people here who need to get up and move around because of their pain," Dr. Chino stated, breaking Bill's train of thought. "So feel free to walk around if you need to. I'm going to sit over here at my desk so that I can take a few notes while we talk. I understand that your doctor asked you to see me. What did he tell you about his reason for the referral?"

Maintaining a firm grip on guardedness, Bill replied, "He really didn't say much except that I needed to see you. And frankly, I'm not sure why I'm here. I've got severe back pain and it's only getting worse. The pain is real, I can assure you. But why he sent me here, I haven't a clue."

There! He had spoken his piece. Bill had let the psychologist know that he wasn't going to be talked into believing that his pain was all in his head. Maybe this would cut the visit short and he could get home in time to watch Jerry Springer. "What?" Bill thought, startling himself. "I'm actually looking forward to watching that crazy show? Has it really come to this? Maybe I *do* need to see a psychologist!"

Sensing Bill's caution, Dr. Chino continued. "Okay, let's start by my telling you about me and what I do."

"Huh?" thought Bill. "He wants to tell me about himself and what he does before we talk about me? This is definitely different. What happened to the paper gown? The (cloth) lab coat? The sunglasses?"

"I'm a clinical psychologist by education, although I don't really work in the psychiatry end of things. Rather, I have focused my training and practice in the area of helping people with chronic medical conditions — specifically, chronic pain. The people I see in my practice have *physical* pain associated with some kind of medical condition. I don't see people with 'imaginary' pain. By virtue of your having been referred to me by your doctor, I suspect that your particular condition is painful enough that it is significantly interfering with your ability to function."

"Today," Dr. Chino continued, "I'd like to provide you with an evaluation that is probably quite different than any you have previously encountered. Without rehashing all of the details you've no doubt been over more times than you'd care to remember, I'll ask about general elements of your medical history. But I'll be focusing more on how the pain has impacted your life and that of your family and on what kinds of things you've discovered that help you to cope with it. In addition, I'll be approaching this evaluation from the perspective of what we know about behavior in normal people, not from the 'mental illness' point of view."

Bill was listening attentively but still had his guard up. "Sounds okay so far. But the first time he asks about whether I've seen my father naked, *I'm outta here!*" he vowed silently to himself.

"In my view, Mr. Dearborn, *I* work for *you*. My goal is to provide you with an evaluation that will yield useful information and, ultimately, treatment options for you to consider. In the process, I'll be asking you a lot of detailed questions. I realize that you have been through quite a lot in seeking treatment for your pain condition and that you don't know me very well. You may therefore have some concerns about whether it is okay to freely discuss your circumstances. I can assure you that I will make every effort to earn your trust. But I want you to know that the quality of the 'product' I will provide to you in terms of conclusions and recommendations will depend almost entirely on the quality of the information you give to me today. At our next meeting, I will be going over all the results with you and then we can discuss your treatment options."

"And while I can't promise to find the answer that will take your pain away," Dr. Chino explained while meeting Bill's attentive gaze, "there's a good possibility that, together, we can find ways for you to gain more control over it and for you to achieve a better quality of life."

So far, Bill liked what he heard. As Dr. Chino spoke, Bill thought to himself, "At least he's honest about not promising me a cure. I know that there are days when I wish I were dead, when I feel that I just can't stand it another second. He's right. I feel that I have no control over my pain — or my *life,* for that matter. And he's not treating me like I'm crazy either. Let's see, what was today's topic? Oh yes, 'Neo-Nazi Transsexuals Seeking Romance with ACLU Attorneys.' Hmm. Maybe I can skip 'Jerry Springer' today."

Warning: Psychological Evaluations Can Be Hazardous to Your Health!

Contrary to the fears of many, referral to a specialist in pain psychology is not about invalidating their experience of pain by "determining" that it is not real. Bill's worries on this front are shared by countless others who have struggled through the healthcare mine field in search of relief. Too often, individuals suffering from chronic pain have been emotionally wounded when told by doctors that they "shouldn't be hurting." When referred to a psychologist, psychiatrist, or other mental health professional, many assume that their experience of pain is regarded as imaginary or not real.

Unfortunately, this assumption frequently proves to be true. There are more than a few doctors — even specialists in the field of pain medicine — who believe that, given no "objective" physical abnormalities, the pain is not real or not "legitimate." When referred to a mental health professional who is not a specialist in chronic pain, the nightmare continues. We have seen it happen many times. The nonpain psychologist or psychiatrist starts the evaluation with the assumption that there is nothing physically wrong with the patient and proceeds to search for the *intrapsychic* cause of the pain. The nonspecialist's thinking process might go something like this:

1. "All physical explanations for pain are known and well understood."

2. "Pain is *either* physical *or* psychological in origin."

3. "This patient has had a thorough medical evaluation and no physical cause has been found."

4. "Since no physical cause for the pain has yet been discovered, there *is* no physical cause."

5. "By default, the pain *must* result from psychological factors. My job is to reveal and explain these factors."

6. "In the event that I do not encounter solid evidence for a psychological cause, I will piece together elements of the patient's history and current presentation in order to provide a plausible explanation for the pain."

For the most part, these are unconscious assumptions on the part of the psychologist or psychiatrist — unconscious in the sense that they are assumed to reflect reality and, therefore, there is no need to even question their validity. But let's take a closer look at these thoughts.

1. **"All physical explanations for pain are known and well understood."** This is a widely held, but unspoken, belief among healthcare professionals, especially arrogant ones. Even though they might deny believing this statement if asked, it is an assumption that nevertheless guides the thinking and actions of many healthcare professionals each and every day. The fact is that there is plenty we do not know about what happens in the body to produce pain. New processes and mechanisms relating to pain are being researched at this moment. The scientific literature on pain is vast — and growing all the time. This assumption is wrong.

2. **"Pain is either physical or psychological in origin."** This notion stems from an old philosophical position called *Cartesian dualism*: the idea that there is a mind and there is a body — and *ne'er the twain shall meet*! As we have seen, modern science is revealing intricate links between

mind and body. Imagine trying to grasp how sounds and images are created on a television set simply by taking it apart and studying the individual parts without also having an understanding of how the sounds and images are first captured and transmitted over the airwaves. The story is incomplete. A full appreciation of the process is impossible. Yet, in a similar way, this is the legacy brought about by our dualist tradition in Western medicine. If we cannot explain an illness by way of physical mechanisms, it, *by default,* must be in the realm of the mind. Not so. In fact, this conclusion should be drawn only in the presence of *positive* evidence for behaviorally conditioned symptoms. It should never be a "diagnosis of exclusion." Unfortunately, it often is.

3. **"This patient has had a thorough medical evaluation and no physical cause has been found."** This is the one thought that is firmly entrenched in the mind of the clinician simply because it frequently constitutes the reason for referral. Because it is usually outside of his or her area of expertise to determine just how thorough and/or appropriate the medical evaluation has been, the behavioral specialist typically has little room — or reason — to actively challenge this assumption. However, it is the wise clinician who withholds judgment on this count, as there are plenty of instances in which the medical work-up is later found to be wanting.

One particularly disturbing example involves Barbara, who was hit by a heavy, malfunctioning door while at work. This caused damage to her cervical spine and resulted in chronic neck pain. Surgery was performed to fuse some of the discs in her neck. Metal plates and screws were surgically placed to stabilize the spine. Immediately upon awakening from surgery, she felt that something was wrong. She began choking and frequently vomited whenever she tried to eat or drink. Barbara was extremely distressed about this (who wouldn't be?) and begged her doctor to help her. The surgeon told her that everything was normal and that her problem was emotionally based. The worker's compensation case manager then sent her to a medical consultant (a physiatrist) who, according to Barbara, said to her upon entering the office, "You will not speak except in response to a question. Otherwise, I'll do all the talking." He, too, concluded that there was nothing wrong with her physically and that her complaints of choking were emotionally based. Despite the fact that her weight had plummeted from 140 to 105 pounds, her complaints were summarily dismissed.

Barbara was then referred to a pain management program by her case manager, even though her primary problems were the choking and her ever-increasing weight loss. An important part of an interdisciplinary chronic pain evaluation is to rule out medical and behavioral circumstances that would substantially inhibit progress toward improved functioning. Unfortunately, the pain program doctors concluded that her complaints of choking and gagging were not the result of organic pathology, but rather were reflective of psychological problems or, worse, malingering. It appeared that this conclusion was based on Barbara's prior medical evaluations which, in fact, were grossly inadequate. Given the acceptance of the previous conclusions, it was an easy step to discount Barbara's own report of suffering in favor of recommending a program aimed at "controlling" her symptoms and getting her back to work. Despite her consistent assertion that something was wrong, she was not taken seriously. In this case, the pain specialists used the previous medical opinions as a springboard to provide appropriate pain treatment at an inappropriate time. One can only imagine how difficult it would have been for her to benefit from pain treatment while constantly gagging, choking, and vomiting — with no relief in sight.

Much to the displeasure of her case manager, Barbara elected not to pursue the pain program, as she felt everyone was on the wrong track. Predictably, she was accused of being "noncompliant" and a "difficult patient." Meanwhile, she continued to choke, vomit, and lose weight each and every day. She even worked out a signaling system with her next-door neighbor. If he answered the phone and no one spoke, it probably was Barbara choking and unable to breathe. He would then bolt next door and rescue her. Eventually, however, she learned to perform the Heimlich maneuver on herself. It came in handy on several occasions — handy in the sense that *it saved her life!* Despite all of this, no one in the system took her seriously. To them, it was "all in her head."

Well, it was *almost* all in her head. As it turned out, they were off by about four inches. More specifically, the problem was proven to be just below the head, in the esophagus. Her surgeon had accidentally cut it during her cervical spine surgery, producing a fistula, or pocket, in her throat. When she attempted to eat, food became lodged in the pocket, producing gagging and infection and wreaking havoc with the musculature in her throat. Liquids leaked into her windpipe and caused multiple episodes of aspiration pneumonia. Fortunately, by taking her complaints seriously, we were able to diagnose the problem and route her to a surgeon who made the appropriate repair (but not without first struggling to obtain authorization from her insurance case manager). Although not cured, this greatly improved her condition. Barbara began eating more normally and started regaining the weight she had lost. Her fear of choking, although not totally gone, subsided. In short, she got better and her suffering was reduced.

In analyzing Barbara's plight, it is clear that the erroneous assumptions discussed earlier were alive, well, and in full swing among those initially in charge of her care:

♦   Potential physical reasons for her complaints of choking were erroneously assumed to be known and ruled out. They were not. One doctor after another relied upon the original surgeon's false conclusion that all was well physically.

♦   Because of this, it was assumed that she was magnifying her symptoms, faking her symptoms, or that there was some presumed psychopathology that produced the symptoms — despite a lack of positive evidence for such psychopathology.

As you may recall, it is not enough to have a lack of evidence for physical causes in order to conclude that symptoms are psychological in nature. Specific evidence for the existence of behavioral factors (i.e., *positive* evidence) must also be present. Even then, the conclusion must be considered tentative, leaving open the possibility that new information could substantially change the conclusion. This perspective is adapted from the scientific method, which teaches us to set up hypotheses and then to test them by collecting and analyzing relevant data. Evidence that would reasonably test such hypotheses is carefully gathered and analyzed. Conclusions are drawn only when positive evidence for a particular hypothesis is consistently observed. Conclusions on the validity of a hypothesis (e.g., "The problem is psychological.") based only on a lack of evidence for alternative hypotheses ("We can't find anything wrong physically.") would be soundly trounced in the scientific world. Yet this occurs on a daily basis in the healthcare world when it comes to treating (or *mis*treating) people with chronic pain. And it is our fellow human beings who are suffering as a result. It doesn't have to be this way. Even though the extensive rigors of science are impractical as applied to day-to-day clinical practice, applying the *spirit* of science within this context is not particularly difficult. But it assumes that the practitioner's motives are truly to unravel the clinical problem before him or her and to alleviate suffering. And it assumes that honesty will prevail over less honorable motives such as making easy money. Unfortunately, these assumptions are not always valid. And when they are not, people suffer.

Pain and the Human Brain

Leading theories of pain used to be similar to a child's connect-the-dots game: assault a part of the body with a noxious stimulus and — zoom — a signal is sent to a particular part of the brain, telling it that something bad just happened. The person says "ouch!" and the analysis is complete. Simple. But a funny thing happened on the way to the 21st century. It was discovered that this analysis was incomplete and much too elementary. Mother Nature apparently conspired to make us really work for an adequate understanding of human pain when concocting this strange creature. The connect-the-dots theory was fine for chickens, lizards, and frogs (remember high school biology?), but wholly inadequate for the species that invented classical music, the microchip, and the Slurpee®.

As discussed in Chapter 3, Melzack and Wall's *Gate Control Theory* of pain essentially argued that thoughts and emotions in human beings play an important role in determining (1) whether pain impulses reach the brain and (2) if they do, how the brain will interpret them. They hypothesized that certain higher order functions of the brain, such as those relating to thoughts and emotions, could open or close a mechanism that operates like a gate in the nervous system. When the "gate" is open, pain signals flow freely to the brain. When closed, it is as if the pain impulse has insufficient change for the toll taker. For example, powerful emotions such as anger, frustration, or anxiety were thought to activate parts of the brain which served to swing the gate fully open (kind of like giving the toll taker a big tip). Alternatively, more pleasant feelings or states of mind resulted in swinging the gate fully or partly closed. ("Reading this *Validate Your Pain!* book is *really* interesting! Let's see…Oh yes, I almost forgot. I'm reading it because of my pain.")

Suddenly, the line connecting the two dots took a detour to the far corners of the human brain and became much more difficult to trace. As if human pain were not difficult enough to understand, thoughts and emotions now became part of the picture. No longer was it a simple matter of "input…output"; it was now more like "input… processing in progress, please wait…output (maybe)." Not a comforting prospect to the obsessive–compulsive pain scientist. After all, many in the physical sciences held the view that the study of human behavior was a lost cause because it appeared to be so random and, frankly, impossible to understand. "Hardly worthy of scientific study. Now Mother Nature throws us this curve in our study of *physical* pain. Wouldn't you know it?"

In real life, our observations of individuals suffering from chronic pain conform closely to predictions from the Gate Control Theory. Those expressing greater emotional distress generally report greater pain. Now it may be argued that of course people with more pain will tend to be in greater emotional distress. Indeed, this is true. However, we have found that as people become more functional, less depressed and anxious, and more satisfied with their lives overall, pain may or may not change in intensity. It usually gets better — but not always. The correlation between pain and emotional distress is, to say the least, imperfect. We know people who are in a great deal of pain but who nevertheless report a pretty good quality of life.

The implication for treatment of chronic pain is that we must pay attention to the whole human being suffering with the pain. If we ignore the social, cognitive, emotional, and spiritual parts of the person, it is as if we have decided to hit the road, embarking on a long journey to that dream vacation to the Liberace Museum in Las Vegas, without knowing if we even have enough change for the toll taker. We stand a good chance of being very disappointed. Alternatively, when we consider these important nonanatomic factors, we are not only more aware of our toll fund but we're also getting to know what makes the toll taker tick. And, of course, it's good to know people in high places.

Psychopathology and the Genesis of "It's All in Your Head"

In the old days, Cartesian dualism (the idea that there is a mind and there is a body — and *ne'er the twain shall meet* — remember?) was in its heyday relative to our understanding of chronic pain in individuals without "objective" physical pathology. "There's nothing wrong physically, so the problem *must* be psychological. The patient is suffering from a sick mind, not a sick body." As we have seen, however, this perspective is wholly untenable when scrutinized closely. Moreover, it is simply counterproductive when applied to the challenge of chronic pain in the real world. Confounding the problem was Western medicine's affinity for basing our understanding of all human behavior on theories and concepts designed to explain not normal behavior but rather *abnormal* behavior (often referred to as psychopathology, the traditional domain of psychiatry). The assumption was that when confronted with a problem of behavior, thinking, or emotions, it was up to the psychiatrist to diagnose and fix the "abnormality." The patient's mind wasn't like ours (i.e., "normal"). She (and the subject of analysis was almost always a *she*) had "psychopathology," or a mental illness, as evidenced by her "irrational" distress and reactions — *as if* she were in pain. To the mental health practitioner well schooled in theories of abnormal behavior, this scenario was an embossed invitation to apply constructs like hysteria, hypochondriasis, conversion disorder, and psychogenic pain — all pointing to illnesses of the mind. It seemed logical at the time. After all, when your only tool is a hammer (theories of psychopathology), you tend to look for the presence or absence of nails (mental illness). Thus, the stage was set for the *psychopathologizing* of chronic pain patients. Remember Barbara's struggle to be taken seriously in the face of her unrecognized life-threatening condition and the repeated medical evaluations which concluded that her symptoms were psychogenic? This tragic case in point is but one in a million.

Behavioral Psychology to the Rescue

In contrast to psychiatry (the branch of Western medicine specializing in the treatment of mental illness), behavioral psychology focused on the discovery of scientific principles that could be applied to the spectrum of human behavior — including "normal" behavior. Thoughts, emotions, and behaviors were neither normal nor abnormal, but instead resulted from a person's exposure to various patterns of environmental consequences to his or her behavior. In other words, behavior that might have otherwise been considered reflective of a mental illness in fact stemmed from an individual responding normally to (adverse) circumstances that shaped the "abnormal" behavior in question.

From the behavioral perspective, a person was no longer seen as being mentally *sick* (a term born of the Western medical tradition). He or she was merely responding adaptively to negative environmental contingencies as predicted by scientifically established principles of behavior. Prune branches at random from a young, healthy, growing tree, and it will probably appear abnormal down the road. Yet the tree itself is perfectly normal in terms of its response to the environment to which it was exposed. In understanding its "abnormal" appearance, it would be folly to search for a genetic quirk or to hypothesize that it responded to a different set of tree growth rules than neighboring trees.

Yet, in a similar way, traditional psychiatric approaches have attempted to explain the psychological states of chronic pain patients by looking inside of them in an attempt to discover the "mental disorder" that produces their behavior. Unfortunately, this is still the prevailing view within Western medicine as well as the larger Western culture. Indiscriminately applied, it invites a judgmental attitude that labels the patient as being somehow different, or even inferior. From there, it's only a short step to blaming the victim. Not a particularly laudable position to take, in our view.

Dr. Wilbert Fordyce, a psychologist and professor emeritus at the University of Washington School of Medicine, is generally credited with having pioneered the application of scientific principles of behavior to the analysis of chronic pain. Instead of addressing pain per se, he introduced the idea of analyzing pain *behavior*. This made sense in that, try as we may, we cannot directly measure a person's experience of pain. We can only infer its existence, intensity, and overall quality from what a person says or does. If one cares to listen, the person's words and actions can tell the story. But once the focus shifted from intangible constructs like mental illness to observable behavior, the door swung wide open to permit the application of scientifically based behavior analysis techniques to the study of chronic pain conditions.

Essentially, the behavioral perspective goes something like this. Pain behavior results from either:

1. Pain (or other neural) impulses within the body, referred to as *respondent* pain behavior, or

2. Reinforcing environmental consequences linked to the behavior in question, referred to as *operant* pain behavior

When you stub your toe on the way to the bathroom in the middle of the night and end up holding your foot, grimacing, and jumping up and down on your good foot — that's respondent pain behavior. You are *responding* to a neural message from the toe which says, "I'd greatly appreciate your being just a bit more careful next time. And thank you for your kind attention in this matter, *ya klutz!*" The idea is that the person is responding to some kind of noxious stimulus in the body. In Western culture and medicine, respondent pain is the primary focus of attention. When someone complains of pain, this is what we usually think of. However, as we have seen, our understanding of respondent pain is far from complete. There's more to the story.

In contrast, *operant* pain behavior is created, strengthened, and/or maintained by what happens as a consequence of the behavior. Suppose the foot-holding, grimacing, jumping-up-and-down-on-the-good-foot behavior came from an actor whose part required a toe-stubbing scene. Upon hearing the thundering applause and reading the rave review of his stellar toe-stubbing performance in the next day's *New York Times,* our actor's subsequent renditions of the scene could best be viewed as operant pain behavior. This is due to the fact that it was caused not by internal neural impulses associated with pain (as in respondent pain behavior) but rather by the pleasing consequences he experienced following the behavior itself. But let's say that the actor wanted to move his career away from slapstick and toward more serious forms of drama, and he wanted help in decreasing the toe-stubbing behavior. If we told him to "break a leg," that would only encourage him. If we gave him a nerve block injection (to treat presumed respondent pain), he would almost certainly drop us from his list of favorite people. It wouldn't work. The pain behavior would persist because we would be treating the wrong thing. Instead, the operant approach would suggest removing the pleasing consequences of the pain behavior. For example:

1. Stop the applause

2. Convince the reviewer not to mention his performance at all

3. Withhold the actor's paycheck

The pain behavior in question would likely dwindle and then finally stop after the first few performances. Notice that these "interventions" focus not on tinkering with the actor's personality, genetics, or other such personal traits but rather on changing the environment's response to the behavior in question. To use the lingo of Western medicine, it is the environment — not the actor — that is "sick" and in need of "treatment."

But before you draw the false conclusion that operant pain behavior pertains only to fakes, charlatans, and thespians, we must consider how the rest of us might come to acquire it. And believe us, you don't have to be weak of mind, spirit, or character. You just have to be relatively normal.

Chronic Pain, Operant Pain Behavior, and the Cat Box

Lou hurt his low back while lifting a heavy box at work. He went through the usual routine: multiple medical exams, X-rays, MRIs, physical therapy, time off work, and, finally, surgery. His hopes for a full recovery were dashed many times over, along with his spirits. He had worked hard in physical therapy and had followed his doctor's advice to the letter. Unfortunately, almost a year after the accident, he was still off work, spending most of his time on the couch watching television. During this time, he became more and more discouraged. Like our friend Bill Dearborn (remember him?), this once active, vibrant man had been reduced to an authority on "The Jerry Springer Show." And this was definitely not what he had envisioned for his life.

Since the injury, there had been many major changes in Lou's lifestyle. During the early phase, he was unable to get out of bed, let alone work or mow the lawn. Perhaps most notable of all, he was "unable" to clean the cat box. Historically, the responsibility for scooping the box had been an irritating point of contention between Lou and his wife, Jodi.

Each repeatedly maintained that it was the other's turn to engage in the prized endeavor. Moreover, neither professed to be especially competent in carrying out the task (nor particularly adept at breathing through the mouth). But given Lou's chronic pain, Jodi was now — by default — the executive director in charge of indoor feline sanitation.

For Lou, the change was subtle, but significant. Even when he was able to get up and move around, things seemed, well, less complicated. Unlike before the injury, he now found himself able to walk past the cat box without the slightest thought of cleaning it. In fact, the cat box never even entered his mind anymore. After all, *he had a bad back*! He couldn't be expected to bend way down there, extend his arm, repeatedly sift the litter, and then lift all that heavy cat poop. Nope. To Lou, cleaning the cat box was *Jodi's* job — *now and forevermore!* When Jodi would observe Lou getting around a bit better, her desperate cries for assistance were met only with complaints of a sudden increase in pain and Lou's disappearance into the bedroom. Classic operant pain behavior.

But to Lou, there was no deception involved. He really did notice that his pain acted up when Jodi would ask for his help. It was as if the neural circuit were hard-wired: Jodi's request bypassed Lou's conscious memories of how he detested cleaning the cat box (as well as his experience of relief when he was "off duty") and proceeded straight to the pain-gate-opening mechanism. Pain suddenly became much more prominent. And when the pain behavior was followed by successful avoidance of the noxious event, it would be strengthened and hence repeated.

Whether it is cleaning the cat box or returning to a less than supportive work environment, few of us are immune to this kind of operant pain behavior. However, it is seldom one or the other — operant *or* respondent pain behavior. In Lou's case, there was a complex mixture of both. There was no conscious ploy to avoid healthy behavior (if you consider grappling with cat droppings healthy). It was all automatic. Lou's improved pain and subsequent movement toward increased healthy behavior served to jeopardize his vacation from a noxious task via Jodi's observing it. This "threat" (fueled by past experience arguing with Jodi about the cat box) increased his anxiety, thus swinging the pain gate wide open. And boom! He hurt more. The result: operant *and* respondent pain behavior all mixed together in one package.

The Behavioral Model: Some Cautions

Although we can thank behavioral psychology for bringing us out of the dark ages relative to understanding chronic pain, the analysis, in practice, is typically one of those unfortunate "either/or" propositions. The pain behavior is the result of *either* neural pain impulses inside the body *or* environmental consequences of the behavior itself. But as we have seen in Lou's case, respondent and operant elements are not mutually exclusive. You can have both fleas *and* lice! In other words, just because environmental reinforcement of pain behavior may be present does not mean that the individual is not *also* responding to pain signals within the body.

In our view, behaviorally based chronic pain rehabilitation programs do a disservice to their patients when they seek to increase healthy behavior and decrease pain behavior *solely* by reinforcing the former and ignoring the latter. Too many such programs are guilty of this. Through the staff's actions, patients learn that good things happen when objective gains occur in, say, exercise performance or reduced pain medication intake via the utilization of other effective pain management techniques. In these cases, staff actions serve to reinforce the "healthy" behavior. Praise and other statements of positive regard are examples of such reinforcement. By definition, reinforcement of these behaviors means that they will become stronger. They will occur more frequently and be more resistant to change. This is a great approach, and we recommend it highly. So far, so good.

The problem comes with the other emphasis in programs based strictly upon the behavioral model: ignoring pain behavior. In practice, pain complaints will be met with indifference by doctors and staff. The rationale behind this approach is twofold:

1. It makes healthy behavior more probable by decreasing incompatible pain behavior. This is based on the assumption that

2. The pain behavior does not result from neural pain impulses within the body but instead is caused by environmental reinforcement.

There's that *either/or* thing again. In our experience with the behavioral pain rehabilitation model, we have had repeated opportunities to question the assumption that the pain behavior was not respondent in nature. In many cases, a strict operant analysis was insufficient to account for the totality of the patient's pain experience.

Recall Barbara, whose choking behavior was deemed to be "psychological" in nature and who was sent to a pain rehabilitation program. If she had been made to stay in the program, it is possible — perhaps likely — that her "unhealthy" behavior would have decreased. She is a bright person and would have easily figured out the rules for getting along in the program. She could have cut her intake of food and water even further, thus decreasing her choking and gagging behavior. Although this would have certainly compromised her health even more, she could have made objective behavioral progress relative to the goals set by the program staff. Also, despite hurting more as a result, she could have pushed herself to exercise and "improved" her objective physical performance. Yet, once she left the program, her "illness behavior" would have returned to its original baseline. Or, perhaps more likely, it would have become worse. Why? *Because the reason for the "illness behavior" was within her body rather than the result of external reinforcement from outside.* Fortunately, she had the wherewithal to refuse the program before it got started. Our point here is that Barbara was evaluated by a behaviorally oriented multidisciplinary pain rehabilitation program and erroneously deemed to be an appropriate candidate. Her illness behavior was judged to be operant in nature when, in reality, there was a life-threatening medical condition that accounted for it. What would have happened had she entered the program? Her symptoms would undoubtedly have been further ignored and her suffering intensified. We have little doubt that, despite being seen as "uncoopera-tive" for refusing to enter the program, Barbara saved her own life by believing her own experience of illness. Sadly, Barbara's case is not unusual. The fundamental error of erroneously ruling out biologically based (i.e., respondent) pain behavior is made frequently.

Cognitive Therapy, Chronic Pain, and *Winnie the Pooh*

Cognitive therapy is a psychological treatment approach based upon the premise that emotional responses stem directly from thoughts, beliefs, and/or perceptions of situations. In other words, you feel what you think.

The cognitive theory of emotions is exemplified wonderfully in the characters of A.A. Milne's *Winnie the Pooh*. As you may remember, each character had a very distinctive personality. Never much out of sorts, the rather simple-minded Pooh approached life in an easy-going, carefree manner. Even when experiencing the tribulations that can come with disguising oneself as a rain cloud while hanging from a balloon and being pestered by relentless bees, Pooh never seemed to get too bent out of shape when his brilliant scheme for purloining honey went awry. An irrepressible "Oh bother" was all he uttered, and then it was on to the next adventure. According to the theory, Pooh's take-life-as-it-comes attitude resulted from his "sometimes-you-win, sometimes-you-lose" outlook. On the other hand, Rabbit's insistent "Which-are-you-going-to-believe, this-*official*-map-or-your-own-eyes?" pattern can be viewed as the product of his assumption that the world should be — mind you, *must* be — predictable, neat, and orderly. When Pooh, the uninvited lunch guest, ate so much that he got stuck in Rabbit's rabbit hole, Rabbit was almost rabid with rageful wrath. Remember? When things did not conform to the way they "should" be, Rabbit was wracked with worry. Eeyore, the despairing, downtrodden, ever-depressed donkey, seemed always to focus on the misfortunes of life, while selectively forgetting the good things. Let's face it, Eeyore was the quintessential pessimist. The result? Chronic depression. Similarly, the anxiety-ridden, perpetually uncertain Piglet was the type who could only see those aspects of life that had the *potential* to yield danger and other unpleasantries. Seemingly incapable of learning from his many instances of somehow, time and again, emerging unscathed, Piglet always anticipated the worst. In the cognitive theory of emotion, his eternal anxiety was the product of this pattern of thinking. But what about the always-effervescent Tigger? Does the cognitive theory of emotion explain his unrestrained exuberance — reflecting *positive* emotions — as well? Indeed, it does. Unlike Rabbit, Eeyore, and Piglet, Tigger's mode of thinking was fraught with denial and was geared toward seeing only the positive. Tigger seemed to bounce all the time. Unfortunately, while attractive on the surface, this thought pattern leaves one ill prepared to cope with the bad stuff when it comes along.

Well, now that we have forever spoiled a well-loved children's story through our dry psychological analysis of its characters, we'd like to redeem ourselves by...Well, maybe it's too late for redemption. But there is a sound application of the cognitive theory of emotion to the problem of chronic pain. Consider the following.

If you are injured and in pain through no fault of your own and you hold the belief that life should be fair, then your anger and resentment are seen to result from that belief. If you tend to forget positive events and remember only bad experiences, then your feelings of hopelessness and pessimism for the future are a consequence of that tendency. If you see the world as being either black or white and your doctors have not cured your pain yet, then your gloomy outlook for the future would be predicted by the cognitive theory.

The cognitive therapy approach would seek to change these "dysfunctional" ways of thinking such as to substitute ones that produce more positive emotions. Instead of insisting that the world must be fair (it isn't), coming to expect that life will take unexpected turns will greatly reduce anger and aggravation. Instead of seeing only the bad stuff in life, the cognitive approach attempts to show individuals how to evaluate things in a more balanced manner. Resentment and pessimism are reduced if this occurs. And instead of perceiving things as being either black or white, good or bad, sick or healthy, one can begin to see shades of gray. Progress toward goals is more readily apparent. Good days are noticed among the bad ones. Pessimism weakens. You get the idea. In short, cognitive therapy has a solid, legitimate place in the treatment of chronic pain.

Caution: Cognitive Therapy Can Be Hazardous to Your Health!

Despite all its merits, the model is based on certain assumptions that, in practice, can prove to be problematic. Most notably, "negative" emotions are seen as resulting from "irrational" or "dysfunctional" beliefs. The question arises: Is it necessarily bad to experience "negative" emotions? We think not. In fact, "negative" emotions are an important part of life. They help us to learn, and they provide a perspective from which to appreciate the good stuff. Unless immobilized by it, the sadness and frustration resulting from one's loss of function seem perfectly appropriate to us. And they certainly do not appear to result from "irrational" beliefs or ways of thinking. Yet, we know people who have undergone cognitive therapy that has sought to eradicate the sadness and frustration by messing around with the underlying thoughts related to their disability. Cognitive therapy is an appropriate method for unsticking an individual who is stuck in the "negative" emotion. For example, it is helpful when people's anger and resentment keep them from adapting to their condition and present circumstances. But when people are not stuck and are merely experiencing natural emotions stemming from their plight, their experience should be acknowledged and validated. Not all "negative" emotions are bad. Not all "negative" emotions should be "treated." Not all cognitive therapists recognize this. Consider the following thoughts or self-statements:

♦ "This pain is *awful*."

♦ "I'll *never* be able to do *anything* again."

♦ "I'm *worthless* because I can't do the things I used to do."

♦ "This pain is so bad I can't *stand* it. I can't *live* with this pain."

Do any of these sound familiar? If you have ever experienced chronic pain, they probably do. They reflect the experience of many who have suffered with it. Now, suppose you went to a doctor who heard you relate the above, and he or she responded with the following:

♦ "Your pain is *not* awful. It's merely uncomfortable and inconvenient."

♦ "Just because you're less able to function with the pain does not mean that you'll *never* be able to do *anything* again."

♦ "Your worth has nothing to do with the things you do. Just because you believe this does not make it so."

♦ "What do you mean you *can't stand it or can't live with it*? The fact is that you've lived with it thus far. It might have been uncomfortable and inconvenient, but it hasn't — and it's not going to — kill you."

Pop Quiz

Check the item that best reflects your anticipated reaction to the doctor's responses.

☐ a. "Thank you, doctor. You know, that makes so much sense. I feel better already!"

☐ b. "I'm sorry, doctor. I am so ashamed of myself for telling you how I feel. I can assure you that it won't happen again."

☐ c. "Uh, doctor? Could you please stand up, turn around, and bend over? I suddenly feel the urge to swing my foot rapidly in your direction."

In this vignette, you have just encountered a rather crass application of cognitive therapy as it relates to chronic pain. In a sense, the doctor spoke the truth, but in the process totally invalidated the person's experience of suffering. There was no acknowledgment of the physical and emotional struggle, the despair, or the sense of isolation due to others not understanding. And, as we have maintained throughout this book, these are essential elements to successful treatment of chronic pain. Yet, it is not uncommon to encounter pain programs that practice cognitive therapy in this rather crude manner. Ignoring pain behavior while simultaneously challenging the experience of suffering can be a devastating combination for people who already feel beaten down.

The bottom line is this: To be of benefit, cognitive therapy must be presented in the proper way. The person's current experience of illness, pain, and suffering must be acknowledged and validated prior to the modification of beliefs and ways of thinking. Respect should be paid to the person's life experiences that created the relevant patterns of thinking. The patient should never be made to feel judged for his or her outlook. Finally, the therapist and patient should openly discuss the process by which thought and belief patterns are created, modified, and maintained. Persuasion via logic won't work. The mere act of reading a book will rarely yield the desired result. Lasting change comes with the right combination of discussion, practicing new thoughts and behavior patterns, and observing their positive consequences. And of course, as is the case with most approaches, cognitive therapy needs to be applied with a healthy dose of compassion and sensitivity on the part of the therapist.

Beyond Behavioral and Cognitive Psychology: The Biobehavioral Model

Generally speaking, the biobehavioral model examines the link between behavioral and biological variables. It incorporates what we know about how biology affects behavior and, just as importantly, *how behavior affects biology*. Consider the following facts:

♦ Humans who repeatedly associate a given odor with taking an immunity-suppressing drug later experience suppressed immune function after simply being exposed to the odor alone. *Behavior affects biology.*

♦ Individuals given training in relaxation techniques prior to surgery require significantly less pain medication postoperatively, heal faster, and are able to go home earlier. *Behavior affects biology.*

♦ During recovery from hip surgery, women with strong religious beliefs walk farther, heal faster, and are less depressed than those without such beliefs. *Behavior affects biology.*

♦ Individuals undergoing stressful circumstances experience elevations in the production of stress hormones and hence have suppressed immune function. They are more likely than nonstressed individuals to become ill. *Behavior affects biology.*

♦ People who talk about, or even write about, their deepest concerns and secrets significantly reduce their frequency of illness and visits to the doctor. *Behavior affects biology.*

♦ As a group, regular church attendees have lower blood pressure and almost half the risk of heart attack when compared with the general population, regardless of other risk factors such as obesity, smoking, and socioeconomic status. *Behavior affects biology.*

♦ Women with metastatic breast cancer who participate in weekly support groups in addition to their regular medical treatment survive twice as long as women who receive standard medical care alone. *Behavior affects biology.*

So, how do we explain these facts? How is it possible that women with breast cancer can actually double their life expectancy just by sitting around talking about their feelings with other women in the same predicament? How can it be that merely talking to another person about one's deepest concerns and secrets can have an impact on the frequency of illness episodes and doctor visits? How in the world can we account for the fact that regular church attendees have lower blood pressure and almost half the rate of heart attacks as nonattendees, even when controlling for other risk factors? Are these results due to poor science? Do they result from a noncritical mentality that relies on wishful thinking to cope with the stress of modern life? Are they the product of the "new age" movement? No. These facts are, for the most part, based on well-controlled studies, some of which have been replicated by independent research groups and reported in scholarly, peer-reviewed journals. So, how do we account for these results?

The answer lies in the human blueprint. The research on stress strongly implies that we are designed to benefit from responding to "internal stimuli" or, in other words, our physical and emotional feelings. There seems to be a definite biological advantage to addressing such feelings through communication and action, while there is a biological disadvantage to ignoring them. Recall our discussion of the human stress response (Chapters 1 and 6) in which we addressed how behavioral events can condition the sympathetic nervous system to stimulate stress hormone distribution, heart rate and blood pressure elevation, vasoconstriction, and muscle tension. These biological events are triggered by what happens to human beings as they go about their day-to-day lives. They are our body's efforts to adapt to challenging circumstances. Behavior affects biology.

Imagine the headlines that would be generated if a new drug or medical procedure were shown to double the life expectancy of women with breast cancer. It would be the lead story on all the newscasts. Medical specialists around the world would incorporate the new treatment into their practices almost immediately. And Wall Street would be scrambling to purchase stock in the company that developed the new approach. So why haven't these findings seen this type of response? The answer is that the biobehavioral perspective is essentially foreign to Western medicine's understanding of health, illness, and disease. The mechanism of action is not readily grasped when one is used to thinking in terms of less complex physical cause-and-effect relationships, such as that between smoking and cardiovascular disease. When thinking of the relationship between behavior and illness, doctors are used to considering more obvious physical factors such as diet and exercise. Yet, chronic stress and the state of one's relationships are as important in their effects on illness as are the factors we usually hear about from doctors and the media. Fortunately, biobehavioral aspects of illness are becoming more mainstream as the research evidence mounts. And we trust that, one-day, they will go on to become a seamlessly integrated part of the medical establishment.

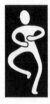

◆ 10

Active Physical
Interventions

Physical interventions in the treatment of chronic pain include physical therapy, chiropractic care, and acupuncture. The common denominator among these forms of therapy is the absence of medication. Many individuals in our society prefer a holistic approach to medical care and view pharmacological intervention with disdain and suspicion. For these folks, a holistic approach is the way to go. If it is effective, and often it is — Hooray! That's wonderful. We applaud their success. However, in cases where success remains elusive, we believe that a trial of pharmacological and/or behavioral intervention should be considered. Our motto is: "Whatever works." We are pragmatists at heart. If the patient is comfortable with the program and is satisfied with the pain relief and level of function achieved, that's good enough for us.

Physical Therapy

Physical therapy is the therapeutic use of physical agents other than drugs. It includes the application of various properties of heat, cold, light, friction, pressure, radiation, water, and electricity. These are classified as passive modalities and will be covered in the next chapter. Physical therapy also encompasses exercise and biofeedback, which, in contrast, are considered to be active. This means that the full participation of the individual is required. In this chapter, we discuss these active forms of therapy.

Preventive Care: Good Posture and Proper Body Mechanics

When it comes to health, an ounce of prevention is worth a pound of cure. Good posture and proper body mechanics are worth their weight in gold. And they don't cost a dime. Just a little self-determination. By standing taller, you will look and feel better. Your self-confidence will improve, and you will convey a more positive self-image. In addition, you can also prevent or diminish all those nagging aches and pains.

What constitutes good posture? Your spine has three natural curves: the cervical curve of the neck, the thoracic curve of the middle back, and the lumbar curve of the lower back. To test whether your three curves are properly aligned, imagine a plumb line beside your body. Your ear, shoulder, pelvis, knee, and ankle on that side of the body should all line up. If they do, your three curves are in optimal position. Proper body mechanics is synonymous with good posture in motion. That means that as you move, your spine's three curves are maintained in their neutral position. The following are important guidelines for posture and proper body mechanics:

◆ **Sitting.** Sit in chairs low enough to place both feet flat on the floor with knees level with the hips. Sit firmly against the back of the chair. Use a lumbar roll to support your lower back.

◆ **Standing.** When standing, rest one foot on a low stool. Alternate the foot resting on the stool every few minutes. If possible, raise or lower your work surface so that your shoulders and neck remain relaxed.

◆ **Walking.** Walk tall, with your head high, chin tucked in, toes straight ahead. Tighten your abdominal muscles to support your lower back. Wear comfortable, low-heeled shoes with good arch support. Control your weight, because a potbelly places extra stress on the lower spine.

♦ **Reaching.** If you have to reach across a level surface such as a bed, place one knee on the bed to support your lower back as you do so.

♦ **Lifting.** Lift objects close to your body. As you lift, tighten your abdominal muscles to support the spine. **Do not** lift with your back, but rather lift with your legs and buttocks. **Do not** twist your torso as you lift.

♦ **Carrying.** When carrying things, be sure to balance the load. That is, put equal weight, such as two suitcases, on either side of the body.

♦ **Sleeping.** The best position for sleep is either on your back with a pillow under your knees or on your side with a pillow between your knees. Use only one pillow under your head.

Do yourself a big favor and follow these simple rules. It's a cheap investment in your health, and it pays big dividends. If you want to replace a slouch with a regal carriage, just remember: according to conventional wisdom, it takes 21 days to form a new habit. So hang in there. After 21 days, beautiful posture and proper body mechanics will seem like second nature.

Exercise

Exercise is one of the most effective treatments for chronic pain. Numerous studies indicate that exercise is much more effective than passive modalities such as ultrasound or massage in bringing about lasting benefit. But the mere mention of the word "exercise" frequently evokes a grimace and a groan from someone suffering with pain and debilitation. "Exercise? When I hurt like this at rest? You've got to be kidding!"

All too often, pain leads to inactivity that leads to deconditioning which, in turn, leads to further pain. It's a vicious cycle. If the person is to get better, this downward spiral must be reversed in a proactive manner. And exercise is the answer.

The goals of exercise are to improve strength, endurance, and flexibility — or range of motion — as well as to alleviate pain. Exercise often reduces the area of pain. It centralizes the pain, decreasing a large, ill-defined area to a smaller, localized one. In addition, it stimulates the production of the body's own natural painkillers, substances called *endorphins*. These substances enhance mood as they reduce pain. Regular exercise is necessary in order to maintain and optimize the benefits.

Exercise as a therapy is based on the belief that the body adapts to the physical stresses to which it is subjected. According to the *Overload Principle,* greater stress must be placed on the body than it is ordinarily accustomed to in order for adaptation — that is, improvement in flexibility, endurance, or strength — to occur. Conversely, if the body is not physically stressed, deconditioning results, and the body loses flexibility, endurance, or strength. This trend inevitably leads to a decrease in function and ability to carry out the activities of daily living, a decline in quality of life, a diminished sense of well-being, and all too often an increase in the "P" word.

A word of caution: You should not embark on an exercise program until you have undergone a thorough medical evaluation by a qualified physician and obtained his or her advice and recommendations regarding the specific exercises to be performed and the intensity at which they can be done safely. This protocol is especially important for those individuals over the age of 35 who have been leading sedentary lives.

Exercise Program: Warm-Up, Workout, Cool-Down

The three key components of any exercise program are the warm-up, the workout, and the cool-down phases. Proper warm-up before exercise is a must. Without it, nerve impulses are sluggish, muscles lack resiliency, reaction time is slow, and the heart and lungs fatigue easily. These conditions are fertile ground for injury. A 5- to 10-minute warm-up phase allows the body to shift from its resting state to the active state. It prepares the musculoskeletal and cardiovascular systems for more intense physical activity.

Each exercise session should start off with a general stretching program to lubricate joints and to warm and lengthen tight musculoskeletal structures such as muscles, tendons, and ligaments. In addition, a warm-up period is required to gradually increase the work performed by the cardiovascular system. This phase may consist of a slow walking, biking, or swimming speed that steadily progresses to a more rapid pace. After about five minutes of this activity, your heart rate should be about 100 beats a minute and your body should be ready for more vigorous exercise.

Flexibility Exercises: Stretching

Stretching is a critical link between the sedentary and active life. It is essential to stretch during the warm-up phase of your exercise program in order to prepare the muscles for movement and to facilitate the transition from inactivity to vigorous exercise. It is also important to stretch during the cool-down phase of the program following the workout phase. Proper stretching promotes flexibility, reduces muscle tension, develops body awareness, promotes circulation, helps to prevent injury, and improves athletic performance.

Caution: Improper Stretching Can Be Hazardous to Your Health

While stretching is easy, it must be done correctly. Poor technique can do more harm than good. Therefore, you must understand and apply the principles of proper, effective stretching in order to be successful and to avoid injury. First of all, stretching should feel good, not bad.

Forget the adage "no pain, no gain." Do not push, push, push to the limits every time you stretch. Do not engage in a personal contest to see how far you can stretch. Do not attempt to defy the laws of physics. Do not strive to become the epitome of elasticity — say, a Raggedy Ann or Andy — you were never meant to be. And for heaven's sake, please do not bounce.

The object of the game is to reduce muscle tension, thereby promoting freer movement. Improper stretching can actually result in the opposite: greater muscle tension and restriction of motion. Here's how. Overstretching and bouncing can cause microscopic tearing of the muscle fibers. This tearing, in turn, leads to the formation of scar tissue in the muscle and the loss of elasticity and flexibility, the exact opposite of the intended goals. It also triggers a protective mechanism called the *stretch reflex*. In essence, whenever you stretch the muscle fibers too far, a signal is sent to the muscles instructing them to contract in order to prevent muscle injury. In other words, the muscles go into spasm. And spasms hurt. So, overstretching and bouncing are no-nos.

The keys to successful stretching are moderation, consistency, and relaxation. The right way to stretch is with a relaxed, sustained stretch, focusing your attention on the muscles at work. Your breathing during stretching should be slow, steady, and controlled. Do not hold your breath while stretching. If a particular stretch position interferes with your natural breathing pattern, then you are not maintaining a relaxed state. To correct this, just ease up on the stretch and continue to monitor your breathing to assure that you are achieving the desired effect. Stretch the particular muscles that will be involved in the workout component of the program. For example, since swimming involves the use of the arms, legs, and trunk, stretching these body parts should be included in the warm-up phase. On the other hand, walking, jogging, and running will require concentration on the musculature of the hips, knees, and ankles.

Begin with an *easy stretch*. Go to the point of mild discomfort but not pain. Then hold that position for 10 to 30 seconds, relaxing as you do. The sensation of tension should subside as you maintain the position.

If it does not, ease up and find a degree of tension that is more comfortable. Repeat this five times per muscle group.

After the easy stretch, gradually move into the *developmental stretch* by moving a fraction of an inch farther until you feel mild to moderate tension. Hold this position for up to 30 seconds. As before, the tension should diminish as you do so. If it does not, ease up slightly and try again. Repeat five times per muscle group.

The benefits of proper stretching are numerous: increased flexibility, reduced muscle tension, improvement in circulation and athletic performance, prevention of injury...the list goes on. Remember: moderation, consistency, and relaxation are the keys to successful stretching. *Don't bounce, and don't overstretch.* Be good to your muscles, and they'll be good to you. (For more information regarding stretching of specific muscles, see Bob Anderson's book, *Stretching*.)

Endurance Conditioning: Aerobic Exercise

Endurance or aerobic exercise is exercise that involves the reciprocal and dynamic use of large muscle groups. It places demand on the cardiovascular–pulmonary system to deliver oxygen to these muscles. *Endurance* is the ability to continue a specified task. Conversely, *fatigue* is the inability to continue a specified task. The biological endpoint of fatigue is maximum aerobic capacity (VO_2 max), that is, the maximal rate at which oxygen may be utilized by the body. It is the rate of oxygen consumption which cannot increase any further despite increasing mechanical work or exercise performed by the individual. Fatigue is a critically important endpoint to reach in both endurance and strengthening training programs to assure that maximum benefit is attained. In fact, studies indicate that muscle fatigue is even more important than the mechanical work performed to assure that conditioning is being achieved.

Examples of aerobic exercise include biking, swimming, cross-country skiing, and jogging. The three parameters of an aerobic program are

Benefits of Aerobic Exercise

The benefits of endurance/aerobic exercise occur within two to four weeks and include:

♦ An increase in maximum cardiac output
♦ A decrease in resting heart rate
♦ An improvement in overall cardiovascular–pulmonary fitness
♦ An increase in work capacity
♦ An increase in aerobic capacity (VO_2 max)
♦ A shortened recovery period following exercise
♦ An increase in the extraction of oxygen both at the lungs centrally and the muscles and organs peripherally (called the increase A-VO_2 difference)
♦ An increase in hemoglobin and blood volume
♦ An improvement in blood glucose control
♦ An increased use of fatty acids as fuel

intensity, duration, and frequency of exercise. The *intensity* of the exercise is reflected in the heart rate, which should be maintained at 60 to 70% of the maximum heart rate (220 minus your age). The *duration* of each individual training session should be at least 20 to 30 minutes or to the point of fatigue. The *frequency* of the training sessions should be four to five times per week.

Endurance or aerobic exercise is all about the delivery of oxygen to working muscles. The ambient air around us is composed of 21% oxygen, the stuff that is essential for life and activity. Muscles love it. The more oxygen, the more energy. The more energy, the more fun exercise the muscles get to engage in, the very activity for which they were designed. Take a big deep breath and think about where the oxygen is going.

Imagine for a moment that you are an oxygen molecule, and you are just dying to get to a muscle so that you can make your essential contribution to the performance of an Olympic long-distance runner. The runner takes a big deep breath, and in you go, entering his system through the nose or mouth. Next, you tumble down an air tunnel or tube called the *trachea* and meet a veritable branch in the road where the trachea divides into two smaller tubes called the *bronchi.* These bronchi, in turn, branch into even smaller ones called *bronchioles.* Before you know it, you arrive in the *lungs,* the spongy organs of respiration, and are sitting in one of millions of little sacs called *alveoli.* This is the site where you, the oxygen molecule, and, of course, trillions of other oxygen molecules enter the bloodstream in exchange for the waste product carbon dioxide. The latter is then exhaled from the lungs into the atmosphere.

So far, it's been quite a ride. The trick is to get into the bloodstream because you, the oxygen molecule, know that oxygen is delivered to muscles and other body parts via the bloodstream. You notice that some of the other oxygen molecules are leaving the lungs and directly entering the bloodstream by diffusing through the capillary membrane. But you're smart. You've been around the block before. You decide to hook up with one of those speedy *hemoglobin* molecules, the ones that give the blood its pretty red color. As one of these molecules cruises by, you latch on, and away you go on the adventure of your life. First you travel to the heart, a muscular organ that pumps blood throughout your body, all day, every day (even on holidays). The heart then pumps the blood out of the heart and away to the muscles and other body parts via blood vessels called *arteries.* Like the heart, arteries have muscles in their walls. These blood vessels branch into smaller vessels

Hemoglobin

Hemoglobin is the iron-containing pigment of the red blood cells. Its function is to carry oxygen from the lungs to the tissues. In the lungs, hemoglobin readily combines with oxygen to form a loose, unstable compound called oxyhemoglobin. In the muscles, oxyhemoglobin releases oxygen in exchange for the waste product carbon dioxide (CO_2). It then carries the CO_2 via blood vessels called veins back up to the right side of the heart, where it is pumped to the lungs and then exhaled from the body.

called *arterioles* and finally terminate in *capillaries,* which are very thin walled, facilitating the transfer of oxygen. You finally arrive at your destination, the gastrocnemius or calf muscle. This runner needs your help. And hopefully, he'll be thankful enough to include your picture on the Wheaties box.

Strengthening Exercises: Isometric, Isotonic, Isokinetic

Strength is the maximum force that can be exerted by a muscle. It can be subdivided into *static strength,* in which no movement occurs, and *dynamic strength,* in which there is movement. There are three types of strengthening exercises: isometric, isotonic, and isokinetic.

Isometric exercise is static exercise with muscle contraction but no movement of the load placed on that muscle. In addition, there is no change in the total length of the muscle. For example, one can increase strength by applying force to an immovable object, such as a brick wall that isn't going anywhere. *Isometric strength* is the maximal force that can be applied against an immovable object and is measured by a static apparatus such as a strain gauge. So, just remember, the next time you try to move a mountain, you are performing an isometric exercise to improve your strength.

Isotonic exercise, on the other hand, is dynamic exercise involving movement. Like isometric exercise, the load, or weight, is constant, but the speed of movement is uncontrolled and therefore varies. As movement occurs, the muscle shortens and lengthens. Examples of isotonic exercise include lifting free weights such as dumbbells or barbells. In addition, the body itself can be used as resistance by moving it against gravity with techniques such as push-ups, pull-ups, and sit-ups. *Isotonic strength* is usually measured by the amount of weight that can be lifted a specified number of repetitions and is referred to as the 1 or 10 repetition maximum (1 or 10 RM).

Isokinetic exercise is dynamic exercise with controlled movement that occurs through a range at a constant number of degrees per second (angular velocity) as the muscle shortens and lengthens. The load applied and force exerted are variable. *Isokinetic strength* is the peak torque generated during movement at a certain preset rate. Equipment to improve or measure isokinetic strength includes the Nautilus® and the Cybex®.

The benefits of strengthening exercise are many. They include hypertrophy or enlargement of individual muscle fibers and a concomitant increase in muscle definition and strength. This is aesthetically pleasing to many and constitutes a serious motivating factor. Not only are muscles strengthened as a result of these exercises, but so are tendons, ligaments, and bones. As a matter of fact, there is an actual increase in mineral content and density of bone. The cartilage between articulating joints thickens as well. Metabolic changes also occur, such as increases in energy stores like adenosine triphosphate, creatine phosphate, and muscle glycogen. In addition, the wall of the left ventricle of the heart thickens (hypertrophies).

An interesting phenomenon occurs, known as *cross-transference of training effects* from the exercised muscles to nonexercised muscles. For example, if the right arm undergoes strengthening exercises, the strength in the left arm improves as a result. The mechanism by which this occurs is neurally mediated. Unlike aerobic endurance exercise, strength training has either no effect on oxidative capacity or an actual *decrease* in oxidative capacity. This is believed to be due primarily to the diluting effect of hypertrophied muscles, which increases the distance that the oxygen has to travel (diffusion distance).

The *DeLorme axiom* states that high-force–low-repetition exercises build strength, while low-force–high-repetition exercises build endurance. The *DeLorme technique* is an isotonic method of building strength. The program consists of progressive resistance exercises with 10 repetitions at 25, 50, 75, and 100% of the maximum weight an individual is capable of lifting. Two-minute rest periods are allowed between repetitions, and the weight is increased weekly as determined by the 10 RM. The disadvantage of this program is that the subject is often unable to carry out the 10 RM at 100% because of fatigue. Therefore, the Oxford technique was developed.

The *Oxford technique* employs the reverse schedule of the DeLorme technique, beginning with 100% of the maximum capability (10 RM). The subject begins at 100% and subsequently does 10 reps at 75%, then 50%, and finally 25%. The subject becomes less fatigued and is usually able to complete the regimen. However, less fatigue is a training disadvantage. Fatigue as the endpoint is critical to assure maximum training effect and is much more important than the amount of mechanical work accomplished.

Approaches more specific to chronic pain sufferers will be outlined in the next few sections, but many believe that an optimum program for most people entails five to seven repetitions per set, three sets per session, four to five sessions per week. The weights should be at a maximum for the number of repetitions to assure full activation of all motor units. A recovery period of two to three minutes between contractions is also recommended.

The maximum rate of increase in strength with maximum exercise is approximately 12% per week, increasing linearly up to 75% of limiting strength. Above 75%, the rate of increase diminishes. This holds true for all muscles, persons, genders, and ages. The length of training time required to increase from zero strength up to maximum strength is about 12 weeks. The length of training before muscle hypertrophy becomes evident is six to eight weeks.

What about maintenance of strength once maximum strength is attained through exercise? Believe it or not, maximum strength can be maintained indefinitely by only one maximum contraction that lasts a mere second about every two weeks, in addition to the usual activities of daily living. A maximum contracture triggers a prolonged stimulus within the muscle for the development of contractile tissue that persists for about seven days. This stimulus is reinforced very little by repetition of a maximum contraction within the next 24 hours.

The rate of decrease or loss of strength in the absence of muscle contraction is about 1 to 5% of the initial strength per day. So the hazards of bed rest or immobilization in a cast are very real.

Cool-Down

Just as it is important to warm up before exercising, it is essential to cool down after a vigorous workout. The body should return to its normal level of functioning gradually rather than abruptly. After running, jogging, swimming, or biking, you should perform that activity during the cool-down phase at a slower pace until your heart rate and breathing are restored to baseline. It is also important, once again, to stretch your muscles, joints, and ligaments.

Programming Exercise to Maximize Success

Has this ever happened to you? You're sick and tired of carrying around those extra pounds and huffing and puffing your way up the stairs. January 1st rolls around, and you finally decide to start an exercise program. Full of determination while basking in the memory of your (rather impressive) athletic prowess during your tenure on the high-school swim team, you hit the gym with a vengeance. But wait. There's something wrong here. You begin to detect a dastardly plot at hand. It becomes obvious that, since your high-school days, they've secretly increased the resistance on exercise bikes. Remember when you could peddle all day and not get the least bit winded? Well, no more. What's worse, they've *underlabeled* the weight settings on the exercise machines. Remember 10 reps at 30 pounds? Forget it. And, perhaps most sinister of all, they somehow recalibrated a mile from 5,280 feet to, oh

— at least *twice* that! Scoundrels! Where's the Bureau of Weights and Measures when you need it?

Of course, the sad truth is that the "conspiracy" lies not outside but rather inside your own body. As we age, we slow down and our energy begins to sag (along with certain parts of our anatomy). Yet, with vivid memories of your stellar swim team glory, you dive into your new exercise program. These memories translate into subconscious personal expectations. "C'mon now — No pain, no gain! Push, push, push." But before you know it, you hit the wall. Wham! You can do no more. "Everyone in the gym has got to be thinking I'm the most pathetic, out-of-shape specimen they've ever seen," you mutter to yourself. Hurting and out of breath, you admit defeat and berate yourself for being such a wimp. The next day, you ache like crazy. You can hardly move. That drive to get fit seems like a distant, laughable memory. "Better take the day off. No exercise today. Maybe tomorrow…"

Sound familiar? This scenario seems to be an almost universal pattern among the human species. The net result is that our laudable intentions go unrewarded — indeed, are literally *punished* — by the consequences of our efforts. Psychologists wouldn't be surprised. Behavior theory says that any behavior (e.g., exercising) that is followed by unpleasant consequences (pain, exhaustion, humiliation, etc.) will tend to reduce the future occurrence of that behavior. It is such a strong tendency that the theory regards this process as a law of behavior. It is not so much a matter of willpower as it is responding to our own personal histories of reinforcement combined with present circumstances. Pushing oneself harder will, in all likelihood, only result in failure.

So what's the solution? It may sound daunting, but it's really quite simple: Use the principles of behavior theory to program your re-entry into the world of exercise. If you want to maximize the probability that you will meet your exercise goals, you will need the following ingredients:

1. **Patience.** We know that we all want results right now. But if you don't have much of this ingredient, expect frustration and large quantities of sedentary inertia.

2. **A record-keeping plan.** It is important that, for each exercise in your program, you keep track of your progress. It will serve as a powerful reinforcer as you progress.

3. **The proper attitude.** You know the phrase "no pain, no gain"? Take a black marker and write it down on a sheet of paper in big block letters. Look at the paper and read it aloud. Now add the phrase "IS NONSENSE!" Next, with a big frown, rip it up and throw it in the recycle bin.

With these basic ingredients, you can formulate a plan to maximize the probability of success. Here's how:

♦ **Step 1: With your doctor and/or physical therapist, determine the particular exercises that are appropriate for you.** Write each exercise on a separate exercise progress record form (a copy of the form used by our patients appears in Appendix B).

♦ **Step 2: Establish a baseline for each exercise.** After a mild warm-up, perform each exercise until you start to notice pain and/or fatigue setting in. Then STOP. Write down your number of repetitions, time, or distance. Do not push ahead with the thought "Oh, I can do 10 more." Remember the "no pain, no gain" routine mentioned earlier. The objective is not to start your program now. Rather, it is to listen to the feedback your body is giving you and use that information to establish your starting point. If you want extra assurance that this plan will work, do this for your first three exercise days.

♦ **Step 3: Set your starting point.** After collecting three days of baselines, establish your starting point. Here's how:

a. For each exercise, take your total number of repetitions, time, or distance (for example, day 1 = 13 reps, day 2 = 9 reps, and day 3 = 10 reps, for a total of 32 reps).
b. Divide that number by 3 to get a daily average, and then round down (32 ÷ 3 = 10.67 reps, rounded down to 10).
c. Multiply that number by 0.8 (10 × 0.8 = 8 reps). That's your starting point, or target, for day 4 of your exercise program.

♦ **Step 4: Establish a winning progression interval** by gradually increasing the amount of exercise over time. But here's the crucial key: *make sure that you are at least 80% confident that you will meet each goal when establishing your daily exercise targets.* One of the greatest sources of failure is pushing too hard, too fast. This typically meets with way too much failure and serves to "punish" your efforts. Instead, increase your target by a small amount every two or three exercise sessions. Write down your targets in advance for the following week.

♦ **Step 5: Adjust your progression interval.** If you do not meet your goal for a given exercise twice in a row, you have set your progression interval too high. Move it back a bit. Remember, you should be at least 80% confident that you will meet each daily target.

♦ **Step 6: Graph your progress.** Plotting your performance on a graph is the best way to see your progress at a glance. Use copies of the exercise progress record form included in Appendix B. Watching your graphs move upward will strengthen your exercise efforts and feed that "willpower thing" that everyone talks about. Although it requires a few more seconds to accomplish, taking this step will definitely be worth the time.

We have used this method with great success in our interdisciplinary pain management program. Time and again, remarkable increases in performance occur. Why? Because the method exploits the behavioral principles that operate for all of us in our daily lives. It maximizes positive reinforcement while minimizing the punishing consequences so often associated with exercise. And that's a recipe for success.

Physical Exercise Summary

There is a plethora of perks for those who exercise regularly: more stamina, greater self-confidence and self-esteem, a decrease in depression, an increase in energy and productivity, improved resistance to illness, and a svelte physique. But hey, who cares? It's a veritable fountain of youth. And it doesn't cost a fortune. Just buy yourself a pair of sturdy tennis shoes and you are set to go. You think face-lifts, body-lifts, and liposuction are going to slow the inevitable tide of aging? Try good old-fashioned exercise. Lose 10 pounds and you'll look 10 years younger. Guaranteed or your money back (just kidding — about the money, that is). Less weight means less stress on arthritic joints like the ankles, knees, hips, and back. Less stress on joints translates into less pain. And, of course, less weight means a smaller body and the genuine necessity for smaller clothes. Voilà! You now have a bona fide excuse to go on a shopping spree for that new wardrobe you've been wanting. You can't go to the ball looking like *this,* now can you, Cinderella? Of course not! Who can argue when your clothes are hanging on you because of all that glorious huffing and puffing you did in the gym? Exercise is the greatest. We rest our case.

Turning Down the Volume with Biofeedback

Pop Quiz

Complete the following statements by circling a or b:

1. If it were too bright in the room, I would...
   a. turn down the lights.
   b. put on a pair of sunglasses.

2. If it were too hot, I would...
    a. turn down the furnace.
    b. put on a bathing suit and fling the doors and windows wide open.

3. If the stereo were too loud, I would...
    a. turn down the volume knob.
    b. put on a pair of earmuffs.

If you answered *a* to each of the above, congratulations. You are within the range of human variation. If you answered *b,* you're probably still dizzy (after screwing in that light bulb) from the ladder turning round and round.

Of course the sunglasses, open window, and earmuff options sound silly. But what if there had never been the need to adjust the light, heat, or volume because it was always done for you automatically? In the absence of a need, there would never have been a reason to learn how to operate the controls. But when something goes haywire and you are suddenly in the position of discomfort — whether it is due to too much light, heat, sound (or pain) — what do you do? Do you reach for the sunglasses, window, or earmuffs? Or do you search for the owner's manual? In a sense, biofeedback is like studying the manual. It teaches us how to work the controls, not of the light system, furnace, or stereo, but of the brain itself.

Unfortunately, in the chronic pain management field, we frequently see an overemphasis on treating symptoms rather than the cause of those symptoms. While pain medications, physical therapy, acupuncture, chiropractic treatment, and massage are often very helpful, they do little to alter the brain's instructions to the body to remain tense. That is why these more mainstream approaches often yield only temporary benefit. When properly used, biofeedback can add a significant — *and lasting* — element of control over the *production* of the physical tension and nervous system activity that aggravate pain.

Biofeedback operates on a simple principle. Feeding back information to an individual about some physiological process (e.g., muscle tension or nervous system arousal) can allow him or her to alter that process. Through experimentation, and with the aid of a skilled practitioner (usually a psychologist or physical therapist), the individual learns to take control over these processes which previously were taken care of automatically by the brain. In a sense, biofeedback involves retraining the brain and putting the control in the hands of its owner. So, instead of putting on earmuffs, the person notes that he or she is uncomfortable and then dials in the proper brain setting by recalling what it took to achieve the desired result during biofeedback training.

Relaxation and biofeedback approaches benefit almost everyone with chronic pain. It is extremely common to see reductions in muscle tension, spasm, and sympathetic nervous system arousal on the order of 50 to 80% during the first few sessions. Pain usually decreases in response to these reductions.

Here's how it works. During the actual training sessions, we make customized relaxation tapes that the individual takes home to assist in daily practice. We also provide a copy of the biofeedback tracing which shows, in graphical form, the physiological changes the person achieved that day. We advise the person to post the tracing on the refrigerator so that he or she will see it and become more aware of changes in tension and nervous system arousal. Within a few weeks of biofeedback training and home practice, the brain becomes more and more familiar with what is required to bring about the desired physiological changes. Then the changes start happening quite automatically in the person's day-to-day life, from moment to moment. There's no more need to listen to a 15-minute relaxation tape each day. The discomfort level decreases and serves to strengthen this new response pattern in the brain and body. Before you know it, the relaxation response becomes generalized to real-life situations. Put down the sunglasses, close the window, and stuff the earmuffs back in the sock drawer. Comfort has been restored by learning how to operate the controls of the brain.

The Interdisciplinary Approach to Treating Chronic Pain

With difficult chronic pain conditions, studies clearly show that a co-ordinated interdisciplinary team approach to treatment works better than the individual practitioner approach. It's true. We've done it both ways. Sometimes referred to as *multidisciplinary,* the term *interdisciplinary* connotes an interaction among disciplines. Rather than working independently, or in parallel, each member of the treatment team is aware of, and works to support, the goals of every other member. The patient's accomplishments in physical, occupational, and behavioral therapies are noted by the physician and each of the other team members. When this occurs, tremendous progress can be made in a relatively short period of time, and the patient doesn't have to contend with the frustrations that come with receiving mixed messages.

Our colleague Dr. William Deardorff published an important study in the journal *Pain* (1991) which compared treatment outcomes for pain patients who had undergone interdisciplinary treatment with those for patients who were unable to participate due to lack of insurance autho-

---

The Interdisciplinary Team

Members of an interdisciplinary team may include some combination of the following chronic pain specialists:

1. Physician
2. Physical therapist
3. Occupational therapist
4. Health psychologist
5. Biofeedback specialist (usually a psychologist or physical therapist)
6. Nurse
7. Case manager
8. Social worker
9. Vocational rehabilitation counselor
10. The patient
11. The patient's family

rization. Otherwise, the two groups were similar. Individuals in the second group continued to receive standard care from individual practitioners. Guess what? Those who continued to receive standard care showed little if any improvement in terms of their physical and emotional functioning, work status, and reliance on pain medication. Alternatively, those involved in the coordinated interdisciplinary approach made amazing progress. Many were able to return to work. Depression, anxiety, and life disruption were all significantly improved. Also, the need for pain medication was reduced by a large margin. Certainly participants' lives were much better. The gains were clear. Patients simply got better when a *coordinated* team approach to treatment was provided.

But it is not enough simply to have representatives from each discipline working with the chronic pain patient. Criteria necessary to make this work include the following:

1. Team members should be educated about and experienced in treating chronic pain conditions. It isn't enough to throw in just any old physician, physical therapist, psychologist, etc. Chronic pain is a specialty. And, as with any specialty, you have to know what you are doing. There is no substitute for training and experience. How would you feel, for example, if a heart surgeon were designated to perform your spinal fusion? Unless you happened to be stranded on a desert island, it would not be acceptable for just any surgeon to perform the operation.

2. Team members should *truly* constitute a team. This means that they should communicate regularly with one another and work toward reinforcing the efforts of every other person on the team.

During his tenure as clinical director of a hospital-based chronic pain rehabilitation program, Dr. Deardorff received a call from an HMO representative inquiring about the multidisciplinary approach to pain management. Apparently, the HMO was not attempting to develop a pain program. Rather, it had an especially difficult chronic pain case and wanted to put a "team" together to treat this particular patient. The representative simply wanted to know what kinds of therapists he should include. Dr. Deardorff explained that, in addition to having certain disciplines represented, the critical elements mentioned above were necessary to make the interdisciplinary team approach work. There was a long pause. The representative thanked him for his time and said good-bye. Obviously, the HMO had no intention of spending the resources necessary to assemble chronic pain specialists or to initiate regular team conferences. It was looking merely at form rather than substance. And it doesn't work that way.

We have seen the unfortunate consequences that can befall chronic pain sufferers when doctors and therapists end up working at cross-purposes due to a lack of communication. One of our patients, Annette, was in a car accident that triggered a severe case of fibromyalgia syndrome. She was under the care of a doctor who assessed her orthopedic condition and concluded that the problem was structural. The fibromyalgia syndrome went undiagnosed. He told Annette that she needed vigorous physical exercise and prescribed a program in which she was to increase her progress at a rapid rate.

Like most fibromyalgia sufferers, Annette was conditioned from an early age to subordinate how she felt in favor of pushing herself to meet others' expectations and/or to maintain a high level of productivity.

The Interdisciplinary Team Approach and HMOs

While we know of only a handful of *nonprofit* HMOs that have developed what appear to be true interdisciplinary pain rehabilitation programs, we have never heard of *for-profit* ones that apply this proven approach. They may be out there, but we're not aware of them if they do exist. Rather, our experience has consistently been that coordinated chronic pain management services are just plain unavailable to people who receive their healthcare from for-profit HMOs. For more about this sorry state of affairs, see Chapter 15: The Managed Care Experiment.

She was an expert at getting things accomplished, even when she didn't feel well. And, true to form, she attacked her exercise program with a vengeance. Her objective progress was stellar. Her physical therapist and the doctor were so pleased. Yet, Annette continued to suffer terrible pain and fatigue. She kept pushing because, in her mind, her efforts were supposed to result in a cure. But the pain and fatigue only got worse. She marinated in her own frustration to the point that she did the unspeakable. She (politely) questioned the doctor as to his diagnostic formulation and treatment approach. This was no easy task for someone who had spent her whole life toeing the line and doing what she was "supposed to" do. Her doctor sent her to us, hoping that we could help.

Shortly after she was referred, the problems became clear:

1. Annette's primary pain diagnosis, fibromyalgia syndrome, had gone unrecognized.

2. Her doctor and physical therapist were inadvertently reinforcing her for a behavior pattern that contributed to the very symptoms everyone was trying to eliminate.

"No pain, no gain" had been the unrelenting motto for all participants. But it was causing Annette's nervous system to be in a chronic state of stress, which only served to fan the flames of her illness. After some education on the merits of trashing the "no pain, no gain" philosophy, we moved quickly to reestablish a greater degree of comfort by making some medication changes and assisting her in learning to listen and *respond appropriately to her body.* Once we all started to communicate and coordinate our efforts, Annette began to feel a lot better. She learned to give herself permission to back off from being "productive" when she was hurting. She essentially learned to be kind to herself. And it paid off. The frequency and severity of her symptoms eased considerably and her overall function improved.

The only ones who weren't real happy at first were her physical therapist and referring doctor. They saw her objective exercise performance drop off dramatically and were very concerned. "She's getting worse," was the initial reaction. And, indeed, Annette stopped pushing herself so hard, consistent with our advice, and her exercise performance *did* decline. But she was relieved. She was reeducated about the role of exercise as it related to her symptoms — that it was not going to bring about a cure and that *mild* exercise was a better approach. She no longer criticized herself for not getting better. Muscle tension and nervous system arousal eased considerably. Headaches, body pain, and fatigue were all reduced. She felt better. By learning to back off in the right way, she was actually able to become more active in the long run.

When we communicated these observations to Annette's doctor and physical therapist, they felt better as well. They were truly worried that the reduction in exercise performance was an indication that she was getting worse. This was based on the assumption that if you feel better, you'll do more. Although this is true for many people, Annette was an expert at concealing her feelings while toeing the line. And even though we knew that this was not good for her, others in the treatment team were cheering her on to push harder. This is an example of working at cross-purposes with the patient caught in the middle. Fortunately, our formulation eventually made sense to Annette's referring doctor and physical therapist, and they started tuning in to her overall progress.

The interdisciplinary team concept seems so elementary that you may wonder why it tends to be the exception rather than the rule. The reason is really quite simple. It requires extra work and a desire on the part of each player to listen to the patient and to each other. Also, insurance companies typically do not pay for the extra time and effort involved. The only benefit is that the patient gets better. And sadly, this outcome variable has come to take a backseat to the almighty dollar. Yet we would be remiss if we did not point out that there are excellent programs that maintain a solid interdisciplinary approach. Programs that are accredited specifically for pain management by the Commission on Accreditation for Rehabilitation Facilities (CARF) are a safe bet. We have developed and accredited two such hospital-based programs in the past and can attest to CARF's commitment to quality. However, CARF accreditation is not a guarantee that you will be listened to or that proper treatment will be forthcoming. There are also practitioners who function outside of an accredited program, but who maintain an interdisciplinary philosophy nonetheless (we are two of them).

Our advice? Do what you can to make sure that your doctors and therapists are communicating and coordinating your treatment with one another — *and with you.* The difference that this makes will become clear very quickly. Your own experience will be the judge.

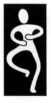

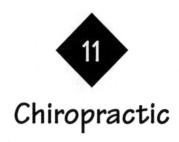

Chiropractic

Chiropractic Care

For the past 90 years, chiropractors and medical doctors have endured a strained relationship, not unlike that of the Arabs and the Israelis. Bloody fistfights (in the rhetorical sense) have characterized their interactions. The subject of spinal manipulation in particular has produced radically polarized views and ignited heated discussions and vicious verbal attacks. This divergence of opinion can be explained, in part, by the fact that the opposing factions treat each other's failures. But there is more to it than that.

Medical doctors claim that they have grave concerns regarding the safety and efficacy of chiropractic care. Scare tactics. They must "protect" their patients from harm by directing them to the paths that lead back to their very own doors — all in the name of altruism and undying devotion. But fact must be carefully sorted out from fiction. Upon careful scrutiny, it can be concluded that it all boils down to that green stuff — pure and simple. It's business as usual, and competition in the marketplace is driving their attitudes and behavior.

Lawsuit: Chiropractic versus the AMA Regarding the Title "Doctor"

On October 13, 1976, four chiropractic plaintiffs filed a lawsuit against the mighty American Medical Association (AMA). In the *Wilks et al. v*

American Medical Association et al. antitrust case (1987), these plaintiffs accused the AMA of orchestrating a long-term, illegal conspiracy to contain and eliminate chiropractic as a competitor based on the calculated and unfair portrayal of the chiropractic profession as "cultist" and "unscientific." The AMA attempted to justify its boycott, while the chiropractors argued that the AMA knew that chiropractic was licensed, effective, desired by millions of consumers, and a competitive threat to the medical profession.

In 1987, after over a decade of litigation, U.S. District Court Judge Susan Getzendanner found the AMA guilty of violating the antitrust laws. She ordered the AMA to:

1. Publish her injunction order to all of its 280,000 members

2. Print and permanently index her injunction order in the *Journal of the American Medical Association*

3. Amend all the rules of the association to allow its members to fully cooperate with chiropractic physicians

4. Pay reasonable attorney fees and costs to the plaintiff–chiropractors (which were in excess of $14 million)

It was more than a slap on the hand. Much more.

But the AMA wasn't done fighting. It got back into the ring for one last bloody round by requesting that the Supreme Court review the case. The chiropractors, in their opposition to this request, sited numerous scientific studies. The findings indicated that chiropractic care was up to twice as effective as medical physician care for nonsurgical, mechanical correction of problems related to the musculoskeletal system. Interestingly, the AMA was tripped up by the very scientific studies that it had previously said were lacking. And, ironically, these studies were used in court to confirm the finding of "guilty" in this antitrust case. The chiropractors also argued persuasively that the "AMA had no justification whatsoever for its direct but private challenge to the 50 state legislatures that license chiropractic. Millions have suffered and continue to suffer because of the AMA's arrogant abuse of power."

The Supreme Court declined the request to review trial court and court of appeals findings that the AMA had been guilty of a "lengthy, systematic, successful, and unlawful boycott" of doctors of chiropractic and their patients. In view of the existing scientific evidence, the AMA's position was objectively unreasonable and made a mockery of any argument that it had acted in good faith. Time is running out on the AMA's ability to bully other providers in our increasingly competitive healthcare marketplace.

Just the Facts, Ma'am

What is chiropractic? And just what *are* the facts regarding its efficacy and safety? Chiropractic is a system of therapeutics based upon the theory that disease is the result of malalignment of musculoskeletal structures, in particular the spinal column. These malalignments lead to abnormal function of the nervous system. Chiropractors attempt to restore the proper relationship between the musculoskeletal and nervous systems by spinal manipulation. While they may use related therapies such as physical therapy, heat, ice, traction, massage, and nutritional counseling when indicated, spinal manipulation is the mainstay of chiropractic care.

Spinal manipulation has been practiced for thousands of years. In the late 5th century B.C., it was described by Hypocrites, the legendary Greek physician who is generally regarded as the "father of medicine." Modern chiropractic practice traces its roots to a grocer in Davenport, Iowa, Daniel David Palmer. In 1895, Dr. Palmer fathered the theory that malalignment of the spine is the primary cause of disease. He claimed to be the first to utilize the spinous and transverse processes of vertebrae as levers, enabling the doctor to nudge the bones back to their normal juxtaposition. His textbook, *The Science, Art, and Philosophy of Chiropractic,* is classic to the profession today. Dr. Palmer described in detail the impingement process (i.e., pressure on a nerve) and its effect on health, according to his knowledge at the time. He rejected the germ theory as well as the humoral theory (that disease results when the four humors — blood, phlegm, and yellow and black bile — are imbalanced). However, he acknowledged that accidents and poisons caused disease and believed that they did so by causing subluxations (partial dislocations), which in turn caused nerve impingement and thereby disease.

Today, doctors of chiropractic are trained in accredited chiropractic colleges. A chiropractor must complete four years of college followed by a rigorous four years of postgraduate chiropractic education (eight years total beyond high school). In many ways, the curriculum resembles that of medical schools in the United States and includes extensive study of anatomy and physiology. During and after completing their formal education, chiropractors must pass national boards (parts 1, 2, and 3) before they can even sit for the state licensing exam that is required in order to practice their chosen profession.

Spinal manipulation is the key therapeutic technique that sets chiropractic care apart from most other medical professions, with the notable exception of osteopathic medicine. Spinal manipulation is a passive mechanical treatment applied to a specific vertebra or vertebral region of the spinal column. There are three main techniques of spinal manipulation: thrust, articulatory manipulation, and isometric manipulation.

Thrusting is also known as impulse or high-velocity–low-amplitude manipulation. It is performed by first identifying the pathological vertebral segment. The patient is then positioned in such a way as to lock the facet joints of the vertebral segments below this level (thereby limiting the motion of the vertebra in question). This vertebra is then passively moved to the limits of motion, and a quick, localized force is applied to the joint in the direction of the restricted motion. Often, an audible click or pop is produced.

Articulatory manipulation is also called mobilization and low-velocity–high-amplitude manipulation. The vertebral joint is passively moved to the endpoint of its range, which is considered to be the pathological barrier to motion. This barrier is then challenged with repeated motion.

Isometric manipulation is a nonthrusting technique. Similar to the thrusting approaches, the patient is positioned in such a way as to remove slack. The patient then exerts small to moderate forces against the resistance offered by the clinician for 5 to 10 seconds. This is followed by a period of relaxation. The procedure is then repeated two or three times. The end result is that the barrier is displaced and the range of motion of the joint increases.

How safe is spinal manipulation? Medical students are cautioned (if not indoctrinated) regarding the alleged dangers of chiropractic. Among these "dangers" is the potential risk of stroke due to cervical spine manipulation. Strokes following chiropractic manipulation are associated most often with damage to the vertebral arteries. These vital arteries course through a narrow passage in the vertebrae of the neck and supply oxygen and nutrient-rich blood to the spinal cord, brain stem, cerebellum, and cerebrum. With age, this channel becomes even narrower due to degenerative changes of the spine. The vertebral arteries are most commonly injured near the junction of the first and second cervical vertebrae, where they angle from a vertical to a horizontal course. As self-respecting medical students know their anatomy, this all makes *theoretical* sense. But what about the actual numbers? Do theory and reality coincide in this instance? Nope. The reported incidence of stroke as a direct result of cervical manipulation is extremely rare and varies from one in 400,000 to one in a million procedures. In a literature review covering 50 years, a mere 107 cases have been documented.

How dangerous is spinal manipulation of the *lumbar* spine? The most serious complication that may occur with low-back spinal manipulation is *cauda equina syndrome*. The cauda equina is a collection of spinal nerve roots that descends from the lower part of the spinal cord (which in the adult ends at the first lumbar vertebra) and occupies a fluid-filled sac in the vertebral canal below the cord. In appearance, the cauda equina resembles a horse's tail; hence the name. The nerve roots of the cauda equina innervate the penis, urinary bladder, bowel, and legs and provide sensation to the groin and anal area. So when the cauda equina is injured, the individual may present with impotence, urinary and rectal incontinence, absence of deep tendon reflexes, saddle anesthesia, and paraplegia (paralysis of the legs). This constitutes a medical emergency that warrants immediate surgical decompression of the nerve roots involved. According to the literature, cauda equina syndrome occurs only once in 500,000 low-back spinal manipulations.

An analysis of the literature between 1911 and 1991 indicates that, overall, the incidence of complications from low-back spinal manipulation is less than one case per year on average. In light of the fact that more than 90 million spinal manipulations are performed annually in the United States, the risk of serious harm as a result of either cervical or low-back manipulation is extremely low. Based on these numbers, avoiding chiropractic treatment for fear of injury would be like refusing to venture outside for fear of being struck by lightning.

Contraindications

Spinal manipulation is not recommended if a patient has a bone tumor, fracture, certain types of herniated discs, progressive neurological deficit, hypermobile joints, rheumatoid arthritis, severe osteoporosis, infection or inflammation of the spine, or bleeding disorders.

Rave Reviews for Chiropractic

Chiropractic care has been relentlessly criticized by the medical profession for having a lack of hard scientific evidence to support its safety and efficacy. But that's old news. The fact is that only about 15% of all *medical* interventions are supported by such evidence, according to David M. Eddy, M.D., Ph.D., professor of health policy and management at Duke University. Today, there is a growing body of research that supports the effectiveness and safety of chiropractic care in the treatment of certain back conditions — research that even the medical community cannot refute.

The Manga Report, an unbiased, independent study commissioned by the Ontario Ministry of Health, represents the largest existing analysis of scientific literature on the management of low-back pain thus far. Not a single clinical or controlled study was found that even suggests — much less demonstrates — that chiropractic spinal manipulation is unsafe in the treatment of low-back pain. While some medical treatments were found to be equally safe, others caused complications. In addition, chiropractic manipulation was found to be not only more effective overall compared with traditional medical management of low-back pain, but also more cost effective. Furthermore, patient satisfaction scores — an important healthcare outcome indicator — were considerably higher for chiropractic care compared with physician management. Based on its findings, the Manga Report proposed a revolutionary idea: that the management of low-back pain be moved from medical doctors to doctors of chiropractic and that hospital privileges be extended to them.

The Manga Report is not alone in its glowing praise of chiropractic care. A study published in the *Western Journal of Medicine* indicated that chiropractic patients were three times more satisfied with their care than patients of family practice physicians. A 1991 Gallup poll revealed that 9 out of 10 chiropractic patients felt that their treatment was effective. Another study published in the prestigious *New England Journal of Medicine* in 1993 indicated a growing trend among Americans toward the use of unconventional or alternative healthcare, including chiropractic, acupuncture, and massage therapy. One-third of all Americans sought alternative healthcare in 1990. In all, 425 million visits were made by Americans to providers of alternative therapy, compared with 388 million visits to traditional Western healthcare providers.

The rise in popularity of chiropractic care is indisputable. Many professional athletes are touting its benefits. Among those singing its praises are

♦ *Joe Montana,* former all-pro quarterback for the San Francisco 49ers. The four-time Super Bowl Champion and three-time Super Bowl MVP said, "I only wish I had tried chiropractic a few years ago when I first started having back pain and maybe surgery would have never happened."

♦ *Ivan Lendl,* world-class tennis professional, said, "I try to go twice a week to a chiropractor, sometimes even more during big tournaments. I feel I am much more tuned-up with an adjustment. I support chiropractic very much. I think it's great for sports, I think it's great for anyone."

♦ *Evander Holyfield,* world heavyweight boxing champion, said, "I do believe in chiropractic. I found that going to my chiropractor three times a week helps my performance. Once I drove twenty miles to see a chiropractor before a fight. I have to have my adjustments before I go into a ring."

Why the trend toward utilizing chiropractic care? Well, for one reason, it offers patients a natural method of healing without the use of drugs or surgery. For many people, this is very appealing. But we believe that there are many other legitimate reasons as well. Almost daily we have the opportunity to speak with patients who have been treated with chiropractic. Overwhelmingly, they express grateful affection for their chiropractors and feel that they have benefited from their care.

Studies comparing the effectiveness of various psychological approaches have concluded that the particular approach employed is often less important in determining success than the therapist's ability to establish a trusting, therapeutic relationship with the patient. As a whole, chiropractors are superb at doing just that. They *listen* to their patients. They *touch* their patients. They *convey concern and compassion* to their patients. Medical doctors could learn a lot from doctors of chiropractic about how to establish a therapeutic doctor–patient relationship — an endangered species in today's world of managed care.

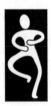

12

Acupuncture

If you want to truly experience the sensation of being on pins and needles, by all means pay a friendly visit to your local acupuncturist. We assure you. Before you leave his or her office, you will feel like a genuine pincushion. But what's the point? (No pun intended — honest.) If you are from Western culture, you may be wondering just what acupuncture is all about. A good place to begin is with a definition. Acupuncture is an ancient Oriental therapy in which small, solid needles are inserted into the skin at varying depths, typically penetrating the underlying musculature. Proper insertion evokes a warm, deep aching, spreading sensation known as *deqi*. It involves the stimulation of specific areas of the body to regulate and balance energy in order to improve health and immunity and to treat existing diseases.

Steeped in Chinese philosophy is the principle of *yin and yang,* a dualistic way of viewing reality. Every aspect of the world, whether material or spiritual, is believed to be composed of two opposing but interdependent forces: yin and yang. Essentially they are opposites that exist only in relation to each other. Together, they form a whole. Examples of yin and yang include light and dark, day and night, hot and cold, female and male, fast and slow, wet and dry, positive and negative, proton and electron, front and back, left and right, liberal and conservative, Sigfried and Roy...Well, you get the picture.

Chinese medicine differentiates between six yin, or zang, and six yang, or fu, organs. *Zang* means firm or solid, while *fu* means hollow. The six

235

yin organs are the heart, pericardium, liver, kidney, lung, and spleen. The six yang organs are the stomach, small intestines, large intestines, gallbladder, urinary bladder, and the "triple warmer." The latter is an association of various functions in the mind and body, rather than an organic reality. It coordinates the three "burning cavities" of the body: the chest (for breathing), the abdomen (for digestion), and the pelvis (for reproduction and excretion). According to Chinese medicine, each organ has not only a physical function but also an emotional, mental, and spiritual function. The mind and soul are believed to exist not only in the brain but also in every cell in the body.

Meridians are energy channels that connect the interior with the exterior, that is, the internal organs with the surface of the body. In addition, they connect one organ with other organs. Through these channels, the life force or vital energy, *chi* (*qi*), flows. According to Taoist doctrine, if the vital life energy, or chi, flowing through the interconnected meridians is either excessive or deficient, tension is created between yin and yang. This may cause pain, discomfort, hypo- or hyperfunction, and eventually trophic changes. The goal of acupuncture is to restore the balance between these opposing forces, thereby restoring harmony, by inserting needles at strategic locations along the meridian.

Acupuncture originated in China over 5,000 years ago. It predates the availability of iron and steel for fashioning needles. It is speculated that acupuncture needles have been made out of bone, stone, and other materials. The earliest textbook on the subject was written in China around 400 B.C. In the West, the first mention of acupuncture was in 1683, and the first documented treatment occurred in 1810. But the practice of acupuncture remained obscure until the early 1970s, when a group of American doctors visited China and witnessed major operations being performed with acupuncture anesthesia alone. This received widespread publicity and evoked a considerable flurry of interest and curiosity about this ancient practice. Subsequently, acupuncture as a form of treatment has grown in acceptance and popularity.

> ## Medical Conditions that Can Be Successfully Treated with Acupuncture
>
> allergies, anxiety, arthritis, Bell's palsy (facial paralysis), bronchitis, bursitis, carpal tunnel syndrome, chronic fatigue syndrome, constipation, depression, diabetes, diarrhea, fibromyalgia, headaches, high blood pressure, infertility, insomnia, low-back pain, menstrual disorders, migraine headaches, neck pain, neuralgia, neurosis, osteoporosis, sciatica, sexual dysfunction, shoulder pain, sinusitis, smoking, sports injuries, stroke, tendonitis, tennis elbow, trigeminal neuralgia, ulcers, weight control, whiplash

Acupuncture has been proven to be an effective therapy not only for pain but also for a multitude of other medical conditions. According to the 1997 National Institutes of Health Consensus Statement, acupuncture, either alone or in combination with Western medical practices, can be effective treatment for back and neck pain, bronchitis, chronic fatigue syndrome, fibromyalgia, infertility, and osteoporosis. Furthermore, the World Health Organization (hardly a fringe outfit) has also recognized the efficacy of acupuncture in treating more than 40 conditions, including insomnia, depression, anxiety, and neurosis.

Mechanisms of Action

Medical research has shown that acupuncture works by means of the body's electrical and chemical systems. Electronic instruments have determined that acupuncture points on the skin have a higher electrical potential compared with the surrounding skin. In addition, Kirlian photography has shown increased bioelectric luminescence at acupuncture points. Stimulation of the points regulates and balances the bioelectric pathways that interconnect with internal organs. Neurochemical studies have demonstrated significant increases in the production and release of endorphins (natural painkillers with a morphine-like structure), enkephalins, and other brain neurotransmitters that lower the body's pain level, improve mood, and augment immune and inflammatory responses. Blood studies done before and after acupuncture treatments have shown significant increases in white blood cells and cortisol, which boosts the body's immunity and suppresses inflammation.

Complications

The National Institutes of Health Consensus Statement noted that one of the main advantages of acupuncture is the substantially lower incidence of adverse side effects compared with surgery, many medications, and other accepted medical treatments for the same condition. It is also cheaper and certainly more comfortable than, say, back surgery. But, as with any medical intervention, there are risks and benefits that should be considered before making a decision to undergo the procedure. Potential complications of acupuncture include infection (although this is minimal when sterile, disposable needles are used), fainting, bruising or local hematoma due to puncture of a blood vessel, pneumothorax due to a punctured lung, and contact dermatitis due to the nickel content of most stainless-steel needles. Cases of spinal cord and peripheral nerve injury have been reported due to migration of a broken needle fragment or an intentionally retained needle. Acupuncture is contraindicated in patients who are pregnant, suffer from bleeding disorders, or are on blood thinners.

Summary

As a result of medical research and public demand, acupuncture has become a viable and respected method of treatment in the United States and elsewhere. Increasingly, people are discovering that this traditional Chinese method of healing is an excellent tool for maintaining optimum health and preventing illness. Pain specialists are also learning to keep an open mind regarding alternative approaches to pain management in the best interests of their patients who frequently suffer from extreme, persistent, and debilitating pain. Perhaps the greatest endorsement of acupuncture by the West is reflected in the approximately 12,000 practicing acupuncturists in the United States today, about 5,000 of whom are medical doctors. To become licensed, an acupuncturist must complete a minimum of three years of training in addition to 60 semester hours of undergraduate work and pass the National Certificate Examination in Acupuncture.

Acupuncture offers a comparatively safe and effective alternative to pharmacological and other approaches to medical management. Its efficacy can be attested to not only by medical research but also by the fact that it has withstood the acid test, that is, the test of time. Acupuncture has survived for 5,000 years not because it doesn't work, but because it does.

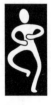

◆ 13 ◆

Passive Modalities

Passive modalities consist of physical interventions that do not require your active participation. Essentially, these are things that are done *to* you, not by you. Included is the application of physical agents such as heat, cold, light, friction, pressure, radiation, water, and electricity. Usually, permanent relief of pain is not achieved by these means. Temporary relief, however, is often forthcoming. Some argue that passive modalities should not be used because the results are only transient. Our position? So what? So it's a band-aid, and later on you'll need another band-aid. Keep a supply handy. Even temporary relief of pain in a person chronically afflicted is welcome and can have a positive effect on both physical and emotional well-being. Who in their right mind would say no to that? Furthermore, periods of diminished pain can be used to facilitate active exercise. And that's a good thing.

The other "minor" factor is that chronic pain patients are often the caretakers of the world. But who takes care of them? We strongly encourage self-nurturance in our patients, whether in the form of a bubble bath, a massage, or a guilt-free period of relaxation in a hot tub. At the same time, we encourage avoidance of potentially harmful factors like unhealthy abusive relationships. Choose your friends carefully. By doing so, you'll suffer less and enjoy life more. (Now what were we talking about? Oh yes. Passive modalities.) The other important issue and potential gain is that chronic pain sufferers often feel victimized by their pain and their circumstances. They feel out of control. We want to put them back in the driver's seat by providing them with the tools and skills to manage their pain. Many of the passive modalities are extremely helpful in this regard.

Bed Rest

The adage "if a little bit is good, a lot is better" does not apply to bed rest. While bed rest for up to 48 hours may be helpful in treating an acute back injury, a longer period of time can actually be harmful, not only to your back but to your overall health as well. This is because significant deconditioning of the cardiopulmonary system and loss of strength are inevitable with disuse, even in a husky NFL football player. What's more, bone density diminishes at an alarming rate after 48 hours. For patients with chronic back pain and pain-focused behavior, prolonged bed rest is not a good idea and provides minimal benefit.

Traction

Traction is the use of a pulling force applied to the body to produce a stretch of soft tissues and to separate joint surfaces. For chronic pain, it is typically applied to the cervical or lumbar spine. The idea is that by applying traction you can decompress segments and bring relief to structures that may be entrapped. But to actually accomplish this, extremely large forces of 40 to 50 pounds in the neck and 200 to 300 pounds in the lumbar spine are required. Wow! Few individuals can tolerate that kind of force!

Cryotherapy

Cryotherapy is the therapeutic use of cold. This is one of the simplest and cheapest forms of therapy. Yet, it can be very effective in managing both acute injuries and chronic pain conditions. Interestingly, sensations of pain and temperature travel on the same pathway to the brain. And, frankly, it can get a little crowded on that road. According to the

Gate Control Theory of pain, one can block the transmission of pain by overloading this pathway with sensations of hot or cold. In addition, the application of cold produces beneficial peripheral effects. Cold causes blood vessels to constrict, slows nerve conduction, reduces cellular metabolism, and decreases muscle spasm. In an acute injury, the application of ice can prevent swelling and reduce spasm, inflammation, and pain. But a word of caution: cryotherapy should be avoided in ischemic conditions (such as peripheral vascular disease or Raynaud's syndrome), severe cold pressor responses (elevation of blood pressure), poor sensation (as seen in spinal cord injuries), cold intolerance, and cold allergy.

Spray and Stretch

In this technique, a vasocoolant spray such as fluoromethane or ethyl chloride is administered to muscles in spasm in an attempt to alleviate pain. It is applied in a sweeping manner at an angle of 35 degrees and a distance of about 18 inches from the overlying skin. This produces an abrupt cooling effect. Then the muscles are stretched. As ethyl chloride spray is flammable and may contribute to the depletion of the ozone layer, fluoromethane is the vasocoolant spray of choice.

Contrast Baths

Contrast baths produce an increase in blood flow to a body part (a condition called hyperemia) by alternating submersion in hot and cold water. This increase is evidenced by a reddening of the skin. Generally, the affected body part is submerged first in hot water for 10 minutes, then in cold water for 1 minute. This is followed by cycles of 4 minutes in hot water and 1 minute in cold water, until a total of 30 minutes of therapy has accrued.

Contrast baths are helpful in alleviating the pain and stiffness associated with rheumatoid arthritis and reflex sympathetic dystrophy. This therapy is most suitable for treatment of the arms and legs.

Heat

Heat, like cold, travels on the same pathway to the brain as does pain. That is the good old spinothalamic tract. Once again, according to the Gate Control Theory, the transmission of pain to the brain can be blocked by overloading this pathway with sensations of either hot or cold. Therapeutic heat is classified as either superficial or deep depending on whether it permeates superficial tissues or deeper structures. Specific heating modalities can also be categorized according to the primary mode of heat transfer into tissues: conduction, convection, or conversion.

Conduction is the transfer of heat energy through matter from a hot object to a relatively cold one by molecular collision. Examples are the hot pack and the paraffin bath, which are both forms of superficial heat. *Convection,* on the other hand, is the transfer of heat energy by movements of a fluid medium such as liquid or air. Examples include hydrotherapy, fluidotherapy, and moist air. Again, all are forms of superficial heat. Finally, *conversion* is the transformation of one form of

---

Superficial Heat

Superficial heat by *conduction* (the transfer of heat through matter from a hot object to a relatively cold one by molecular collision) includes:

- ♦ Hot packs
- ♦ Paraffin baths

Superficial heat by *convection* (the transfer of heat energy by movements of a fluid medium such as liquid or air) includes:

- ♦ Hydrotherapy
- ♦ Fluidotherapy
- ♦ Moist air cabinet

Superficial heat by *conversion* (the transformation of a form of energy into heat energy) includes:

- ♦ Radiant heat

energy, such as mechanical energy, into heat energy. All forms of deep heat and only one form of superficial heat (radiant heat, exemplified by heat lamps) operate by conversion.

General indications for heat treatment include pain, muscle spasms, arthritis, bursitis, myofascitis, tendonitis, superficial thrombophlebitis, joint contractures, hematoma resolution, and collagen vascular disease. Contraindications include acute inflammation, trauma or hemorrhage, bleeding disorders, insensitivity (as in spinal cord injury), inability to communicate the effects of heat (e.g., comatose patient), scar tissue, atrophic skin, edema (swelling), ischemia (diminished blood supply), and areas of malignancy (cancer).

Hot Packs

Hot packs heat superficial tissues by conduction. Suspended on racks in hot water, they are removed only when needed. The packs are applied to the designated body part and then wrapped in an insulating cover such as six to eight layers of towels. This maintains the temperature within the therapeutic range for approximately 30 minutes. Electric heating pads, circulating water heating pads, and hot water bottles are alternatives to hot packs. But beware. Many of these devices do not cool spontaneously. To avoid burns, exposure should be limited to 20 minutes. Heat can produce temporary as well as permanent mottling of the skin. The advantages of hot packs include patient acceptance, ease of use, low cost, and minimal maintenance.

Paraffin Baths

Paraffin baths heat superficially by conduction. A container is filled with a hot mixture of mineral oil and paraffin. While the temperatures are considerably higher than that of water-based therapy, they are safe and well tolerated for a couple of reasons. First, an insulating layer of wax forms on the body parts being treated. Second, the mixture has a low heat capacity.

Paraffin treatment may be administered by one of two methods: the dip method or the continuous immersion method. During the *dip method,* the hand, as an example, is repeatedly dipped into the paraffin and then removed. Between dips, there is a brief pause that allows the paraffin to solidify. After approximately 10 dips, the hand is wrapped in a plastic sheet and a towel for about 20 minutes. In the *continuous immersion method,* the body part remains immersed in the paraffin bath for 20 to 30 minutes. Paraffin baths are primarily used to treat contractures, arthritis, and scleroderma.

Hydrotherapy

Hydrotherapy produces superficial heat by means of convection. The most common forms are the Hubbard tub and the whirlpool bath. Pumps agitate the water, providing gentle debridement and massage, as well as heat. Tanks vary in size from those designed for a single extremity (e.g., an arm) to those large enough to accommodate the entire body. The therapeutic temperature that is set depends on the patient's condition and the treatment goals. Because the water is in constant motion, no insulating layer of cooler water forms on the surface of the skin. Therefore, more vigorous heating occurs than would be the case with stationary water of the same temperature.

Hydrotherapy is effective for wounds and burns, mobilization of joints after the removal of a cast, muscle spasms, arthritis, and diffuse myalgias (aching muscles). This form of treatment is expensive and requires vast amounts of water and large areas of floor space.

Fluidotherapy

Fluidotherapy heats superficially by convection. Jets of hot air are blown through a pad of fine solids such as glass beads. This produces a warm, dry, semifluid medium into which an extremity can be immersed. Although this form of treatment has been available since the 1970s and has enjoyed considerable popularity, the benefits derived from dry, hot temperatures with low heat capacity remain somewhat controversial. The conclusion that fluidotherapy is a more effective heating agent compared with hydrotherapy or paraffin baths is not supported by scientific research.

Moist Air Cabinet

The moist air cabinet also provides superficial heat by convection. This method is versatile in that either a body part or the entire body may be treated. Water-vapor-saturated air that is temperature controlled is blown on the designated area.

Heat Lamps

Heat lamps produce radiant heat, the only form of superficial heat that operates by conversion. They are cheap to buy and easy to apply. All you need is an ordinary incandescent light bulb to produce large amounts of infrared energy. It's true, folks. Specialized bulbs such as tungsten and quartz are not necessary. Heat lamps often use a 250-watt bulb placed 16 to 20 inches from the skin. The maximum temperature attained and the rate of heating are controlled by adjusting the distance between the lamp and the body part being treated.

Deep Heat

Deep heat is also known as diathermy. It includes shortwave, microwave, and ultrasound. The primary mode for heat transfer into tissues for all forms of deep heat is conversion, that is, the transformation of one form of energy into heat energy.

Shortwave diathermy is the therapeutic application of high-frequency currents. In essence, radio waves are used to heat tissues. Both water-

---

Deep Heat

Deep heat, or diathermy, by conversion (the transformation of a form of energy into heat energy) includes the following modalities:

- ♦ Shortwave diathermy
- ♦ Microwave diathermy
- ♦ Ultrasound diathermy

---

rich tissues, such as muscle, and water-poor tissues, such as fat, can be effectively heated depending on the particular application. Vigorous pelvic heating is also possible using rectal and vaginal applicators or probes. This may be effective in treating pelvic myalgias and, in conjunction with antibiotics, pelvic inflammatory disease and prostatitis. Yet for some strange reason, people are often reluctant to use these invasive probes (hmm...go figure).

Metallic implants, including cardiac pacemakers, surgical implants, and intrauterine devices, are contraindications for shortwave diathermy for several reasons: they may malfunction, they may be destroyed, or they may become selectively heated, resulting in a burn to the patient. All external metallic objects, such as jewelry, should be removed. To avoid the occurrence of a burn to the skin, accumulation of sweat beads must be prevented. Dry terrycloth towels are therefore used to absorb excess perspiration. Pregnancy is also a contraindication because of possible damage to the fetus. In addition, due to the potential danger to the immature skeletal development, shortwave diathermy should not be used in children. Also, stray radiation is an occupational hazard for the therapist.

Microwave diathermy is a form of electromagnetic radiation that utilizes frequencies of 915 and 2,456 megahertz for medical use. As with other electromagnetic waves, microwaves travel at the speed of light and can be propagated through a vacuum. Microwaves can be absorbed, refracted, reflected, or scattered. Unlike shortwaves, they can be relatively easily focused for therapeutic purposes. Compared with both shortwave diathermy and ultrasound, microwaves penetrate less deeply.

Microwave diathermy is used primarily to heat relatively superficial muscles and joints. This is based on the fact that they are selectively absorbed in tissues with high water content, such as muscles, and therefore allow selective heating of these tissues. However, the fat overlying these muscles may absorb a significant portion of the beam. Microwave may also speed the resolution of hematomas.

Like shortwave diathermy, the impact of microwave diathermy on bone growth is not well established. Therefore, use in children should be avoided. Because water is selectively heated, treatment over fluid-filled cavities, blisters, moist skin, and swollen tissues can produce dangerously high temperatures. Since microwaves can produce cataracts, both the patient and the therapist should wear goggles. Although microwave leakage can occur, therapists use microwave equipment so intermittently that exposure levels in most situations seems acceptable.

Ultrasound is defined as sound at frequencies above the limits of human hearing. Frequencies below 17,000 hertz (cycles per second) are usually called *sound* and are detectable by the human ear. Frequencies above this level are designated ultrasound and are inaudible. Both sound and ultrasound are propagated in the form of longitudinal compression waves that require a medium for transmission. Ultrasound transmits energy that can be focused, refracted, and reflected. The therapeutic effects of ultrasound are due to the conversion of this energy to other forms of energy, in particular heat. For a number of reasons, including issues of standardization, ultrasound treatments in the United States are limited to 0.8 to 1 megahertz.

Ultrasound is the most commonly employed deep-heating agent and the most effective. It selectively heats interfaces between tissues of different acoustic impedance. The temperature distribution produced by ultrasound is unique in that it causes relatively little temperature elevation in the superficial tissues and has greater depth of penetration in the musculature and other soft tissues compared with shortwave and microwave diathermy. For example, ultrasound can raise the temperature in the hip joint to therapeutic levels without deleterious effects on overlying tissues. In contrast, both shortwave and microwave are incapable of doing so even if they have produced superficial burns in overlying tissues.

Ultrasound has been found to be effective in the treatment of subacute tendonitis and bursitis, degenerative arthritis, joint contractures, postherpetic neuralgia, plantar warts, and skin ulcers. It may also be helpful in bringing about the resolution of hematomas.

Ultrasound is contraindicated over joint prostheses, pacemakers, and fluid-filled cavities such as the eye and the pregnant uterus. Areas of vascular insufficiency should be avoided because the blood supply may not be able to meet the increased metabolic demands imposed by the heat, and therefore necrosis might result. Likewise, areas of malignant tumors should not be exposed to ultrasound as tumor growth may be accelerated. Infection is a contraindication because the spread of microorganisms may be enhanced. The heart should not be directly exposed to ultrasound because the heart's action potential and contractile properties may be altered. In addition, the brain, cervical ganglia, and spinal cord should not be treated with this modality. Finally, areas of hemorrhage should be avoided as ultrasound may increase bleeding.

Phonophoresis

Phonophoresis is the application of ultrasound to medication combined with a coupling medium. This medication is placed topically over the body part to be treated. The ultrasound forces the medication into the tissue and enhances the therapeutic effect. Among the medications administered in this manner are the local anesthetics lidocaine and carbocaine, corticosteroids, phenylbutazone, and chymotrypsin. Conditions that meet with varying degrees of success when treated with phonophoresis include arthritis, bursitis, tendonitis, contractures, keloids, plantar warts, skin ulcers, and herpes zoster.

Electrotherapy

Electrotherapy is the use of any type of electrical current to promote healing and pain relief. The notion that electricity has medicinal value is not of recent origin. In fact, many centuries ago, ancient Greek and Roman physicians prescribed treatments with electric eels for their pain patients. Can you imagine? Thank God for new technology! Among the 20th century forms of electrotherapy are TENS, H-Wave®, and iontophoresis.

TENS

TENS, or transcutaneous electrical nerve stimulation, is the modern-day equivalent of the eel. (My, how times have changed!) Electrodes are placed directly onto the skin over the area of pain, along pathways of specific nerves, and/or on acupuncture points. Electrical stimulation is then delivered in a pulse-like fashion. (A vast improvement over the eel!) In essence, TENS acts as a counterirritant. According to the Gate Control Theory of pain, the electrical input preoccupies the sensory highway to the spinal cord and brain, thereby blocking the transmission of pain. In effect, it "closes the gate."

High-intensity, low-frequency (less than 10-hertz) pulses release endorphins, bringing about relatively long-lasting analgesia. Like the pain relief associated with the use of opiates, this effect can be reversed with naloxone, an opiate antagonist (blocker). Such stimulation also inhibits the spinothalamic tract, the pathway that carries sensations of pain and temperature to the brain. This particular effect is not reversible with naloxone.

Low-intensity, high-frequency (greater than 50-hertz) pulses alter the A-delta component of the compound nerve action potential in peripheral nerves, thereby producing short-term analgesia. This effect is not naloxone reversible. The relief of pain at these settings is facilitated by high levels of the neurotransmitters dopamine and serotonin and inhibited by high levels of norepinephrine.

Transcutaneous Electrical Nerve Stimulation

TENS has been used successfully for both acute and chronic pain conditions. Studies indicate that TENS is effective in 12 to 60% of chronic pain patients. Success rates depend on a number of factors, including the type and location of electrodes, the pattern and frequency of electrical stimulation, the condition being treated, and the experience of the personnel applying the unit and instructing the patient in its use.

Manufacturers of TENS units have improved the efficacy of this device by allowing multiple variations of current, waveform, and stimulus pattern to be set by the user or prescriber. Complications, which are rare, include contact dermatitis (you know, a rash) around the electrodes and interference with cardiac pacemakers.

In the elderly, certain factors mitigate for and against the use of TENS. Altered liver, kidney, and neurological functions as well as concomitant disease may preclude the use of many medications. These patients may also have difficulty engaging in active physical therapy. As a result, TENS is an attractive alternative method of pain control. On the other hand, the elderly are also more likely to live alone and to have cognitive problems (such as early dementia) that could interfere with their ability to understand and use this device.

Follow-up studies of patients who initially felt that TENS was effective are very encouraging. Ninety percent of these patients continued to use the device for pain control two years after the initial prescription. This suggests long-term benefit.

H-Wave®

H-Wave® therapy is a unique form of transcutaneous electrical stimulation that consists of a portable unit with two channels which deliver bipolar electrical stimuli via four electrodes placed on the skin. It is believed to be especially successful because of the particular waveform it utilizes. This waveform is felt to be biocompatible, which means that it is readily accepted by the body with minimal resistance. While almost all other electrical stimulators use a static waveform, the H-Wave® delivers a biphasic, exponentially decaying waveform. (Decay time is the amount of time it takes for a signal to go from its peak amplitude to zero baseline.) Because H-Wave® stimulating current decays, it is active for a longer period of time, allowing the recruitment and activation of greater numbers of motor units. It causes therapeutic muscle contractions that are nonfatiguing.

H-Wave® has been used successfully to manage both acute and chronic pain conditions, such as neck and back pain, fibromyalgia, and peripheral neuropathies. It reduces the pain and paresthesia (pins-and-needles sensation) associated with neuropathies. In addition, it has been found to be effective in the treatment of edema and diabetic ulcers. H-Wave® accelerates healing of wounds by reducing edema and the formation of adhesions. Reliance on pain medications and injections by patients using the H-Wave® tends to decrease, thus further improving their quality of life.

Patients seem to gain optimum benefit when they use the H-Wave® on both high and low settings. On high-frequency settings, which increase endorphins, the H-Wave® unit slows the sodium pumps of the A-delta and C pain fibers, thereby producing a nerve block. The anesthetic effect produced is equivalent to that produced by the local anesthetics lidocaine and Xylocaine®. To date, the H-Wave® is the only electrical medical device to be registered as anesthesia with the Food and Drug Administration.

On low-frequency settings, H-Wave® reduces edema. When injury occurs, blood proteins and other large particulate matter permeate the capillary walls and infiltrate surrounding tissues, causing edema or swelling. This edema causes pain by stimulating nociceptors and by putting pressure on nerves. In addition, edema can delay healing. The

H-Wave®, on low-frequency settings, produces comfortable, nonfatiguing muscle contraction that improves circulation and enhances lymph flow. This, in turn, aides the evacuation of pain-producing peptides such as bradykinin, prostaglandins, and histamine and other proteins.

Some practitioners report that with use of the H-Wave® there is a decrease in costly trips to the emergency room as well as a reduction in the amount of narcotics taken by patients to manage pain. In one study, the continued use of H-Wave® over a prolonged period of time (average 1.7 years) strongly suggests long-term benefit. The incidence of side effects for this noninvasive therapy is low and includes contact dermatitis due to the electrodes or gel.

Iontophoresis

Iontophoresis is a method of delivering medication in the form of ions through the skin by the application of a direct electrical current. An *ion* is a constituent of a molecule that consists of an atom or group of atoms that carries an electric charge. Some ions carry a positive charge and are called *cations,* while other ions carry a negative charge and are called *anions.* When the medication applied is positively charged (such as the local anesthetic lidocaine), the electrical current must also be positive in order to drive the medication into the tissue (since like charges repel). Likewise, when the medication applied is negatively charged (such as a corticosteroid), the current must also be negative.

Many ionic pharmaceuticals are available, including fluoride, lidocaine hydrochloride, epinephrine hydrochloride, methylprednisolone, sodium succinate, and several antiviral drugs and antibiotics. Iontophoresis is especially effective for the treatment of local conditions near the surface of the skin. These include carpal tunnel syndrome, tennis elbow, tendonitis, bursitis, myofascial pain, neuritis, postherpetic neuralgia, muscle or ligament strain, and arthritis (joint inflammation). Tooth sensitivity can be successfully treated with fluoride iontophoresis. In addition, idoxuridine iontophoresis has been effective in the treatment of aphthous ulcers and herpes simplex virus.

Contraindications include allergies to the medications; inflamed, irritated, infected, or broken skin; and cardiac arrhymias or pacemakers. In the case of these cardiac conditions, no electrical current should be applied, especially across the chest.

The advantages of iontophoresis are many and include the absence of systemic toxic effects and the lack of dependence upon the gastrointestinal system for absorption. Both food and acid in the stomach can profoundly affect the amount of drug that enters the system. Furthermore, iontophoresis is noninvasive and, as such, is pain free. No needles are necessary (a big plus for the needle-phobic). Perhaps the biggest bonus of all is that the medication is delivered directly to the affected area, thereby maximizing the potential benefit.

Heliotherapy

Heliotherapy refers to any treatment involving light. As an example, laser light may be applied directly to injured tissue to promote healing and to relieve pain. In the United States, infrared helium–aluminum–arsenide or visible helium–neon lasers are most commonly used. No appreciable change in skin temperature occurs. Overall, studies report relief in about 80% of patients.

Massage

If you've ever questioned the therapeutic effects of touch, take a trip to your local massage therapy salon. You are in for the treat of your life. There is nothing like a great massage. It's a little bit of heaven. No doubt about it. Massage is the regulation of muscle tone through reflex and mechanical action to reduce stiffness and pain and to improve circulation. It is generally thought of as an art rather than a science.

There are different massage techniques designed to produce different effects. One of the principle forms is *stroking* (or *effleurage*). This technique is performed by moving the hand over the surface of the skin. The primary purpose is to remove deposits or edema. Stroking may be superficial or deep. In *superficial stroking,* the direction of applied force is unimportant. But in *deep stroking,* it is critical, as the latter is designed to enhance circulation. To accomplish this, the pressure movements are from the particular body part toward the heart.

Another form of massage is *compression* (or *petrissage*). It includes kneading, squeezing, and friction. These techniques are designed to mobilize tissue deposits and to stretch adhesions. *Kneading* is a motion in which the soft tissues are picked up between the fingers and manipulated in an alternating manner so that there is motion within the muscle itself. *Squeezing,* on the other hand, is performed with larger portions of muscle, squeezing the part either between the two hands or between the hand and a solid object such as a table. *Friction* is a rapid, circular motion performed by placing a small part of the hand, such as the palm, the thumb, or the fingertips, on the area. The pressure applied is steadily increased during this treatment.

Finally, *percussion* (or *tapotement*) is a form of massage that consists of alternating movements performed to produce stimulation. Specific forms of percussion include *hacking* (sounds bad, feels good), which is usually done with the outer borders of the hands; *clapping,* which is done with the palms of the hands; and *beating,* which is performed with clenched fists.

The greatest contraindications to massage are infections and malignancies because both may spread through the tissues due to the breaking down of barriers. Skin disease is also a contraindication because of possible contraction by the masseur. Massage should be administered cautiously in patients who are debilitated, suffer from burns, or have thin skin. Finally, massage is contraindicated in thrombophlebitis because blood clots may break off and travel to the heart and lungs, a potentially life-threatening situation.

The benefits of massage are many and include pain relief, diminished muscle spasms and stiffness, decreased edema, and enhanced circulation. But it is not a substitute for an active exercise program. Massage does not, will not, and cannot improve muscle strength. This will only occur when muscles contract actively against resistance. However, massage does prepare the body for strengthening exercises and can enhance performance.

Magnets

Despite all the hoopla about the therapeutic effects of magnets, there is currently very little supporting evidence that stands up under scientific scrutiny. Still, the number of believers among both patients and practitioners is growing by leaps and bounds. Some of their stories are compelling. One doctor, the director of a critical care unit in Ohio, became a convert when he was touched in a personal way by the benefits of neuromagnetic therapy. His wife had been seriously injured in a car accident and had tried conventional medical treatment unsuccessfully. In fact, her care had been managed by his anesthesiology colleagues, who were pain specialists. Trials on multiple medications had resulted in inadequate pain control and unpleasant side effects. The pain seemed to have a life of its own. That is, until she tried magnets. Within 10 days, her pain had decreased 80%. After 30 to 60 days, the pain was reduced 100%. Because of his wife's phenomenal experience, this doctor has taken up the banner to actively promote magnet therapy. Another doctor who manages a pain clinic reported that she has tried magnets on hundreds of chronic pain patients with "near miraculous results in many cases." Although anecdotal, these examples suggest that magnets deserve a closer scientific look.

If they are effective, how do magnets work for pain control? No one knows for sure, but there are a number of theories. Magnets have a positive and a negative pole that work together to complete the magnetic circuit. Invisible "flux lines" of energy exit from the negative pole and are drawn to the positive pole. This creates a magnetic field. (Gauss is a unit of measure that indicates the strength of a magnetic field.) Magnet therapy may increase blood flow by dilating blood vessels and attracting oxygen. Magnets may attract iron in the blood to stimulate circulation. They may alter the pH balance (acid–base) of body fluids.

They may block pain signals along nerve pathways to the brain. They may alter the movement of calcium ions to promote the healing of fractures. They may draw calcium away from arthritic joints. Ultimately, it will be up to the scientific studies to determine if and how they work.

Contraindications include cardiac pacemakers and defibrillators. Women in the first trimester of pregnancy should first consult their doctor before using magnets.

Magnets should not be placed near videotapes, audiotapes, magnetic strip cards, computers, watches, calculators, or any portable electronic device.

The magnet business is now a multibillion-dollar industry that has impacted the lives of millions of people worldwide. While no medical claims are made that these products are useful in the treatment or cure of any disease, they are believed by many to promote restful sleep, warmth, and reduced discomfort and pain. No. The research isn't there. Not yet, anyway. But the case reports are piling up. Besides, there are plenty of patients who couldn't care less about what the scientific gurus say. They feel better, and that's the main thing. Our recommendation to the magnet lovers is this: Enjoy your magnets. They won't hurt anything. And who knows? They may even help. In the meantime, the jury is still out.

Orthotic Devices

Orthotic devices are frequently thought of as corsets or braces to support the spine. In actuality the name refers to any device designed to rest or stabilize a body part, any body part. The specific orthosis is named for the joint or area it is designed to support. For example, an AFO is an ankle–foot orthosis, a WHO is a wrist–hand orthosis, an LSO is a lumbosacral orthosis, a KO is a knee orthosis, and a TKO is a technical knockout in boxing (which, by the way, has nothing to do with the subject at hand). These devices can provide pain relief by splinting the involved area and by assuming partial function of the supporting muscles. Unfortunately, there is a downside to the use of orthosis, especially with chronic pain. Prolonged use can lead to weakness and atrophy of the involved muscles. Using a back brace, for example, can lead to weakness of the very muscles that are designed to support the spine. The potential consequence is greater back pain. For that reason, we generally recommend that orthotics be used for limited periods of time. When possible, their use should be accompanied by an exercise program to keep muscles strong.

Summary

No. Passive modalities may not win the war, but they sure can help in the raging battle against chronic pain. A certain amount of pain relief can go a long way in providing a person with the energy, will, and motivation to pursue the more active therapies, as well as personal interests and hobbies. The end result is an improvement in quality of life. Our advice to patients, doctors, therapists, and insurance companies: Don't shortchange measures that yield temporary pain relief. They represent a critical step on the road to wellness.

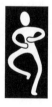

Surgery and Other Desperate Measures

Many chronic pain conditions ultimately lend themselves to surgical intervention. Many do not. Back pain is one of the most common causes of pain for which surgery is warranted. In addition, it is the leading cause of disability in the United States among individuals between 18 and 55 years of age. The vast majority of back pain — 80% — is simply due to back strain. Most acute back injuries will resolve with a short period of bed rest (up to 48 hours) followed by an appropriate exercise program and a little time. Within two to three weeks, 70% of individuals afflicted with back pain will improve substantially. Within three months, the number of individuals who experience significant improvement has usually risen to 80%. So, if you are unfortunate enough to have a back injury, you'll be happy to know that the odds are in your favor. The chances of improvement without surgical intervention are about 90%. The important message is that, in almost every instance, you should not rush into surgery.

Overall, it is estimated that Americans spend $16 billion on back pain each year. Ten percent of the injuries represent 80% of the costs. The range in cost is extremely variable. At the low end is a few pennies worth of aspirin. At the high end, the sky is the limit. Back surgery, always an expensive proposition, should be the last resort. Over half of the back surgeries performed in this country are unnecessary. To state the obvious, you can never undo surgery. Although there are certainly indications for immediate surgery, in most instances — 99% of the time — back surgery is elective. In other words, you won't become paralyzed or die prematurely if you fail to undergo an operation. Therefore, surgery can and should be postponed until a course of conservative treatment has proven ineffective.

To Cut or Not to Cut? That Is the Question!

Few things are black and white in medicine, but there are some clear-cut indications for back surgery. One of the least controversial is cauda equina syndrome, a condition in which the patient may experience numbness in the feet and around the vagina and anus, loss of bowel control and sexual function (erectile impairment), diminished sensation of the need to urinate, and difficulty initiating urination. This suggests the impingement of nerve roots, usually from a herniated disc, and constitutes a medical emergency. The proper action to take is to go directly to an emergency room to be evaluated by an orthopedic surgeon or neurosurgeon. *Do not* wait for an appointment. If not treated promptly, permanent nerve and muscle damage may result, along with a lifetime problem of bowel and/or bladder incontinence.

Tumors of the spine are an indication for surgery, whether malignant or benign, because as they grow they may encroach on the spinal cord. This is of particular concern in the cervical (neck) and thoracic (upper back) areas, as the spinal cord ends at the first lumbar vertebra, where it gives rise to the cauda equina. A benign tumor of the lumbar spine that involves one or more nerve roots is not an absolute indication for surgery. The question is whether or not the patient is able to live with the pain and loss of function. If surgery is done, the nerve root may be damaged in the process of removing the tumor.

Infection of the vertebrae (osteomyelitis) or discs (discitis) may also warrant surgery in some cases. Frequently, patients with these conditions are initially misdiagnosed with a soft tissue injury such as muscle strain. The length of time between the onset of infection of the spinal column and the diagnosis ranges from 6 to 12 weeks or longer. The clue that points to a diagnosis of spine infection is throbbing, aching pain that occurs at night while the patient is lying down. This is called "rest pain."

How does an individual get an infection in the spinal column? Unfortunately, this is not completely understood. We do know that there are certain groups of people who are immunocompromised (have a weakened ability to fight off infection). Patients with AIDS, cancer, or diabetes, for example, are more susceptible to infection, as are individuals who chronically abuse drugs or are maintained on steroids for either legitimate medical purposes — such as the treatment of rheumatoid arthritis or chronic obstructive pulmonary disease — or for cosmetic or competitive reasons (such as bodybuilding). Minor dental or genitourinary procedures performed on these individuals may introduce germs into the bloodstream that travel to the spine, where they set up housekeeping and wreak havoc.

To diagnose an infection of the intervertebral discs or vertebrae, the physician may order blood tests, a bone scan, and/or an MRI. In addition, a biopsy may be obtained in order to identify the organism responsible and the appropriate drug to eradicate it. To effectively treat a spinal infection, the medication (antibiotic, antifungal, or antituberculosis agent) usually must be administered intravenously. Surgery is sometimes necessary to clean out the affected area. Fortunately, in most cases, conservative treatment is successful without the need for an operation.

Foot drop is another emergency that warrants immediate medical attention. When walking, the individual is unable to flex his or her ankle in order to raise his or her forefoot, so the foot drops and the toes drag. This may occur as a result of a herniated disc or from severe spinal stenosis. The condition should be evaluated by an orthopedic surgeon or a neurosurgeon without delay.

The role of surgery in the management of lumbar disc herniation and radiculopathy remains open for debate. Studies by Jeffrey Saal, M.D., demonstrate that these patients can often be successfully treated by nonsurgical methods. In fact, their return-to-work rates and sick-leave time were superior to those individuals who were treated surgically. However, there may be certain circumstances where surgery offers advantages over nonsurgical management. One such circumstance is when the herniated disc is associated with lateral spinal canal stenosis (narrowing). If the lateral canal stenosis is not surgically corrected, the patient has a high likelihood of persistent pain and disability.

The time line for expected improvement in the patient with a herniated disc and radiculopathy *without* lateral stenosis during a course of conservative management must be closely monitored. During the first month of treatment, a reduction of pain and an improvement in function of 30 to 50% should be expected. By the end of the second month of treatment, an improvement of up to 80% should have been achieved. At eight weeks, progress should be carefully assessed. If the patient's recovery rate is delayed with conservative treatment, he or she should undergo evaluation by a competent, conservative spine surgeon for possible surgery. The patient should be informed that, given the lack of progress in the first two months, surgery will probably be more effective in bringing about a successful result than will continuing with conservative treatment.

Other indications for surgery include severe scoliosis (lateral curvature of the spine) or kyphosis (humpback) that compromises the ability of the heart and lungs (cardiopulmonary system) to function effectively. An unstable spine should, in most cases, be stabilized surgically by a fusion with or without instrumentation. In addition, surgical procedures may be performed to interrupt pathways and centers of the brain and spinal cord that transmit, receive, or interpret pain messages, thereby alleviating pain.

Back Surgery

There are two main types of back surgery: *fusion,* which involves fusing two or more vertebrae together in order to stabilize the spine, thereby preventing painful movement, and *decompression,* which is the re-

Overview of Spinal Surgeries to Reduce Pain

1. Spinal fusion
2. Decompression
    a. Discectomy
    b. Percutaneous discectomy
    c. Microdiscectomy
    d. Laminectomy
    e. Laminotomy and foraminotomy
3. Spinal cord stimulation
4. Intraspinal drug infusion
5. Sympathectomy*
6. Rhizotomy*
7. Epidural adhesiolysis*
8. Chymopapain injection or chemonucleosis*
9. Cordotomy or (tractotomy)*

* See Appendix C.

moval of pressure on nerves in the spinal canal. As you will see, there
are various ways of accomplishing fusion and decompression. In addition, there are a number of other surgical procedures performed on the
back to alleviate pain.

Spinal fusion is an operation in which the surgeon attempts to stop
painful motion between two or more vertebrae. Using bone obtained
from the patient's hip or from a bone bank, the surgeon grafts bone
alongside two or more vertebrae. Over time (usually four to nine
months), the unstable vertebrae and the bone grafts grow together,
that is, fuse, into a solid bridge, thereby restricting unwanted motion
at that level. An alternative method is to use metal implants (plates,
rods, screws, wire) alone or in combination with a bone graft. Many
surgeons believe that this type of instrumentation should be considered in cases where fusion is required at multiple levels or in patients
who have had a previous fusion which failed. Another indication for
instrumentation is smoking. Smokers have a significantly lower chance
(60%) of obtaining a successful fusion compared to nonsmokers (85%).

Cigarette smoking is such a hazard that many surgeons refuse to attempt a fusion until the patient stops smoking for a minimum of four to six weeks.

A fusion may be performed from an anterior approach or a posterior approach. In the former, the spine is approached from the front and requires an incision in the abdominal or flank (side) area. Essentially, the abdominal organs are moved aside to provide access to the spine. The posterior approach is done from the back. In rare instances, both an anterior and posterior approaches are appropriate. Patients who have had prior failed surgeries, who are smokers, or have had previous complications such as infection may benefit from this dual approach.

The recovery period following a fusion is longer compared to other spine surgeries and is associated with considerably more postoperative pain. Usually, a brace must be worn for a period of three to four months. Patient compliance in wearing the brace when out of bed is believed to improve the chances of obtaining a solid fusion by up to 10%. Formal rehabilitation following a spinal fusion usually does not begin until two to three months after surgery. Prior to that, a walking program is recommended.

The indications for a spinal fusion are instability due to spondylolisthesis (the forward slippage of one vertebra over another) and postlaminectomy instability due to a pars fracture. Leg pain, in and of itself, is not an indication for fusion.

The risks associated with a spinal fusion include a failure of the vertebrae to fuse, infection, blood clots, nerve or blood vessel damage, problems with anesthesia, reherniation, failure or breakage of instrumentation, and hip pain due to the bone graft harvesting.

In recent years, there have been several national news reports regarding complications associated with the use of hardware such as pedicle screws, plates, and rods. Consumer groups have asked the Food and Drug Administration to ban the use of steel screw implants, arguing that screw recipients are twice as likely to need further surgery compared to patients who undergo spinal fusion without screws. They also report that a third of these patients develop complications such as infection and leg weakness due to nerve damage.

In response to these concerns, Dr. Hansen A. Yuan of the State University of New York at Syracuse analyzed data regarding the surgical use of pedicle screws. The study involved 314 surgeons and 3,498 cases. It was notable not only for its large sample size but also because of the media flap concerning the safety of these devices. The bottom line was that, in sharp contrast to the recent media reports that pedicle screws were associated with poor outcomes and complications, pedicle screw fixation was found to be as safe and effective as other means of achieving spinal fusion, both instrumented and noninstrumented. In fact, in some respects, the outcome achieved with pedicle screws was clearly superior.

Questions regarding such instrumentation should be addressed with your surgeon if you have been recommended for such surgery. In addition, we believe that it is imperative that you obtain a second opinion from a qualified spine surgeon.

Discectomy is the decompression of nerve roots by the removal of all or part of a herniated disc. Since surgery has come under close scrutiny, it has been shown that discectomy does not beneficially change the course of degenerative disease of the spine unless it is associated with neurological impairment.

Percutaneous discectomy is the surgical removal of part of a herniated disc using a suction device or laser. The procedure is typically done on an outpatient basis. In order to prevent nerve damage, the patient is kept awake as the surgeon, guided by fluoroscopic X-ray, uses a probe to remove portions of the offending disc through a small incision that can later be covered with a band-aid. Following surgery, the patient usually recovers rapidly and is able to return to sedentary work within two to three days. The primary indication for percutaneous discectomy is disc herniation associated with radicular symptoms of the extremities that has persisted for six or more weeks.

Complications are rare. Risks include discitis (disc infection), recurrent disc herniation, and nerve or blood vessel injury. Symptoms recur in up to 30% of patients within six months of the procedure. The advantages of this procedure compared to the traditional discectomy are less tissue trauma and early recovery.

Microdiscectomy is performed through an operating microscope and requires only a small incision (1 to 1½ inches). Partial removal of the lamina (laminotomy) is necessary in order to gain access to the herniated disc. The patient is hospitalized for the procedure, which is done under general anesthesia. The indications for a microdiscectomy include a herniated disc associated with radicular pain that is unrelieved by conservative treatment, progressive neurological loss resulting in a decline in ability to perform daily life activities, spinal stenosis associated with herniated disc, and recurrent disc herniation.

Because microdiscectomy is less invasive compared with an open surgical discectomy, recovery time is usually shorter and postoperative pain is relatively mild. In addition to the risks associated with percutaneous discectomy, there may be rare complications associated with general anesthesia. Furthermore, blood clots may develop in the legs; these clots can potentially break off and travel to the lungs (pulmonary emboli). The chance of recurrent herniation following microdiscectomy is about 4%.

Laminectomy is an operation in which the entire lamina of the vertebral arch and associated ligaments are removed at a given level in order to permit access to the spinal canal. The indications for this procedure are severe spinal stenosis or a large herniated disc that is causing cauda equina syndrome. The goal is decompression. In some cases, this may include decompression of the spinal cord as well as the nerve roots, depending on the severity of the lesion. The recovery time following surgery is usually prolonged: four to six months or more. Postoperative rehabilitation, especially physical therapy, is usually initiated three weeks after surgery and may continue for six weeks or more. The risks associated with laminectomy are the same as those associated with microdiscectomy. However, because of the longer operating time, the incidence of complications is considerably higher. There is a 4 to 6% chance of disc reherniation, requiring another surgery.

Laminotomy is the surgical removal of part of the lamina in order to gain access to the spinal canal. This is essentially what is done during the course of microdiscectomy.

Foraminotomy involves making a larger opening in the intervertebral foramina to relieve nerve root pressure. The foramina is the natural opening in the spinal canal through which the nerve roots exit. Just as a tight ring on the finger can cause painful swelling, a narrowed foramen can cause pressure and pain on exiting nerve roots. The risks associated with laminotomy and foraminotomy are the same as those associated with microdiscectomy.

Spinal cord stimulation (SCS) is a reversible, nondestructive technique in which a programmable device is surgically implanted for the suppression of chronic, intractable pain of the trunk or limbs. Through this device, low-voltage electrical stimulation is applied to the spinal cord to block the transmission of pain signals to the brain. The SCS system consists of three parts: a lead, an extension, and a power source.

The lead is a set of electrodes through which electrical stimulation is delivered to the spinal cord. Under fluoroscopic guidance, leads are placed in the epidural space, which is located between the bony spine and the spinal cord. The procedure is carried out with the patient lying prone (on his or her stomach), with a flexion roll placed under him or her to facilitate entry of the lead. The position of the lead is critically important in SCS and requires the cooperation of both the physician and the patient during implantation. The goal is to place the lead at a level along the spinal cord that causes a tingling sensation in the same distribution as the patient's pain. The extension is a conducting wire that carries the electrical pulses from the power source to the lead. The power source produces the electrical pulses for SCS by a combination of a battery and special electronics.

In order to determine whether or not SCS will be effective in reducing pain in a particular patient, a test trial is done for a couple of days using a temporary power source. A successful trial is defined as a reduction in pain of 50% or more. If the trial is deemed successful, a permanent power source is added to the system, which may be implanted in the skin or worn externally. In either case, the surgical procedure is brief and is considered minor by the medical community.

Following implantation of the spinal cord stimulator, the activity of the patient is restricted by the doctor for a period of several weeks while the system becomes stable. Abrupt movements in particular are prohibited. Break-dancing is generally discouraged. After this initial period, the patient may actually be able to resume a more active lifestyle than was possible before the procedure due to improved pain control.

How does spinal cord stimulation work? Theories abound. Among them is Melzack and Wall's Gate Control Theory of pain. According to this theory, dorsal horn (sensory) cells of the spinal cord (the "gate") could be affected by both input from the periphery and input from the brain, thereby modifying the pain experience. This revolutionary idea was instrumental in triggering the development of SCS as well as other treatment modalities that utilize electrical stimulation to reduce pain. These include transcutaneous electrical nerve stimulation, peripheral nerve stimulation, and deep brain stimulation. High-frequency, low-amplitude electrical stimulation dramatically inhibits most dorsal horn cells of the spinal cord, thereby blocking the entry of pain messages to the central nervous system (spinal cord and brain). In addition, it is thought to produce analgesia by activating endogenous opiates, natural painkillers found in the body. Chronic pain sufferers are known to have lower levels of serotonin and endorphins in the cerebral spinal fluid compared with the general population. According to the theory, neural stimulation increases both chemicals. Other physiologic responses to SCS include an increase in the delivery of oxygen to the tissues. This is extremely beneficial for patients with peripheral vascular disease and results in a reduction not only of their pain but also in the incidence of foot amputation.

Specific conditions in which SCS may be effective include ischemic pain (pain due to insufficient oxygenation of the affected tissues) due to peripheral vascular disease, arachnoiditis, spasmodic torticollis, phantom limb pain following an amputation, peripheral neuropathy, postherpetic neuralgia, reflex sympathetic dystrophy, and radiculopathy associated with both intraspinal scarring and failed back surgery syndrome.

According to the guidelines established by the Health Care Finance Administration (HCFA), SCS should be used only as a last resort for patients with chronic, intractable pain when other treatment modalities such as physical therapy, behavioral treatment, surgery, and medication have been exhausted and found to be ineffective. In addition, HCFA guidelines indicate that there should be documented pathology to substantiate the subjective complaint of pain. For example, a myelogram documents lumbar arachnoid fibrosis in a particular patient who complains of severe back pain. The patient must have undergone careful diagnosis and screening by a multidisciplinary team, including a psychologist. Behavioral factors that may contribute significantly to the pain condition, including drug addiction, must have been ruled out. The facilities, equipment, and professional personnel required for proper diagnosis, treatment, and follow-up must be available. Finally, the patient must have undergone a successful trial with temporarily implanted electrodes prior to permanent implantation of the spinal cord stimulator.

Contraindications to SCS as a therapeutic option include infection or uncontrolled coagulopathy (bleeding disorder) at the time of implantation, psychological instability, untreated drug addiction, absence of an objectively documented cause for the pain, presence of a demand cardiac pacemaker, imminent need for an MRI, patient aversion to electrical stimulation or to an implant, and an unsuccessful test trial.

Improvements in SCS devices, techniques, and patient selection over the last two decades have enhanced the safety and efficacy of the procedure and expanded the role of SCS in the treatment of chronic, intractable pain that has failed more conservative or conventional treatment. Because it is invasive and costly, it should not be a first-line therapy. SCS is safe, and its benefit/risk profile compares favorably with alternative procedures. Approximately 60% of patients report 50% or greater reduction in their pain.

Intraspinal drug infusion therapy was first introduced in 1979 as an alternative method for the management of severe, intractable pain. In this method, a pump is implanted that reduces pain by administering small doses of morphine directly to the spinal cord. The pump may do so either epidurally (outside the dura mater, the outermost membrane covering the spinal cord and brain) or intrathecally (into the subarachnoid space beneath the arachnoid membrane, which is the middle membrane covering the spinal cord and brain). The epidural route of morphine administration provides pain relief that is 10 times more potent than that of the intravenous route. Analgesia produced by the intrathecal route is even more impressive: 100 times greater than that of the intravenous route. In addition, there are fewer side effects, such as nausea or drowsiness. However, the complication rate is more than 50% and increases with the duration of treatment.

Intraspinal narcotic infusion therapy should be considered in patients with severe, diffuse, chronic pain that has been unresponsive to more conventional treatment. The success rate is dependent on careful patient selection. The candidate's physical and mental status must be evaluated and found to be within normal range. In addition, the patient should have narcotic-sensitive pain as determined by a trial of epidural or intrathecal narcotics. This trial is imperative prior to implantation and should result in a pain reduction of at least 50%.

The intraspinal drug infusion system consists of two parts: a catheter and a pump. The spinal catheter is inserted through a needle into the spinal canal. The other end of the catheter is placed under the skin and connected to the pump. The catheter delivers the morphine from the pump to the spinal canal. The pump is surgically placed under the skin, usually in the lower abdominal area. It is a round metal disc that weighs about six ounces and measures three inches in diameter and one inch in thickness. This pump stores and releases prescribed amounts of morphine into the spinal canal. It is refilled on a routine basis by inserting a needle through the patient's skin into a port in the center of the pump. After the procedure, the patient must follow up with the physician regularly every 4 to 12 weeks for medication adjustments and pump refills.

Intraspinal drug infusion of narcotics is contraindicated in patients who suffer from opioid-insensitive pain, generalized sepsis or localized infection at the proposed site of implantation, a bleeding disorder, significant psychological problems, or who refuse this mode of therapy.

Side effects and complications occur in more than 50% of patients during long-term spinal opioid treatment. Possible side effects include urinary retention, pruritis (itching), sedation, pain from the injection, nausea, vomiting, constipation, euphoria, depressed mood, and decreased respiratory rate and blood pressure. Potential complications include technical failures (such as catheter disconnection, kinking, or dislocation), catheter or port occlusion, leaking reservoir, localized infection, meningitis, or the development of a seroma (tumorlike collection of serum in the tissues) around the implanted device. In patients with intrathecal catheters, leakage of cerebrospinal fluid, causing a spinal headache, is the most frequent complication. Fistulas may develop. Cerebrospinal fluid leakage either resolves on its own without intervention or may be treated with an epidural blood patch.

Research indicates that fewer than one in 1,000 patients becomes addicted to morphine administered by intraspinal drug infusion. As you may recall, the term "addiction" refers specifically to compulsive drug-seeking behavior and the use of pain medication for emotional gratification. Because patients in severe pain use morphine for pain control and not emotional gratification, they rarely become addicted. Benefits include (1) good to excellent pain relief in 50 to 80% of patients, (2) smaller drug dosages, (3) decreased nausea and drowsiness due to the medication, (4) improved sleep, (5) a more active lifestyle, and (6) a reduced need for oral pain medication.

The need for intraspinal drug infusion therapy is rare. It is estimated that only about 1% of cancer patients require this kind of treatment in order to control their pain. Because of the availability of this modality, there has been a decline in the number of neurodestructive procedures performed to alleviate cancer pain. Recently, this form of therapy has been expanded to treat selected patients suffering from severe, intractable pain of nonmalignant origin.

Intraspinal drug infusion therapy is very expensive. The initial cost of the pump itself is about $10,000. Including installation, the start-up cost is well over $20,000. Monthly maintenance runs around $500, and the ongoing daily cost of the medication must also be considered. Some providers and payers believe that a patient's life expectancy should be more than three months in order to justify the cost of the treatment.

Brain Surgeries

Frontal lobotomy is an operation in which white matter fibers of the frontal lobe of the brain are severed via holes drilled in the skull. This surgical procedure was originally devised to alleviate severe, intractable psychiatric disorders. It was based on experimental observations of a calming effect in animals following the procedure. The operation was then performed on members of the chronic pain population with the hope that it would reduce pain and suffering. The major benefit was a reduction in anxiety and depression. Minimal if any effect on pain perception occurred, but the impact of the pain on the patient's mood and functioning was diminished.

Prior to the advent of modern drug therapy, frontal lobotomy was an accepted treatment for schizophrenia. Today, however, the procedure is considered to be a last resort. The abusive overuse of this operation during the first 25 years of its widespread acceptance led to a rebound in the United States, rendering it difficult to perform any "psychosurgery." Its descendant, the cingulotomy, can be effective for pain relief in some patients.

Brain Surgeries to Reduce Pain

1. Frontal lobotomy
2. Cingulotomy
3. Hypophysectomy*
4. Thalomotomy*
5. Deep brain stimulation*

* See Appendix C.

Cingulotomy is the creation of precisely placed lesions in the cingulum of the frontal lobe of the brain for relief of intractable, diffuse pain. The cingulum is one of the major pathways that transmit information between the frontal lobe and the limbic system, a part of the brain that plays a key role in emotional behavior. The goal is to interrupt this pathway, thereby reducing pain perception and suffering. The procedure is generally reserved for cancer patients rather than those who suffer from severe, chronic nonmalignant pain.

Cingulotomy provides short-term analgesia in 80 to 100% patients. When patients survived longer than three months, only about a third continued to experience pain relief. Neuropsychological testing of patients before and after cingulotomy has documented an improvement in IQ scores, probably due to a decrease in depression. Most studies have reported no deaths or major neurological complications. However, side effects such as apathy and flattening of affect occur in 10 to 30% of patients.

Other Surgeries to Reduce Pain

Revascularization is the restoration of an adequate blood supply to a body part by means of a blood vessel graft. Because oxygen is carried to the various body parts by hemoglobin in the blood, it stands to reason that any process which diminishes blood flow, such as athero-

---

Other Surgeries to Reduce Pain

1. Revascularization
2. Abdominoplasty
3. Breast reduction
4. Peripheral nerve stimulation*
5. Neurectomy*

* See Appendix C.

---

sclerosis (hardening of the arteries), will also decrease tissue oxygenation, thereby causing ischemic pain. Bypass grafts are designed to create a detour around a diseased or blocked artery. These grafts can be constructed from a vein in the patient's body or from artificial material. One example of such a procedure is the coronary artery bypass graft, which is performed to improve the blood supply to the heart, thereby relieving angina (chest pain due to ischemia). Bypass grafts are also done frequently in the legs.

Reconstructive abdominoplasty, commonly known as the "tummy tuck," is a surgical procedure that is frequently performed for cosmetic reasons. What a lot of people don't know is that it can also be done to alleviate chronic low-back pain. Abdominal muscles play a critical role in supporting the lumbar spine, especially during lifting. Many people have weak, overstretched, and incompetent abdominal muscles that can no longer do the job for which they were originally designed. This may happen, for example, when an obese individual loses a lot of weight. It may also occur in women following pregnancy when these muscles fail to regain their normal length and tone after delivery. Chronic lower back pain may develop as a result. In some cases, reconstructive abdominoplasty can be very effective in relieving these symptoms.

Breast reduction for macromastia (or large, heavy breasts) is associated with a number of pain complaints due to biomechanical factors. These include headaches, neck pain, shoulder pain, painful bra strap grooves, ulnar neuropathy (numbness and tingling in the little fingers), and back pain. In one study, 97% of patients with macromastia reported pain in at least three of these areas preoperatively. Following mamma-plasties (breast reductions), all patients experienced less pain; 25% reported complete elimination of pain. Most of these patients reported an improved self-image, became more physically active, lost weight, and reduced or discontinued the use of pain medications.

Guidelines for Choosing a Doctor in General, A Surgeon in Particular

If you were planning to buy the best possible car for you and your family, you might start by poring over *Consumer Reports.* You would probably check the safety records, statistics, mileage, and repair histo-ries. After obtaining the critical information — critical as defined by you, the consumer — perhaps you would narrow your choices to the top three or four. Then you would probably cruise down to the local auto dealer to take a look around.

If a given car catches your eye, you might first size it up from a dis-tance. Do the style and color appeal to your senses? If so, you no doubt would take a closer look. You might walk around the car, study it from all angles, and kick the tires a time or two. If you know anything whatsoever about engines (many of us can't make such a claim), then you would probably take a look under the hood.

Next, you would open the door of the vehicle and get in. Perhaps you would put the key in the ignition, start the car, and listen to the sound of the motor hopefully purring to life. Then you would take a spin around the block a few times, followed by a test drive on the freeway. How does the car handle? Does it have any zip? Is it easy to maneuver in and out of traffic? Are the neighbors likely to become envious? You know, the usual questions.

As you drive along, you'd take a few deep breaths and enjoy the aroma of a brand new automobile. You might run your hand over the upholstery. You'd turn on the air-conditioning or the heat to see if it is working properly. And you just might turn the radio to your favorite station.

Picking out a new car is, no doubt, a big decision that warrants studious attention. But we think that picking out the right doctor for you and your family is even more important and deserves at least as much time and consideration. According to the People's Medical Society, a national medical consumer group in Allentown, Pennsylvania, over 80,000 people in the United States die each year from medical negligence. Another 300,000 suffer serious injuries, often leading to permanent disability. The take-home message is: *Choose your doctor carefully.* Don't just "let your fingers do the walking." The yellow pages as a definitive source can be improved upon. You have a right to know about your doctor's credentials. You have a right to know about his or her education, experience, and outcomes. You have a right to know whether or not your doctor is board certified. Remember. Your doctor works for *you.* Not the other way around. You are the consumer. Be an informed one.

In our opinion, everyone should have a competent and compassionate primary care physician. The 50 million people in the United States who are enrolled in a PPO or HMO do have a primary care physician, because it is a requirement. Primary care physicians include family practitioners, pediatricians, and internists. These physicians are generalists who are trained to treat a wide range of problems and who know when to refer you to a specialist. They can often spare you from unnecessary procedures, including surgery, by obtaining a second opinion.

National board certification is a good indicator that a doctor has the training and experience to practice in a given specialty. To verify certification, you can call the American Board of Medical Specialties (800-776-2378). But beware. Medical boards evaluate medical knowledge and test-taking capability, not performance as a physician. Moreover, there are sound-alike boards that do not have high standards and do not require doctors to take an examination to be "certified." Although it can be difficult to sort all of this out, it is worthwhile to take heed.

You as the patient and consumer should consider other factors as well and be assertive in your own self-interest. You may wish to run a background check on a doctor. If so, you can call the state medical board and ask whether or not the board has ever disciplined the doctor you are considering. After all, he or she may be making decisions that affect the health and well-being of you and your family. A visit to the courthouse can yield detailed information on malpractice claims against a physician. However, you will be limited to learning of suits filed only in your county. If a physician is a recent transplant to your area, that may give you pause. Any number of physicians flee a given geographic area because of legal difficulties.

The National Practitioner Data Bank in Washington, D.C., compiled by the federal government, is the only central clearinghouse in the country. The data bank possesses nationwide listings of malpractice judgments and disciplinary actions. Unfortunately, at this time, the information is available only to state licensing boards, insurance companies, physicians, and hospitals. Congressional efforts thus far have failed to open this information up to the public.

If you are choosing between a number of HMOs and PPOs, select the one that has the greatest number of physicians in each specialty. Choice is very important in assuring that you will be satisfied with the healthcare that you receive. It goes without saying that, in today's world, a physician must be a provider for your healthcare plan in order to be your potential physician. Time spent evaluating a physician who is not on your plan is time wasted unless you are seeking out-of-plan care and are prepared to finance it yourself. Ask with what hospitals the doctor has admitting privileges. If a doctor has privileges only at a hospital that has a questionable reputation or is located a long way from your home, you may want to think twice.

Word-of-mouth recommendations can be very helpful, particularly if they are from family or close friends who may be able to shed light on a doctor's personality and reputation. Nurses are an excellent source of helpful information, as they are often privy to the inside scoop. And, of course, a personal interview with a potential doctor may be very helpful as well. Only in a face-to-face encounter will you be able to evaluate a doctor's personality and style of communication. Does he or she listen to your concerns and convey a kindly, competent manner? If a physician doesn't listen to you or behaves in a rude, arrogant, or intimidating manner, trust your instincts and head for the door. There are plenty of doctors who *do* listen respectfully. Keep in mind that the number one reason for malpractice suits in this country can be traced to poor communication on the part of the doctor.

There are other warning signs as well. Approximately 10% of physicians in this country have problems with substance abuse. If a doctor seems to be mentally impaired, get out and keep looking. Doctors who order endless tests and procedures that yield no useful answers that affect care are also to be avoided. So are doctors who continue to provide ineffective treatment and fail to make appropriate referrals to specialists. This is a major problem for many individuals suffering from chronic pain.

In the interest of self-preservation, never use doctors for medical problems that are not within their area of expertise. If, for example, you have been told that you may need back surgery, see a spine specialist, not a general orthopedic surgeon. A spine specialist may be either an orthopedic surgeon or a neurosurgeon who has gone through a spine fellowship after completing his or her residency. And, by all means, get a second opinion from an equally qualified surgeon. Inquire about the surgeon's rate of success for the surgery being recommended. Ask how many operations of the type recommended he or she performs annually. Ask to speak with some of his or her patients who have undergone the procedure. What is the best-case scenario and what is the worst? What is the cost–benefit ratio? Will physical therapy be ordered after surgery? Will you have to wear a brace, and if so, for how long? When can you expect to be able to return to work? What kind of limitations does the doctor expect? Will he or she treat the pain or will you just have to tough it out?

These questions are fair game. You, the consumer, have a right to know what to expect before undergoing surgery. And the answers should be provided in an understandable, straightforward, manner. If you are not satisfied with the explanation, it's the perfect opportunity to utilize your assertiveness skills and ask questions. A great deal of research has shown that becoming knowledgeable about what to expect from your upcoming surgical experience *will* make a significant difference. (For more information on choosing healthcare providers, see the practitioner checklist in Appendix A.)

Preparing for Surgery

Everyone — the patient, the doctor, the family, and the insurance company — wants a successful surgical outcome. Who wouldn't? Yet many people are surprised to learn that outcome is dependent upon more than just the skill of the surgeon.

Juan, a 41-year-old heavy equipment operator, injured his back when he fell eight feet from his loader onto the ground. He had three children and a wife to support but was no longer able to work. After a struggle with the state worker's compensation system, he was granted disability payments and medical treatment for his injury. Following an evaluation by an orthopedist, back surgery was recommended. Although Juan wanted very much to get his pain under control and to return to work, he was extremely wary of surgery as he knew a man who underwent such an operation and wound up worse off than before. He also lacked an understanding of what was wrong with his back and what the surgery would entail in terms of his length of recovery, physical limitations, and the ultimate outcome. Then there was the most chilling thought of all: What would happen to his wife and children if he died on the table?

A week later, Juan received a telephone call from his insurance case manager. She informed him that he was to undergo back surgery on December 30th, just 10 short days away. This took Juan by surprise, and he expressed his reservations about the surgery. In response, the case manager informed him that the operation had to be undertaken prior to the end of the year and that if he did not comply with this plan, his disability benefits would be cut off. Juan was afraid but felt that he had no choice in the matter. Like it or not, he was about to face major back surgery.

Juan was born and raised in Mexico. He quit school in the sixth grade in order to go to work to help support his rather large family of 10 children. At 21, he immigrated to the United States, obtained citizenship, and landed a job as a manual laborer with a large construction company. During his 17 years with the company, he worked his way up to the position of heavy equipment operator. A soft-spoken man, he loved his job, was well respected, and made a decent wage to support his growing family. In his mind, he had arrived.

And then it happened: a freak accident in which he fell from his loader and injured his back. With only limited education, unable to work, and a belief that making waves only brings trouble, Juan politely asked what benefits were available to him. After all, he had a family to feed. He immediately noticed that his employer and the worker's compensation case manager responded coldly to his questions and at times even treated him with hostility. It was as if they thought that he was faking his pain and disability in order to get a free ride. Juan felt his only choice was to go along with what he was told to do, despite his significant misgivings.

On the evening of December 30th, and after a less than joyous Christmas, Juan reluctantly went to the hospital. His surgery was to take place the next morning. He struggled with restlessness, fear, and anxiety. Sleep did not visit him that night.

The sounds of the recovery room began to penetrate Juan's consciousness following what was a routine back surgery. The effects of the general anesthesia were starting to wear off when he heard a nurse telling him to take some deep breaths. Suddenly, Juan became short of breath. He struggled to get air into his lungs. Images of his wife and children flashed through his mind. He feared the worst — that he was going to die. "How are they going to survive when I'm gone?" he thought. Juan began to panic as he gasped for air. His heart raced as the nurse yelled for assistance in restraining her highly agitated patient. Now he was breathing too deeply. The excess oxygen led to hyperventilation and dizziness which, coupled with the anesthesia, made Juan feel even more out of control.

Although he did not know it at the time, he was experiencing a full-blown panic attack. The mixture of awareness that his ability to breathe was somehow disrupted, coupled with his preexisting fear that the surgery might disable or even kill him, added to the loss of personal control that comes with general anesthesia, yielded a recipe for such an attack.

After a few minutes — minutes that seemed like an eternity — Juan began to recover from the abject panic that had befallen him. As the anesthesia wore off, his awareness and sense of control slowly returned. This, in turn, eased his anxiety and lowered the demand on his sympathetic nervous system. His breathing and heart rates descended to more normal levels. But he remained confused as to what had happened to him and became extremely fearful that such an experience might occur again.

Recovery from surgery was slow and there were complications. No matter how hard he tried, he simply could not get that nightmare in the recovery room out of his mind. When he finally managed to fall asleep, he would frequently awaken, gasping for breath. His heart would race and his skin would be cold and clammy. All this was coupled with a profound sense of anxiety and dread. And there was the pain. Apart from the normal postsurgical pain, his back didn't feel much better at all. He required large doses of pain medication which didn't seem to help very much and made him lethargic. Despite this sedative-like effect, it made Juan feel even more anxious because it reminded him of what it felt like to awaken from the general anesthesia after the surgery. The chronic pain and anxiety led him to believe that, instead of helping him, the surgery only added to his problems. And nobody seemed to understand what was wrong with him. After all, the postsurgical X-rays showed that the operation was "a complete success." According to the doctor, the fusion "appeared solid." There was "no reason" why he should still be hurting.

When he came to us for an interdisciplinary pain evaluation, his records revealed not a word about his misgivings prior to surgery, his having felt pressured to follow through with the surgery, his difficulty breathing and resultant panic attack in the recovery room, his episodes of anxiety following surgery, or his fear of reinjury, which he felt would lead to another terrifying operation. He scored at the 100th percentile on the anxiety scale and he was clinically depressed — factors known to produce a chronic stress response in the body. A biofeedback evaluation showed extremely high sympathetic nervous system arousal which reacted with an even greater stress response to discussion of his surgical experience. In summary, Juan's nervous system was in a state of chaos. He was taking large quantities of pain medications, in part to quell his anxiety and quiet his nervous system.

Given these details — obtained simply by asking the patient about his own experience — it is not surprising that his postsurgical X-rays and CT scans were of little help in understanding his continued suffering. After all, his panic attack, chronic anxiety, elevated muscle tension, fear of reinjury, and depression were all invisible to the radiographic studies of his spine. Yet, they explained why he responded so poorly to the surgery. In the absence of this kind of understanding, it is easy to blame the poor outcome on the patient and attribute it to a lack of motivation to get better. Some would even accuse Juan of faking his debilitated state in order to get a free paycheck. These kinds of unfair accusations are made all too often, especially in the world of worker's compensation. And it is a tragic mistake in that a suffering individual is accused of malingering, all because of the shortsightedness of those given the mandate to "help" him or her. The good news is that there is a great deal of research showing that surgical outcome can be significantly enhanced by certain behavioral interventions. The bad news, however, is that these interventions are rarely prescribed. But being aware of their availability will arm you with options to discuss with your doctors before being wheeled into the operating room.

Behavioral Interventions and Surgical Outcome

What if we were to tell you that a few simple behavioral procedures, provided prior to surgery, can significantly improve the following:

♦ Emotional stress

♦ Physical stress

♦ Pain

♦ The need for pain medication

♦ Clinical recovery

♦ Behavioral recovery

♦ Length of stay in the hospital

Does this sound like a come-on pitch from an annoying telemarketer (calling just as you're sitting down to dinner)? Well, don't despair. The fact is, the improvements in outcome listed above are well founded in the research literature and are available in most areas. Yet, most surgeons are completely unaware of these findings, and consequently they are rarely considered. What are these interventions? They are summarized below. For an excellent book on what you can do to prepare for surgery, we highly recommend *Preparing for Surgery: A Mind–Body Approach to Enhancing Healing and Recovery* by our colleagues Drs. William Deardorff and John Reeves II.

1. **Procedural information.** This intervention involves providing the patient with detailed information about what will happen leading up to, during, and following surgery. Often, this includes a rundown of what is wrong in the body and what the surgeon seeks to correct. Providing detailed procedural information prior to surgery was associated with improvement in seven out of seven outcome variables listed above in a recent statistical review (meta-analysis) of the scientific literature. Most good surgeons do a thorough job of providing this information to the patient. But if you find

yourself unable to describe these kinds of details to another person, it's time to start asking questions. You'll be doing yourself a big favor.

2. **Behavioral instruction.** This refers to the discussion of specific actions that the patient can take to aid in his or her recovery. Examples include when to take which medications, when to start resuming which kinds of physical activity, how to monitor the surgical wound, and what to do in response to pain or anxiety. Again, the good surgeon will cover many of these issues in preparing his or her patient for the operation. However, detailed instruction about how to respond to psychological symptoms is usually lacking, even though it is an important contributor to improved postsurgical recovery. In fact, behavioral instruction has been associated with improved outcome in all seven of the outcome variables listed above.

3. **Relaxation.** When patients are given training in how to relax, they are significantly less likely to experience emotional stress, physiological stress, and pain, compared with patients who have not received such training. They will also, as a group, require less pain medication, have a better overall clinical recovery, and go home sooner from the hospital. You may recall that, within the context of pain management, relaxation refers to more than simply watching television or reading *People* magazine. This skill, when finely honed, produces profound beneficial changes in the nervous, circulatory, endocrine, and immune systems. With this in mind, it's no wonder that exposure to this skill is statistically related to improved surgical outcome, as successful healing is dependent on all of these systems working efficiently together. Although easy to learn, relaxation training is almost never considered, let alone provided. Ask about it. If your surgeon just stares back at you with a clueless gaze, insist on a referral to a qualified health specialist (usually a health psychologist) who can provide the training.

4. **Cognitive interventions.** These refer to a variety of behavioral procedures aimed at controlling unpleasant psychological states such as fear, anxiety, and depression. Typically, the patient's concerns are addressed through discussion with a behavioral health professional. The patient is taught how to modify his or her thinking in such a way as to reduce unwanted emotions. Such interventions have been statistically linked to improvement in emotional stress, pain, pain medication intake, and overall clinical recovery.

5. **Sensory information.** Interventions in this group focus on providing the patient with detailed information regarding what he or she will likely encounter in terms of physical and emotional sensations, during and after surgery. Again, many surgeons will convey some information of this nature, although it is rarely detailed or specific. In the relatively few investigations that provided sensory information as a formal intervention, improvements were limited to behavioral recovery and length of stay.

6. **Emotion-focused interventions.** Several studies have examined the effects of discussing with the patient how he or she is feeling emotionally. By supportively attending to his or her needs, improvement in physiological stress and length of stay has been observed across studies.

7. **Hypnosis.** Only a few studies have looked at whether hypnosis affects surgical outcome. The results have been inconclusive. This is not to say that hypnosis is ineffective in improving the postsurgical course. The relative lack of research and/or the variety of hypnotic procedures investigated may not allow for statistical evaluation across studies.

Juan's experience was a case study in what not to do in preparing a human being for surgery. As it turned out, his insurance case manager was responding to her supervisor's admonition to get as many expensive procedures taken care of before the end of the year so as to satisfy

Behavioral Interventions
Shown to Enhance Surgical Outcome

Type of Intervention	Outcome Variable Improved by Intervention
Procedural information	Emotional stress Physiological stress Pain Pain medication intake Clinical recovery Behavioral recovery Length of stay in hospital
Behavioral instruction	Emotional stress Physiological stress Pain Pain medication intake Clinical recovery Behavioral recovery Length of stay in hospital
Relaxation	Emotional stress Physiological stress Pain Pain medication intake Clinical recovery Length of stay in hospital
Cognitive interventions	Emotional stress Pain Pain medication intake Clinical recovery
Sensory information	Behavioral recovery Length of stay in hospital
Emotion-focused interventions	Physiological stress
Hypnosis	No consistent benefits across studies Length of stay in hospital

the accountants. Hence the rush to schedule surgery for December 30th. This nonclinical factor contributed to some extremely complicated, and unnecessary, clinical problems. The price paid in terms of dollars and human suffering has been immense. As for Juan, we were unable to weaken the grip of fear in his life, despite our best efforts. He remains disabled at home, with little hope of significant improvement in his quality of life. Not all stories have a happy ending. But perhaps Juan's experience will help others to muster the requisite assertiveness to insist on getting what they need to ensure a positive surgical outcome.

By the way, we were never paid for treating Juan due to a technical billing error on our part. Although minor (the bills were not sent out in a "timely manner"), the error provided Juan's insurance company an excuse to deny any and all payment. Despite our efforts to work things out, we were told that we were not going to be paid. Period. How gratifying to know that we were able to contribute to the insurance company's bottom line — *NOT*!

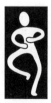

The Managed Care
Experiment

The worst sin towards our fellow creatures is not to hate them, but to be indifferent to them; that's the essence of inhumanity.

—George Bernard Shaw
Anderson, in
The Devil's Disciple, Act 2

The opposite of love is not hate, it's indifference. The opposite of art is not ugliness, it's indifference. The opposite of faith is not heresy, it's indifference. And the opposite of life is not death, it's indifference.

—Elie Wiesel
U.S. News and World Report
October 27, 1986

A funny thing happened on the way to the 21st century. Biological, medical, and behavioral science made the most incredible discoveries in the history of the world. These discoveries translated into applications that healed the sick, eased suffering, and saved lives. Vicious maladies that once haunted the human species, causing untold misery, were now tamed. People suffering from agonizing pain could be helped to feel better. The biomedical and behavioral technologies for controlling pain, usually involving a coordinated interdisciplinary approach, became more widely understood and accepted within the medical community. There was no question that a compassionate society would put this important knowledge to good use. Or was there?

In response to rapid escalations in healthcare costs, the managed care movement was born in the 1980s. For insurance companies, the idea was to change the way healthcare was "delivered" so as to keep costs down. The solution was to alter the incentive system for doctors and hospitals. Instead of giving them free reign, why not "manage" the care they give by making payment contingent upon their following a narrow set of criteria? Take away the incentive for providing "too much" care and substitute one for providing *just enough* care.

For this concept to succeed, however, insurance companies needed leverage. In the old days, everyone would have been appalled if an insurance adjuster ever questioned a doctor's treatment decisions. It simply wasn't done. But what if the concepts and methods of big business could be applied to healthcare? What if employers and patients were made financial offers they couldn't refuse in the form of significantly lower health insurance premiums along with the promise of the same "high-quality" healthcare they were used to? Maybe you couldn't continue to see Dr. Welby (who had taken care of you since you were a baby), but you were "free to choose" from the list of "qualified" providers (qualified in the sense that they had agreed to accept less money for their services and abide by the corporate rules). For this to work, the insurance companies had to attract a larger and larger proportion of healthcare "consumers" to their health maintenance organization (HMO) "product lines." And with an increasing "market share," they gained more leverage with "providers" (doctors and hospitals).

Into the 1990s, HMOs indeed did grab a larger and larger proportion of the market share. And with this exponential rise came an increased concern among doctors and hospitals that soon they would be left out in the cold with no patients to treat — *and no income.* Their response?

> Better get on board; the train's already left the station. Although
> I used to get $75, I guess I'll have to learn to live with $20 for an

office visit. It probably won't even cover my overhead, unless, of course, I spend only 6 or 7 minutes with each patient instead of my usual 15 or 20.

Yup, "managed" care had arrived. Yup, the rise in healthcare costs came to a screeching halt. And yup, we could all breathe a sigh of relief that sanity finally prevailed. Right?

Wrong, Wrong, Wrong!

For those old enough to remember what healthcare services were like prior to the mid-1980s, consider the following questions:

♦ Have you noticed any changes in the way your doctor relates to you?

♦ Are you spending less time with him or her than you used to?

♦ Does it seem harder to get your questions answered?

♦ Does it seem like doctors don't know you or your condition as thoroughly as they used to?

♦ Have you had the sense that the doctor isn't really listening to you or taking your problems seriously?

♦ Does he or she seem less concerned than doctors in the past about how your medical problems are affecting your life?

♦ Is it more difficult to get in to see your doctor in a timely manner? Or...

♦ Are you often seen by a nurse or physician's assistant instead of a doctor?

♦ Have you had trouble getting a referral to a specialist?

♦ Does it seem more difficult than in the past to obtain necessary X-rays, lab tests, or procedures?

- Have you had to leave the hospital before you thought your were ready?

- Have you had to change doctors due to a change in insurance plans or because your doctor was dropped from the provider list?

- Have you had to substitute a less effective medication for one that was prescribed because the one that worked wasn't on the insurance company's list of approved drugs?

- Over time, has it become more difficult to get your medical bills paid by your insurance company?

- Are denials more frequent than they used to be?

- Have you received an insurance denial for services that were deemed necessary by your doctor? If so...

- Did your condition worsen as a result? If so...

- Did you die? (Don't laugh; plenty have.)

- Does it seem like the *care* has been taken out of healthcare?

- Overall, are you less satisfied with your healthcare now than you were 15 or 20 years ago?

If you answered no to each of these questions, chances are either you pay cash for your healthcare or you haven't gotten sick. We are willing to bet that the vast majority of you have encountered one or more of the problems referenced above. (We certainly have, not only as "providers" but also as "consumers" of healthcare for ourselves and our families.) Has managed care lived up to its promise to deliver the same high-quality service at a lower cost? The answer is a resounding NO!

Mom, Apple Pie, and the Free Market

The concept of health insurance is really quite simple. It amounts to a business contract. In return for a fee, the insurance company agrees to pay for part (or all) of the healthcare services provided to the patient.

As with any contract, the terms are specified in a written document signed by each party. Also, as with any business, the party receiving money in exchange for providing the service is entitled to make a profit. After all, that's the American way. So, what's the problem? Well, in theory, nothing. But in practice — everything.

For-Profit HMOs: Making Money at Any Cost

In a free market, competition drives quality. Recall what happened in the 1980s when consumers became dissatisfied with the quality of American cars. The Japanese automakers clobbered the Big Three because their cars were better and less expensive. This hit the American manufacturers where it hurt, and all of a sudden, there was a dramatic shift toward producing higher quality cars. But it took the emergence of an attractive alternative to turn things around. This is an example of competition working to the advantage of the consumer.

But how much choice does the typical employee have when it comes to deciding on a health insurance plan provided by the employer? (Forget, for the time being, the fact that record numbers of workers are offered no insurance at all. That brings up a whole other set of ethical questions.) In larger companies, employees are usually offered a choice of Plan A (Cadillac), Plan B (Chevy), or Plan C ('73 Dodge Dart). And they pay accordingly. In smaller companies, however, it's the '73 Dodge — take it or leave it. And who decides what kind of plan to offer the employees? The employer. And what is the leading consideration in deciding which plan to offer the employees? Cost to the employer. This is business, and the goal is to make money, remember? Thus, the most "economical" plan (almost always a for-profit HMO) is the most attractive to cost-conscious companies. And when the sales pitch promises substantially reduced cost *with no compromise in quality* (almost always a lie), what benefits manager could resist?

But where's the competition here? If an employee is dissatisfied, he or she can file a complaint with the employer's benefits manager. But what incentive would there be for the employer to complain to the

Nonprofit versus For-Profit HMOs

Lest we commit the error of painting with too broad a brush, we must point out that HMOs run the gamut from good to terrible in terms of the care they provide. A 1997 study by the Healthcare Finance Administration (the federal agency that administers Medicare) measured consumer satisfaction with Medicare HMOs by examining disenrollment rates. In looking at those with the highest rates (where more than 50% of subscribers canceled) and lowest rates (where less than 6% bailed), it was discovered that 70% of the worst plans were for-profit whereas only 10% of the best were for-profit. Put another way, people leave the for-profit HMOs in droves compared with the nonprofit ones.

Similarly, *Consumer Reports* magazine (1996) surveyed its subscribers and ranked HMOs according to consumer satisfaction. Of the 13 worst, 92% were for-profit. But of the 11 best, *none* were for-profit. Clearly, people are much more dissatisfied with HMOs that are set up and operated to make money.

Reporting in the prestigious *New England Journal of Medicine* (1998), healthcare commentator Robert Kuttner reported that

> ...nonprofit plans are more efficient. They characteristically spend more than 90 cents of the premium dollar on health care...whereas expenditures by the most aggressive HMOs are in the range of 70 or even 60 cents on the dollar.

That leaves a gap of 25% between for-profit and nonprofit HMOs — premium dollars that are channeled into the pockets of shareholders and the executives to whom they pay obscenely high salaries and other compensation. Meanwhile, the chronic pain patient continues to suffer because the doctor's appropriate and effective treatment regimen is deemed "unnecessary" — often by someone possessing only a high-school diploma.

insurer? If enough employees complained and threatened to strike because of their lousy healthcare coverage, then that might create an incentive. But we're not aware that strikes occur over single-item issues like the particular health plan offered to employees. (Besides, the proportion of workers represented by unions is not what it used to be.) Given this, the employee is left with either accepting the employer's health plan or giving it up and purchasing one on his or her own at a substantially higher (nongroup, nondiscounted) cost.

But isn't it in the HMO's self-interest to provide needed services, to keep everyone healthy in order to contain its costs? After all, the more sick its "members" are, the more it will have to spend on subsequent medical care. In theory, yes. In practice — *no!* If you have been with a particular employer for more than a few years, you have probably seen insurance companies come and go when enrollment time comes around. Many (if not most) people have probably changed insurance companies two or perhaps three times. Given this trend, what incentive does an HMO have to spend money to keep its members healthy when some other company will, in all likelihood, step in after a year or two to reap the benefits?

The only possible incentive involves doing the right thing and living up to the promises made in the sales pitch. (We happen to believe that the sales pitch is ethically more valid than the actual written contract when it comes to keeping promises.) Sadly, however, the almighty dollar seems to have become the ultimate arbiter when it comes to deciding what's right and wrong within for-profit corporate healthcare. The prospect of living up to the promise of complete, timely, and compassionate healthcare (have you seen the ads?) doesn't stand a chance when pitted against the incredible pressures to keep the quarterly profits moving higher. Forget free market competition as it applies to the managed care movement. If your criterion for success is complete, timely, and compassionate healthcare, it doesn't work. But if it is the transfer of money from the patient to corporate executives and stockholders, then it works pretty well. The score? Right — 0. Wrong — 1.

The Death of Honor

Following a car accident, Cathy developed spasmodic torticollis, an extremely painful condition in which her muscles were in a state of constant contraction, causing her head to be tilted and shoulder raised. She went through surgery and other difficult invasive procedures, all to no avail. Formerly a head nurse, she was no longer able to work and had to go on disability. Her life was devastated by this vicious condition — so much so that she actually planned to commit suicide at one point. Thankfully, her attorney and a couple of her doctors stepped in to help. Although tenacious, her pain came under better control and she was able to start rebuilding her life (which included a new baby granddaughter a year later).

Cathy's monthly medication bill was in excess of $600, and her financial resources were all but depleted. When she heard a local (for-profit) Medicare HMO's claim that she could receive the same "high-quality" medical care and have all of her medications covered, she decided to investigate further. She saw that Dr. Davis was on the list of "providers" and signed on.

On the very day that the new plan started, she learned that Dr. Davis had been abruptly dropped from the list. Apparently, the HMO had decided to cancel its contracts with all existing pain physicians and hire *one person* — an anesthesiologist who provided anesthetic nerve blocks — to take care of all of its members' pain needs (a profit-enhancing move perhaps?). Never mind the research findings and collective knowledge of pain management experts that indicate the need for a more comprehensive interdisciplinary approach. Effective treatment of chronic pain was simply going to be a "luxury" unavailable to this HMO's members. Nevertheless, Cathy would have to get an appointment with her new primary care physician in order to get a referral to the new pain "specialist." But she had already had several unsuccessful anesthetic blocks in the past, and it had been established that she needed other types of medical pain management services.

Because her medications would be running out and she needed to make sure that there would be no interruption to the regimen that had been so carefully worked out with Dr. Davis, Cathy immediately called to get an appointment with a primary care physician (whom she did not know). To her horror, she was told that the first available appointment was five weeks away. When she explained her circumstances — that her pain condition would be totally neglected for those five weeks, she was told that she would just have to wait.

The HMO salesman, whose company was known for its aggressive marketing approach, had painted a pretty rosy picture. Cathy could see specialists, get all her medical care without any trouble, and have all of her medications paid for to boot! She could even change primary care physicians at any time (provided she chose from the list). If for any reason she wished to return to her regular Medicare policy (not that she would ever want to), no problem. Just call and cancel. Regular Medicare would resume the following month. The salesman never mentioned anything about delays in getting in to see a doctor or that the provider list was subject to change without notice. On the surface, there was no downside. Only a fool would pass up this opportunity. Yet, on the very first day of her coverage, the terrible reality became clear. And she wanted out.

In a state of near panic, Cathy called to disenroll from the HMO plan. The woman on the other end of the phone seemed unconcerned about Cathy's plight. In fact, she seemed rather indignant that Cathy had a complaint. The woman tried to talk her out of canceling, but Cathy wouldn't budge. The next morning, she got a call from another (rude) HMO representative, apparently a more senior person, who also tried to convince her not to disenroll. Cathy held her ground, and the representative finally accepted her decision, albeit begrudgingly.

A few weeks later, it was determined that Cathy needed to undergo surgery for an unrelated condition. Knowing that regular Medicare would soon kick in, Cathy purchased a secondary insurance policy that would pay for the portion of the bill not covered by Medicare. The new policy was to begin the following month. As planned, she underwent the surgery and continued to see Dr. Davis for her pain care. Then, a few months later, she started getting notices that Medicare was not paying her medical bills *because she was still under the HMO plan*! She had not been disenrolled after all. And predictably, the HMO refused to pay because none of her care had been "preauthorized." Never mind that the HMO continued to accept payments from Medicare to take care of Cathy. Never mind that she had clearly communicated her wish to disenroll. And never mind that the salesman's promises amounted to nothing more than snake oil. No. Cathy had not played by the rules, and therefore, the HMO was not going to take responsibility for her bills. Besides, there was "no record in the computer" of her request to disenroll.

Some 20 or 30 phone calls later, Cathy felt absolutely beaten down. She was unable to get anywhere, even after contacting the HMO president's office. She said, with tears streaming down her face, "Everyone was

---

Before You Dial 9-1-1...

In the fall of 1999, one of the nation's largest HMOs announced that its subscribers would be well advised to dial its 1-800 number prior to heading to the emergency room via ambulance in order to make sure that their symptoms represented a true emergency. Otherwise, the subscriber might be stuck with the bill. The reason? Too many people were taking a siren-assisted trip to the E.R. when a "true" emergency did not exist. And it was just too darned expensive. Indeed, many people have complained that their HMO refused to cover the excursion after the fact — after the condition was found by E.R. doctors to be nonlife-threatening. Talk about Monday morning quarterbacking!

So, the scenario might go something like this: You are suddenly gripped with horrible chest pain. You become short of breath. It's not going away so you reach for the phone to dial 9-1-1. But suddenly you remember your HMO's advice to call its 1-800 number first to avoid a possible denial of coverage. Despite your excruciating pain, abject terror, and feeling of impending doom, you remember that the number is on your insurance card in your wallet. "What a relief. I found the card. Now, if only I could make it over to the phone..."

You manage to pound out the 1-800 number. After several rings, a recorded voice asks you to listen to the following eight options

mean — everyone! They talked to me like I was a criminal. And I treated them all with respect. (Indeed, that was Cathy's nature.) That salesman lied to me! I know now to put everything in writing — no matter what."

Now, the skeptics out there may say that Cathy only got what she deserved. She should never have relied on the sales pitch or verbal confirmation over the phone that her membership would be canceled. Instead, she should have sent written instructions for cancellation via certified mail and made contemporaneous notes as to whom she spoke with and what they said. Perhaps she should have also had her attorney

in order that your call can be properly routed and informs you that, for quality control purposes, your call may be recorded. The pain has gotten worse and you've become severely light-headed. Yet, you manage to listen to the phone menu and make an appropriate selection. (Thank God the emergency option was among the first three!) The phone rings again and another recorded voice comes on the line: "Using the telephone keypad, please enter your membership number, followed by the pound sign." Somehow, you manage to press the right number of keys (but it's a crapshoot as to whose account number you actually entered). "Thank you!" the voice says exuberantly. "All available representatives are currently assisting other customers. Your call is important to us. Please stay on the line and your call will be taken by the first available representative."

Then the commercials start: "Keeping families healthy for over a year and a half, our company prides itself on fast, efficient, and courteous service. You can count on us to..." You look at your watch and are shocked to see that its hands have disappeared! Unfortunately, your senses have become so blurred that you're actually looking at the wrong wrist. (And those blurry numbers are really freckles.) After what seems like an eternity, a real live human voice comes on the line: "This is Tami...How may I help you?... Hello?...This is Tami...Is anybody there?...Hello?..."

present while speaking with them on the phone. Oh, and maybe a video production team should have been there as well to film the conversation, along with a notarized copy of the morning paper to document the date. *Baloney!* Such notions are inventions of our litigation-oriented society and have nothing to do with what is *truly* right and wrong. There was nothing at all honorable about the way Cathy's HMO handled this situation. For them, honor died at the hands of greed. While it is true that honest mistakes are made in business, these were not honest mistakes. All the more reason that, when mistakes were discovered, Cathy's HMO should have:

♦ Treated her with kindness and respect

♦ Been honest and owned up to how it represented itself during the sales pitch

♦ Assessed Cathy's unique healthcare needs and made sure they could be met on day one

♦ Clearly advised Cathy as to what actions were needed in order to disenroll

♦ Paid for the medical care provided to her, whether or not she had any proof of her verbal request to cancel. Just because the HMO could technically get away with sidestepping its responsibility does not mean that it was justified in doing so.

In short, the HMO representatives should have relied on the lessons learned in preschool, not business school. Shame on them.

Penny-Wise, Pound-Foolish

In their rush to produce attractive quarterly profit figures, many insurance companies routinely deny necessary treatment. Although offending companies will vehemently deny this accusation and insist that the well-being of the patient is *always* the guiding consideration, this is a load of crap (and tobacco "isn't addicting," remember?). The abuses documented by the media, Web sites, and congressional testimony leave no doubt that this is occurring — not inadvertently, but purposely.

One of our patients, Aaron, had been injured on the job when a ladder broke, sending him plummeting to the ground. He injured his feet and legs. Within a week, a diagnosis of reflex sympathetic dystrophy (RSD) was made and a treatment plan was submitted to the worker's compensation carrier for authorization. If properly treated early on, RSD can often be stopped in its tracks. But if left alone, it can gain momentum and turn into a permanently painful and disabling condition.

The treatment plan was denied. Instead, the carrier immediately routed Aaron to a doctor of its choice (at a state-run rehabilitation facility) who, without making a firm diagnosis, sent him for physical therapy. On the first day, Aaron was told that if he refused to go along with the program, his disability benefits would be cut off. Not a great way to build a positive prognosis in our view. But predictably, the physical exercise regimen served only to pour fuel on the fire, and despite severe pain, Aaron was never prescribed any pain medication. None. His pain and suffering were repeatedly invalidated. Meanwhile, his feet and legs started to swell and burn with pain. When he threatened to see an attorney, the case manager "assured" him that such a move would only complicate matters and tried to talk him out of it. But Aaron did so anyway. After seven months with no proper diagnosis or treatment, he was finally allowed to see a medical pain specialist who confirmed the diagnosis of RSD and recommended an appropriate plan. Again it was denied. In a gamble to get an opinion that might save it some money, the carrier sent him for three additional independent medical evaluations, all out of state. In addition to the expensive evaluations, the carrier had to pay for the flights and lodging for Aaron and a case manager who accompanied him. If it could get at least one doctor to invalidate the link between his condition and the work injury, the carrier would be off the hook and save buckets full of money in the long run — or so it thought. Unfortunately for the carrier, it lost its wager. Each doctor came to the same conclusion: RSD caused by the work injury. That made four opinions for RSD and one for — well, we're not sure.

By this time, it was too late. Tragically, Aaron's RSD had become so severe (the worst case we have ever seen) that no amount of treatment would cure it. It was now a permanent part of Aaron's life. Upon learning that his RSD might have been cured if treated early, he went ballistic. His anger was palpable, and he was not afraid to express it. The decisions made by the nonphysician case manager — decisions motivated by saving a few dollars — had radically changed the course of his life. In addition to living out the rest of his days in severe pain, he would never work again. Despite all of this, he never received so much as an apology. (Whereas most of us were taught by our mothers to say "I'm sorry" when we realize that we have caused someone harm, it seems that today's legal advice overrides mom's. The prevailing strategy is almost always to deny responsibility. If you don't, you stand a chance of losing money.) Though strenuously contested by the worker's compensation carrier, the court deemed that the carrier would be responsible for monthly compensation (since he could not work) and all future medical expenses relating to the RSD — for the rest of Aaron's life.

Now you might think that the court's decision would lay to rest any future difficulties in getting treatment authorized by the carrier. Guess again. Treatment is, to this day, often denied until Aaron hauls out the court ruling and waves it around for a while. Even then, he routinely has to wait for weeks in order to see a specialist or to get a procedure approved. It is a constant struggle for both Aaron and his doctors. And the struggle translates into more aggravation to Aaron's nervous system, more pain, and diminished quality of life. The bottom line? Because of uncaring, penny-pinching decisions made early on, everyone lost (and is still losing). And the score (for those keeping track)? Right — 0. Wrong — 2.

ERISA: The HMO Sanctuary

In 1974, Congress passed ERISA, the *Employee Retirement Security Act,* which was subsequently signed into law. It was intended to protect working Americans from fraud and mismanagement in their benefits plans. In essence, it held that you could not sue your employer-sponsored health insurance company. Unfortunately, Congress in 1974 did not anticipate the sweeping changes that were to affect healthcare in the 1980s and 1990s. The notion that aggressive corporate profit incentives could ever supersede the Hippocratic oath would have seemed laughable in 1974. But they did.

To their horror, Americans came to realize that managed care organizations (MCOs) could wreak havoc on their lives with federal government-sanctioned impunity. MCOs could hoodwink the public into be-

---

Thanks to ERISA, Managed Care Beats the Rap

Florence Corcoran's obstetrician ordered her into the hospital due to her high-risk pregnancy. Even with a second opinion that backed up this decision, Ms. Corcoran's HMO case manager, who sat in an office thousands of miles away, overruled the doctors and denied the hospitalization. To save money, the HMO hired a nurse to visit Ms. Corcoran at home for 10 hours a day. Monitoring equipment to evaluate the baby's condition was also denied. Unfortunately, the baby went into distress when the nurse was not there. The baby died. Ms. Corcoran's wrongful death suit against the HMO was "preempted" because the 1974 federal ERISA law specifically forbids employee-sponsored insurance companies from being held liable for damages. Although her hands were tied, Judge Carolyn Dineen King ruled that "...the basic facts are undisputed, [but] the result ERISA compels us to reach means that the Corcorans have no remedy, state or federal, for what may have been a serious mistake...[ERISA] eliminates an important check on the thousands of medical decisions routinely made. With liability rules generally inapplicable, there is theoretically less deterrence of substandard medical decision making" (Source: *Corcoran v. United Healthcare, Inc.*, 965 F.2d 1321 [5th Cir. 1992]).

But what's really amazing is the fact that, instead of hanging their heads in shame, HMO lawyers frequently wave the judge's legal decision around in order to dissuade others from trying to sue.

Echoes of Nuremberg:
An Insurance Medical Reviewer Comes Clean

"As a physician, I caused the death of a man. Once I stamped 'DENY' across his authorization form, his life's end was as certain as if I had pulled the plug on a ventilator. Although this was known to many people, I have not been taken before any court of law or called to account for this in any professional or public forum. In fact, just the opposite occurred: I was 'rewarded' for this. It bought me an improved reputation in my job, and contributed to my advancement afterwards. Not only did I demonstrate I could indeed do what was expected of me, I exemplified the 'good' company doctor: I saved a half million dollars."

—1997 testimony of a former insurance
medical director and medical case reviewer
before the California legislature and the U.S. Congress
(Source: http://www.consumerwatchdog.org)

lieving that its medical needs would be well taken care of, pocket the premiums, and deny life-saving care, all the while knowing that (because of a prized loophole) they could never be held legally accountable for their dishonorable actions. Forget higher level morals and ethics. There was simply no *legal* incentive to put patient welfare above profit on the corporate priority list. Employer-sponsored HMOs (and other insurance entities) could not be sued for damages. It was cold. It was calculated. And it brought about untold misery to countless patients and those who cared about them.

As the horror stories piled up, it became clear to members of Congress that paying attention to this matter would boost their reelection prospects. Legislation pertaining to patients' rights began cropping up in 1997 and 1998. Some had substance. Many were just for show. But guess who spent untold millions on lobbying Congress to defeat those with merit? That's right: the health insurance industry (especially HMOs). It actually persuaded the Republican party to defeat the Democratic-sponsored *Patients' Bill of Rights Act of 1998* — which would have reversed the ERISA loophole and allowed MCOs to be held legally accountable — on the grounds that, because it "encouraged" people to sue their insurance companies, it would drive premiums through the roof. In addition, the health insurance industry maintained, it would only serve to benefit lawyers. Never mind that a study by Muse Associates of Washington, D.C. indicated that premiums would increase at most 0.2% (2 cents for every $10) if the bill passed. And never mind that, in one fell swoop, it would remove the incentive to deny needed care to the 150 million Americans whose health insurance was covered under ERISA. The Republican Congress defeated the bill 217 to 212 in a partisan vote. But it *did* manage to pass its own "The Patient *Protection* Act" by a vote of 216 to 210. The name sounds awfully reassuring — until you discover that it conspicuously *left the ERISA loophole intact*! Insurance companies can still deny needed care and sleep peacefully knowing that they won't have to face a lawsuit. (Oh, and we can also apparently sleep better knowing that we are

---

A Nobel Peace Prize Recipient's View on Managed Care and ERISA

"I have been shocked to learn how a cabal of business can distort the legal process to free themselves from responsibility in a system of profit-driven madness. From my perspective, the worst aspect of market health care is the abandonment of fundamental medical principles. Central to the doctor–patient relationship is the expectation that the physician will put the need of the patient first, over and beyond personal interest or interest in a third party. By contrast, market medicine is organized, like any other business, to generate profit. HMOs are far more concerned with the loss of revenue and market share and the value of their stock than the well-being of the sick. ERISA's shield of immunity provides profit-driven companies the ability to generate profits at the expense of patients and fundamental medical values."

—Dr. Bernard Lown
1985 Nobel Peace Prize Recipient
(Source: http://www.consumerwatchdog.org)

keeping those "greedy" lawyers from "taking advantage of us.") The score? Right — 0. Wrong — 3.

"Sorry, Pain Management Is Not a Covered Benefit"

In many (if not most) managed care organizations, effective, high-quality interdisciplinary chronic pain management services are simply not available. Very often, we have been told that treatment for chronic pain is not a "covered benefit" under the plan. Indeed, some specifically exclude pain management in the policy itself. Other times, however, the patient has no way of being forewarned that he or she will be left out in the cold. Though not specified in written policies, this is true for many who receive coverage through the worker's compensation system.

On one notable occasion, one of our physician colleagues worked hard to convince a worker's compensation case manager (who had no medical training) to refer an injured worker to Dr. Chino for behavioral assessment and treatment of her chronic pain. The case manager told the doctor that she had never authorized this for any patient in the past, but she was willing — reluctantly — to approve the referral. After seeing the patient, Dr. Chino noted in his report that she had a significant amount of anxiety and depression due to the chronic pain and subsequent disruption to her life. He indicated that these conditions needed to be taken into consideration when planning treatment for her chronic pain. Not at all unusual in such cases. However, the case manager, upon reading the report, went nuts. The reason? The psychological symptoms constituted "new" conditions (i.e., new in the sense that none of the patient's previous doctors — physicians and surgeons — had ever mentioned them despite their having been present for some time since the injury). This being the case, the insurance company would now be responsible for treating them. To the case manager, that meant spending more money. She may have been unaware of the studies showing that, in the long run, appropriately attending to psychological conditions related to pain ends up saving tons more money than is spent on treatment. But even if she were aware of them, we're pretty sure it wouldn't make a difference. Needless to say, the case manager denied authorization for Dr. Chino's proposed treatment plan — a plan that would have significantly improved the injured worker's pain condition, suffering, and the probability that she would return to work. What's more, the referring physician got an earful. The case manager told him — in no uncertain terms — that she would "never again" allow another patient in her charge to see a psychologist. Wow! A pretty blatant display of ignorance, arrogance, and total contempt for the patient's feelings and legitimate medical needs, wouldn't you say? And yet, the case manager held the patient's fate in her hands.

Drunk with Power? Insurance Adjusters and Their Authority to Overrule the Doctor

We have noticed, time after time, that getting necessary pain treatment authorized is an arduous, contentious endeavor. It's simply no fun at all. Although there are exceptions to the rule, many insurance adjusters and case managers with whom we have spoken really do seem to enjoy their position of power. We assure you that we are not being paranoid here. It is as if they delight in sizing up the clinical situation and then overruling the doctor when the proposed treatment plan does not conform to what they think it should be. This is insane! But it happens — routinely. In fact, we have spoken to some former adjusters who confirm this view. They have told us that, indeed, there exists a culture in which:

♦ The patient is the enemy and is out to cheat the system.

♦ The less you spend on patient care, the better you are doing your job.

♦ There are good doctors and bad doctors.

♦ Doctors who view patients as the enemy are good.

- ◆ Doctors who are patient advocates are bad.

- ◆ Doctors who downplay the extent of illness or injury are good.

- ◆ Drs. Davis and Chino are bad.

Although there are some really fine, caring insurance adjusters and case managers, they typically don't last very long. Some just quit because they cannot handle the ethical conflict. Others are canned. This is because they are seen as being "wasteful" and, worse, "too soft" on patients, who, after all, are only out to "defraud the system." While it

---

The Stanford Prison Experiment

In the 1960s, Stanford University psychology professor Phillip Zimbardo conducted a controversial study that evaluated the extent to which we humans respond to the influences of our social environment. The basement of the psychology building was transformed into a mock prison. Dr. Zimbardo randomly assigned male college student volunteers the role of either prisoner or guard. These were normal, well-adjusted young men.

Although the experiment was to run for at least a week, Dr. Zimbardo had to call it off after only a few days. Why? Because the participants' responses to their social roles were way above and beyond what was expected. Within hours, the "guards" became downright sadistic in their treatment of the "prisoners." And the "prisoners" began to break down emotionally — apparently forgetting that they were free to leave the experiment at any time. This experiment showed us that social expectancies are extremely powerful in molding behavior and can completely override one's sense of right and wrong.

Now look at what has happened in managed care. See a resemblance? We do. Those (medically untrained) individuals who are given the role of case manager are empowered to dictate the fate of the patient. Meanwhile, those trained to take care of people (doctors, therapists, nurses) are at the mercy of the guards — er...*the case managers.*

is true that there are some unscrupulous people who go to great lengths to cheat the system, it is a grievous and inexcusable mistake to regard all injured workers in this way. Yet, this truly appears to represent the dominant view among adjusters and case managers within the worker's compensation insurance arena. (For those seeking support and guidance for their worker's compensation or personal injury problems, check out http://www.prairielaw.com.)

Get a Lawyer When You Need One

We are among the last people on earth who want to see disputes move into the legal arena in order to be settled. We would much prefer that people talk with one another in good faith and settle disputes amicably. But in the absence of good faith on the part of an MCO, you just may need help from a good attorney.

One of our patients, Mary, was a registered nurse who had the misfortune of injuring the joints in her wrists in a work-related accident. Her worker's compensation case manager sent her from one doctor to another hoping that at least one would invalidate the link between the work accident and her disabling condition (the same strategy that misfired with Aaron). They all agreed that her condition was work related. By chance, another doctor happened to make a tentative diagnosis of rheumatoid arthritis affecting another part of her body. Once the insurance company saw this, it immediately ceased all of her medical and disability benefits. The adjuster used this one statement, made by one physician, to conclude that the problem in her hands was due not to a work injury but rather to the rheumatoid arthritis. Mary was shocked. But unlike Aaron, she did not fight the decision. Aaron was seething with anger. Mary was beaten down with depression from her pain and debilitation. She ended up on Social Security disability at the age of 46.

Mary could have used a lawyer who would stand up against this kind of shameless abuse. But we understand that her depressed state of mind (also a work-related condition because it stemmed from her pain and inability to function) made the prospect of a legal fight unthinkable for her at the time. The score? Right — 0. Wrong — 4.

The Squeaky Wheel

According to the old saying, the squeaky wheel gets the grease. If you're not getting adequate care for your pain condition, make plenty of noise. It will probably get you labeled a "difficult patient," but it may also get you what you need. In today's managed care world, being quiet, polite, and deferential will only serve to funnel more money into the pockets of corporate executives, stockholders, and maybe even your doctor — *all at your expense.* We hate to say it but, in the world of corporate healthcare, it's a dog-eat-dog world out there. We wish it weren't so. But it is.

Ask your doctor about your diagnosis and his or her treatment plan. This should be clearly stated. The idea is for both of you to know where things stand and what treatment options are indicated — *whether covered by your insurance plan or not.* There should be an ongoing dialogue between you and your doctor about how the pain is affecting

---

The HMO Gag Rule

Now outlawed in most regions, HMO lawyers dreamed up one of the most dastardly inventions ever seen in healthcare: the gag rule. It was a clause in the contracts of participating doctors that, in essence, forbade them from saying anything negative about the organization. For example, a doctor would be in breach of contract if he or she truthfully disclosed to a patient that needed diagnostic or treatment services were not available within the HMO. What possible reason could there have been to require that participating doctors sign such a clause? Could it be that HMOs were well aware of how crummy their care was and knew that, unless threatened, ethical doctors would be unwilling to subordinate the needs of the patient to those of the stockholders by keeping quiet? Bingo!

your life and what you can do about it. A seven-minute office visit is insufficient to cover this important element of your care. (Unfortunately, that is the average amount of time doctors spend with each patient in an HMO setup.) If you are in an HMO (or other managed care situation) and you suspect that your doctor is withholding needed diagnostic tests, treatment, or his or her opinion as to what is really going on with your pain, insist that an outside opinion be authorized. Contact the HMO patient advocate. File an appeal. Also, write to your employer, your state insurance commissioner, and your congressperson. Send copies to your HMO. If your appeal is successful, see an outside physician that is board certified in pain medicine. If your pain has become chronic, you should also see a behavioral pain specialist, usually a psychologist (and preferably one with board certification in health psychology). The bottom line is that it is simply wrong for you to suffer when effective treatment is available.

Pop Quiz

Check all that apply.

Who among the following would probably rather eat a worm than defend the HMO gag rule?

☐ a. Your HMO attorney's college ethics professor

☐ b. Your HMO attorney's pastor/priest/rabbi/spiritual advisor

☐ c. Your HMO attorney's mother

☐ d. Your HMO attorney

Managed Care, Medical Research, and the Rain Forest

In addition to the human toll, for-profit managed care has set the stage for another tragedy in the making: the demise of medical research. In addition to federal research grants, many of the great discoveries in clinical medicine have been brought about by the support of teaching and research hospitals across the country. Supporting training and research is an expensive proposition but has traditionally brought prestige and attracted the brightest of the bright to participating medical centers. This arrangement has been of immeasurable value to our world in many ways. Not only has it led to cures for terrible diseases, but it has also allowed for our doctors-in-training to gain the experience necessary to effectively heal the sick and save lives.

But research and teaching hospitals vie for the same healthcare dollars so aggressively sought after by the corporate for-profit hospitals. And HMOs have become known for squeezing every ounce of profit from hospitals in the form of bidding wars. The hospital that will agree to provide the most services at the lowest price wins the competition. Those that don't have contracts will go broke and fold.

The combination of for-profit HMOs and for-profit hospital corporations has led to the devastation of the once prominent nonprofit community hospital. With its mandate to care for the poor and destitute, its expenses were greater, and hence, it could not compete with the corporate hospitals that had no such mandate. A similar plight has threatened to befall teaching and research hospitals because of their worthy (and expensive) mandates. The result? These valued elements of our society are in danger of extinction — all so that a few can get rich.

This outrageous situation is not unlike the destruction of the world's rain forests. In order to reap short-term financial rewards, corporate entities have bought up ever-increasing amounts of rain forest land to convert it to grazing pasture for the production of beef. This action renders a severe blow to the earth's ability to produce oxygen and scrub out carbon dioxide, thus endangering all future generations of life. To make matters worse, producing grazing land in this way will not sustain cattle for more than a few years. The result is the permanent devastation of a wonderful system (the rain forest) that was developed and honed over millions of years but which is being rapidly destroyed so that a few can make a quick buck.

Likewise, it seems that the wonderful system of teaching and research hospitals that has yielded so many benefits to us all is being severely compromised so that corporate executives and stockholders can increase their wealth. There is absolutely no concern for the greater good. This is not only unethical. It is downright *immoral*. By the way, the score is now a frightful: Right — 0. Wrong — 5.

The Managed Care Experiment: Failure to Thrive

The managed care experiment seems to have run its course and is now showing signs of financial failure. Although it initially lived up to its cost-containment and profit-generating promises (by its aggressive capture of the market share, deep reductions in reimbursement to doctors and hospitals, and ruthless rationing of services), the chicken has finally come home to roost. Once the darlings of Wall Street, for-profit HMOs are now going broke and dropping like flies. Why? Because financially, they can't deliver on their other promise: *to take care of people.* In their zeal to capture more and more new members, they miscalculated the amount of money it would take over the long run to give stockholders and executives healthy dividends, even while simultaneously providing patients with shockingly *unhealthy* levels of care. When HMOs go out of business, their members are left out in the cold. They have to scramble to secure other coverage. And you know what? Once provided at bargain basement prices, HMO premiums are now almost indistinguishable from the formerly more expensive traditional plans. And for your increased premium you still can get the same lousy care. What a deal!

If Congress enacts legislation that eliminates the ERISA loophole and free market forces continue to play, we will probably see the demise of for-profit managed care plans. As it stands, the "fittest," most aggressive plans will continue to squeeze doctors and hospitals for even greater reductions in fees while finding perhaps even more creative ways to limit care. Undoubtedly, this will translate into the ruination of even more lives.

In the end, we will probably come full circle when the profit-driven managed care experiment collapses under its own greedy weight. When that happens, we will all look back and see that, like the rain forest, so much damage was done — all to benefit the few who got obscenely rich in the process. And we will be no better off than when we started. God must be more than a bit upset about the way profit-driven HMOs have treated His children. But in the final analysis, we are certain that He will see to it that Right triumphs over Wrong.

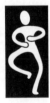

The Doctor's Dilemma

Saving lives is not a top priority in the halls of power.
Being compassionate and concerned about human life
can cause a man to lose his job.

—Myriam Miedzian
Boys Will Be Boys, Chapter 2 (1991)

The Doctor

Practicing medicine in these days of rapid change in the healthcare
delivery system is an increasingly arduous task with diminishing re-
turns. The milieu is adversarial on every front. The patient is frequently
pitted against the physician and the physician against the insurance
companies. The medical–legal system is teeming with "hungry" lawyers
who see the physician as a potential source of revenue in an increasingly litigious society. Worse yet, the physician is at odds with himself
or herself in attempting to meet the increasingly impossible demand of
delivering quality care while containing costs. For these and other
reasons, many physicians are seeking to leave the medical profession.

Most physicians chose to go into medicine, at least in part, to alleviate
pain and suffering. As superior students with high academic standards,
they naturally want to maintain the same high standards in the care of
their patients. Unfortunately, finite resources and a premium placed on
cost containment by the healthcare system have rendered this noble
goal increasingly difficult to attain.

In fact, the hand of the physician is soundly slapped if he or she is "unnecessarily" thorough. The assumption is not that he or she is conscientiously addressing the medical needs of the patient, but rather that he or she is milking the system at worst or being wasteful at best. Clearly, the demand is not for excellence in healthcare but rather for mediocrity, for passable work. Required to compromise deeply entrenched values, the physician suffers from *ego dissonance*: The "A" student must practice "C" medicine.

What happens if the well-intentioned physician decides to buck the system and commit the "unpardonable sin" of placing his or her patient's well-being first? The physician will suffer significant repercussions. He or she loses provider contracts with given insurance companies because he or she won't play ball. This process is known as being "deselected" from a provider list. When this happens, patients are instructed to go elsewhere for care. In some situations, this has meant a loss of up to 50% of a physician's income.

Typically, the physician receives notification of having been "deselected" without explanation from the insurance company. There is no forewarning that a given behavior must be modified or rectified, and there is no recourse. This loss of control and autonomy has contributed to the sense of despair and rage experienced by the vast majority of physicians practicing medicine today. However, most remain publicly silent for fear of contributing to their own economic demise via deselection.

Physicians are weary of walking the fine line between containing costs and delivering quality medical care. The malpractice burden is uniformly placed on the shoulders of the physician. Medical tests and treatments recommended are often denied by the third-party payor. Yet, if the patient suffers as a result of not having the test or receiving the treatment, it is the physician who is held liable. Where is the justice?

The double bind of the physician practicing medicine today is widely underrepresented and misunderstood. The current situation in healthcare is untenable. The future does not look bright for conscientious physicians who, long ago, made a decision to go into this demanding profession to help their fellow human being.

The Patient

You may be asking yourself, "Does the doctor's dilemma affect me, the patient?" The answer is an unequivocal yes. The sad truth is that the doctor's plight can and does impact the quality of medical care in this country. For example, you may be denied evaluation or treatment for a given medical condition that your doctor deems necessary, because the insurance company refuses to pay for it. We can assure you that there are cases on the books where denial of such care has led to unnecessary death.

Your inability to choose your own healthcare provider can interfere with the establishment of a therapeutic doctor–patient relationship and may erode your confidence in the care that you are receiving. Indeed, the mere fact that a doctor is an approved provider for a given insurance company may be a bad omen. There is no reason to believe that because a doctor has survived the screening process to become a "selected" provider, he or she is necessarily competent, dedicated, and compassionate. None whatsoever. What it does mean is that the doctor will generally play by the insurance company's rules, not necessarily in accordance with that "old-fashioned" icon of a bygone era: the Hippocratic oath. As a result, your health may be seriously jeopardized.

Recently, one of us (CD) received a call from an insurance claims adjuster stating that the employer of two injured workers seen the previous week was irate because both were placed on temporary medical leave from work until they could receive proper treatment. As chronic pain specialists, we know that an acute injury that is not treated effectively early on can significantly increase the chances that a chronic pain problem will arise, leading to more disability and higher healthcare costs in the long run. The well-reasoned recommendation for temporary leave stemmed from this knowledge. As a result, however, the employer (who is self-insured) didn't like the decision, and the care of both patients was transferred to another doctor who apparently was more willing to play ball.

This clearly was a decision based on economics. In the eyes of the self-insured employer, taking the workers temporarily off duty so that they could undergo treatment translated into the employer having to spend more money on healthcare and provide a paycheck without services rendered by the employees. At first glance, it looks like the employer is saving money by denying authorization for care. But the studies clearly show that it pays to take care of a worker as soon after an injury as possible. Fewer dollars are spent in the long run and the employee is less vulnerable to future injuries. Unfortunately, the prevailing attitude is that such employees are out to take advantage of their employers and are looking for a free ride. Those doctors willing to play ball, usually to protect their own financial security, reinforce this notion by inappropriately sending injured employees back to work prematurely. Thus, an adversarial relationship develops among all players. And the studies also show that ill will between employer and employee is the single most powerful predictor of future disability.

One of the patients mentioned above, Bill, had contracted polio as an infant. It affected his right arm and both legs. He suffered from chronic pain and weakness. Despite the strikes against him, this heroic man worked full time as a floor supervisor, a job that required him to be on his feet eight hours a day. He had made a life for himself, was married, had a child, and had just purchased a new home.

When I (CD) saw Bill, he was in a great deal of pain. He told me that he had fallen down the stairs at work and had injured his back and right leg. Since then, he had been walking with a cane because of the weakness, pain, and his fear of falling again. His job as a floor supervisor required that he walk constantly during his shift. Yet, he could barely walk the length of the examination room. In addition to his severe pain, Bill was suffering emotionally, fearful that he would lose his job because of his injury. On top of that, he was afraid that he would lose his new home because he would be unable to make the mortgage payments. Bill was miserable.

The other patient, I'll call him Roberto, had injured his back lifting wet linens. He sat on the exam table propped up with his arms in an effort to decrease his excruciating back pain. He had great difficulty getting from a sitting to a standing position, and he walked with a pronounced limp. Despite my attempts to be gentle, he could barely tolerate my examination because of his discomfort.

Both Bill and Roberto had been seen by another physician prior to my seeing them, and both had been placed on light-duty status by him. Roberto had been given work restrictions that consisted of no sitting, standing, or walking for more than five minutes and no bending or lifting whatsoever.

Do you think that the physician really felt these men should be working? Obviously not. But because of the onus of placing any injured employee on temporary medical leave, he chose to set severe restrictions instead, in hopes that the employer would realize that, for the time being, they could not fulfill the requirements of their jobs.

Someone at the company administering the employer's health plan evidently was unhappy with that physician's recommendations and had transferred the care of both patients to me, hoping that I would play ball. That someone was even more unhappy with me when I placed them temporarily off work — *where they belonged*! Once again, he or she responded by transferring the case to yet another physician, who perhaps was willing to sell his or her soul for financial gain at the expense of these unfortunate human beings. In the current system, my extensive medical knowledge and experience were preempted by a nonmedically trained person looking (probably in vain) to save a few dollars. In essence, medicine is increasingly being practiced by such nonmedically trained individuals whose ultimate allegiance is to the stockholder, not the patient. This is wrong.

I never saw these two gentlemen again, and I never received another referral from that employer. But I can assure you that the physician who was willing to play the game and send all such patients back to work full-time without restrictions, regardless of their physical limitations, will be flooded with referrals. It is not only the patients who will lose in such a system. The employers will end up spending far more for healthcare and lost productivity in the long run. They either haven't read the studies, haven't been in business long enough, or aren't paying attention to their long-term healthcare expenses.

Is there corruption in this system which was designed to take care of our healthcare needs? You bet there is. Not only is there corruption, there is a cover-up, especially designed to conceal the truth from us so as to keep the profits rolling in. The doctor's dilemma results from ignorance and a twisted set of priorities among those holding the purse strings. And it is hurting us all.

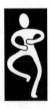

Stacking the Deck
in Your Favor

So you're saddled with chronic pain and you want to make the most of your life here on earth. How do you do that? The fact is, all too often, the pain controls the person rather than vice versa. It determines what you do, where you go, and how often. How do you regain control of the pain and your life? As you will find out, lifestyle habits are a big key to success. But so is appropriate attention to the three components of each and every one of us: the mind, the body, and the spirit. To assure success, it is important to find ways to nurture each vital part. This chapter is designed to provide practical advice on how to get back into the driver's seat and become the master of your own destiny.

Lawyers

Does everyone need a lawyer? Definitely not. There are many doctors, claims managers, and employers who are genuinely concerned about their patients or employees and want them to receive proper treatment. But unfortunately, there are others who are not so noble.

If you have been injured at work and the claim is denied, if you aren't getting approval for treatment that you believe you need, or if you are getting the runaround, you may want to consider retaining the services of an attorney who will fight for your rights. The downside of doing so is that it can be costly. The upside is he or she will direct you away from doctors who are known "hired guns" for employers or third-party payors and toward doctors who are honest, dedicated, competent, and compassionate. A good lawyer, like a good doctor, is worth his or her weight in gold.

Eat Right

There's a lot of truth to the saying "garbage in, garbage out." And it doesn't just apply to computers. It applies to our bodies as well. We *are* what we eat. A proper diet can contribute to an overall sense of well-being, which is often lacking in people who suffer from chronic pain. Eating a well-balanced diet can strengthen a sense of self-control over one's body and life in general. Experts agree that most of us eat too much saturated fat, cholesterol, sugar, and salt (sodium) and not enough starch and fiber. The rule of thumb is that about 60% of our diet should be carbohydrates (rice, pasta, bread, vegetables, and fruits), 30% fat (limiting saturated fat such as butter to 10%), and 10% protein. By governmental decree, food labels now provide the number of grams of fat in a serving as well as the percentage of the recommended daily value of carbohydrate, fat, and protein. So, does this mean that, in order to assure ourselves of a nutritious, well-balanced diet, we are doomed to a life with a calculator every time we sit down to the table to eat? The answer is no.

Fortunately, the U.S. Department of Agriculture has spared us such a dismal existence by issuing the user-friendly Food Guide Pyramid, which translates the 60% carbohydrates, 30% fat, 10% protein guidelines into servings of specific types of food. This pyramid has essentially replaced the basic four food groups. The key difference between the two is that meat is no longer the centerpiece of a meal. Instead, the Food Guide Pyramid advocates that the bulk of our diet consist of rice, pasta, or other grains, along with fruits and vegetable because these foods are low in fat and unwanted calories and high in fiber, carbohydrates, vitamins, and minerals. (Their production also happens to be a lot kinder to our environment.) A multivitamin every day, though not necessary, may be helpful in assuring that you are receiving the essential nutrients, but it should not substitute for a balanced diet.

Too much salt in the diet can be hazardous to your health. High salt intake can lead to hypertension and congestive heart failure in some individuals. In addition, research shows that there is a strong relationship between the incidence of stomach cancer and diets consisting of large amounts of salty, smoked, and pickled foods. In 80% of cases, cancer means pain. So beware! There are exorbitant amounts of salt in junk and processed foods. As a general rule, they should be avoided.

A good way to decrease the salt in your diet is by substituting lemon, garlic, herbs, and spices. Herb blends work well in shakers on the table. Instead of putting salt in the salt shaker, for example, try a combination of basil, rosemary, tarragon, and marjoram to flavor chicken or turkey. In another shaker, try a blend of savory, sage, cumin, coriander, ginger, and thyme to season pork. For Italian dishes, use a mixture of parsley, oregano, and basil, with a pinch of cayenne pepper and fennel. Classic herbs for fish are dill, chives, lemon thyme, tarragon, and chervil. Herb blends can also be used to make a delicious dip when combined with plain yogurt or low-fat sour cream. Be creative. Use your imagination. Finding satisfying substitutes for salt can be a lot of fun. The possibilities are endless.

Keep Fit

It's not good for a car to sit indefinitely in the garage. The battery loses its charge. Rust sets in. The tires go flat. To be assured that your car runs properly, it is advisable to take it for a spin regularly. Likewise, your body will function better if it gets a workout on a routine basis at least three to five times a week. Your physical therapist can set up an exercise protocol for you that is tailored to meet your needs. But be sure to obtain medical clearance from your doctor before engaging in a fitness program.

Maintain Proper Body Weight

While the greatest health problem worldwide is malnutrition and starvation, most of us, by an accident of birth, have the luxury of living in a culture where food is available in abundance. Therefore, it comes as no surprise that 30% of Americans are overweight, 9% severely so. In general, the term obesity is defined as 20 to 30% over the average weight for an individual's age, sex, and height. Being overweight is associated with a plethora of medical conditions including high blood pressure, elevated cholesterol, stroke, heart disease, adult-onset diabetes mellitus, breast and prostate cancer, uterine and endometrial cancer, gallstones, back pain, osteoarthritis, gout, varicose veins, sleep apnea, and carpal tunnel disease. Pain is an unwanted visitor that accompanies many of these problems.

For those of you with pain in the back, hips, or legs, think about what it would be like to carry around two full bags of groceries all day long. Fatigue and increased pain are the predictable result. If you are 20 pounds overweight, you are doing the equivalent every day. Imagine what a relief it would be to put down those groceries or to shed those unwanted pounds.

In order to maintain ideal body weight, calories ingested should not exceed calories burned. Overeating and a sedentary lifestyle both promote obesity. Diet (the dreaded "D" word) and regular exercise are the keys to success. One pound of fat is equal to 3,500 calories. Dietary fat provides nine calories per gram, alcohol provides seven calories per gram, and both carbohydrates and protein provide four calories per gram. It doesn't take a mathematical wizard to see that curtailing your intake of fat provides more than twice the benefit of cutting down on carbohydrates or protein.

Basal metabolic rate is the rate at which an individual burns calories in the awake and rested state. It decreases 2% per decade in men and 3% per decade in women. So, obviously, then, weight gain is an inevitable part of the aging process unless you actively fight the battle of the bulge. How do you do that? Stop eating so much. Start exercising more.

If you walk one mile a day, you will burn 100 calories. If you walk one mile a day, 365 days a year, you will burn 36,500 calories. If during that same year you cut down your eating by only 100 calories a day, you will lower your yearly caloric balance another 36,500 calories. Two hundred calories per day times 365 days equals a total reduction of 73,000 calories. And 73,000 calories times 1 pound per 3,500 calories of fat equals 20.85 unwanted pounds lost in a year. Not bad for a minor adjustment in one's diet and a daily walk in the park.

Medications to Aid in Losing Weight

Many people in our culture want a quick fix for their weight problem. However, a ton of research indicates that there is no enduringly effective quick fix. The best answer to reaching and maintaining ideal body weight lies in the establishment of a proper balance between caloric intake and caloric expenditure.

Chromalyn picolinate is a mineral that improves glucose tolerance (blood sugar) and reduces blood serum cholesterol levels. A few studies have suggested that this mineral may help reduce body fat without cutting caloric intake. In a study of athletes, those given chromium picolate lost 22% of their body fat in six weeks, compared with only 6% in the control group. In another study, subjects who were given 200 to 400 micrograms of chromium picolate per day lost an average of 4.2 pounds of fat and gained 1.4 pounds of muscle. However, the majority of studies failed to show any benefit at all.

Get Your Daily Dose of Sunshine

Sunshine is one of Nature's treatments for depression, a common companion of chronic pain. Ultraviolet rays stimulate a small structure in the brain called the pineal gland, which regulates the circadian (day/night) rhythm.

At night, the pineal gland secretes melatonin in response to darkness. The light of day, as it passes through the eye to the pineal gland, has

328 Validate Your Pain! Exposing the Chronic Pain Cover-Up

the opposite effect, suppressing the production of melatonin. This fluctuation of melatonin regulates the day/night cycle.

Seasonal affective disorder (SAD) is a common problem that is caused by the disruption of circadian rhythm. People afflicted by SAD are sensitive to the lengthening periods of darkness that occur in the fall and winter months of the year. This results in an increase in the production of melatonin and, with this increase, a mood disorder characterized by depression, irritability, and tension. In addition, these individuals frequently experience an increase in appetite and a craving for carbohydrates. The physiological reason for this craving is that carbohydrates accelerate the production of serotonin by the pineal gland. Serotonin plays an important role in alleviating depression. In fact, it is the key mediator affected by Prozac®, one of the most popular and effective antidepressant medications on the market today.

SAD affects about 1% of the general population and is three times more likely to affect women than men. It is more prevalent in the temperate climates of the north. In fact, latitude (the distance from the equator) is the most important geographical determinant of the severity of symptoms. The farther north one is from the equator, the more diffuse the sunshine. The less sunshine, the higher the rate of SAD. Bummer.

Sunshine has many benefits. It helps to regulate circadian rhythm, alleviates depression, enhances sex drive, and it doesn't cost much (last time we checked). Just walk outside and get your free dose. But take heed. One can get too much of a good thing. Dermatologists warn us to avoid exposure to sunlight, especially during midday, when the sun's rays are most direct, because of the risk of skin cancer. All things in moderation.

Sleep

Here's the last pop quiz:

Pop Quiz

Circle the right answer.

Insomnia sucks!   TRUE   FALSE

If you answered true, you have achieved a perfect score. Nice job. If you answered false…(oh, never mind).

Nine out of 10 "experts" (our patients) agree that insomnia sucks. In fact, of those nine, eight agree that it sucks big time. Quite aside from the statistical studies, they have experienced insomnia from the inside. No amount of stratified sampling or statistical analysis can substitute for what it feels like to spend night after night tossing, turning, getting up, lying down, pacing, taking pain medication, and watching infomercial reruns while everyone else on the planet is fast asleep. Insomnia sucks.

We are truly amazed at how much sleep is lost among those with chronic pain conditions. How can it be that a person who is used to sleeping 8 hours every 24 can exist for days, weeks, months, and even years on only 3 to 4 hours of *interrupted* sleep? Yet we hear this routinely. While the studies tell us that individuals with chronic sleep disorders usually underestimate how much sleep they truly get, there is significant sleep loss nonetheless. If you have ever lost a night's sleep, think about what the next day was like. Chances are, you felt pretty sluggish and lacked your usual zest for your day's activities. Usually, however, you can make up for a night or two of insomnia with a few nights of normal sleep. But what if it has been weeks or months with night after night of disrupted, poor quality sleep? What happens to one's ability to function? What happens to one's motivation to pursue previously enjoyed activities? What happens to one's ability to concentrate, to work, to become enthralled in a good book, to cope with everyday hassles and stresses? Look down the drain. It's all there.

The Sleep Reconditioning Protocol

The sleep reconditioning protocol, outlined below, is a proven method for combating insomnia. For those who are chronically unable to get a good night's rest, remember — *and consistently follow* — these important guidelines:

1. **Don't sleep anywhere but in your bed.** Although you may be able to sleep on the couch or in your recliner now, you'll have a hard time reconditioning yourself to sleep in your bed if this habit is not broken.

2. **Use your bed only for sleeping** (exceptions are made for certain other bed-related activities). Avoid reading, watching television, or arguing in bed (especially if you are alone). The goal is to avoid any association between your bed (and bedroom environment) and feelings of restlessness, irritability, and/or frustration.

3. **Go to bed only when sleepy.** Do not turn the lights out with the thought that you must get to sleep. Unlike almost all other activities, the harder you try, the more likely you are to fail.

4. **If not asleep in 20 minutes, get up and out of bed.** Go to another room. Watch television or read a book. Avoid subject material that is particularly stimulating (for example, page-turners like *Validate Your Pain! Exposing the Chronic Pain Cover-Up*).

5. **Stay away from any beverage that contains caffeine** (e.g., coffee, many teas, and soft drinks). Some patients have reported making a pot of coffee at 3 A.M. when they cannot sleep. Not a good idea if getting back to sleep is the goal.

The sleep–wake cycle is age-linked. On average, the newborn sleeps from 16 to 20 hours a day (ah, the good old days), the 10-year-old from 9 to 10 hours per day, and the adolescent sleeps about 7 to 7.5 hours per day. A decline to 6.5 hours per day occurs in late adulthood. The range in healthy adults is from 4 to 10 hours. Increased mortality is associated with individuals who sleep less than 4 hours or more than 10 hours every 24. But there is wide individual variation in the length

6. **Return to bed only when you feel sleepy.** If not asleep in 20 minutes, get up and out of bed again. Repeat #2 through #4 as often as necessary.

7. **Awaken and get out of bed at about the same time every day** (even on weekends). This is necessary if you are to "decondition" your insomnia. Don't worry about how little sleep you got the night before. Try not to justify sleeping into the late morning (or afternoon) because you didn't sleep much last night. The goal here is to reset your body's "internal clock" so that it gets used to sleeping at night.

8. **Do not nap during the day.** A nap will zap your ability to sleep at night. Stay awake by keeping busy.

9. **If you find that you cannot sleep without sleeping pills, you probably need additional help in getting control of your insomnia problem.** Sleep medication, other than the antidepressants and antihistamines, should be used only on a short-term basis. When used for prolonged periods, medications such Dalmane® and Restoril® may actually promote insomnia by disrupting the natural sleep cycle. A health psychologist can probably lend some helpful assistance to get things back on track.

In following the above guidelines, it is very important to be consistent night after night. They will not help much if you follow them for only a few nights and then revert to old habits. It may take five to seven days, perhaps less, to see results. Most people find that they actually get less sleep the first two or three days. This is to be expected. But if you stick with it, your efforts will more than likely pay off. So if you want to stack the deck in favor of the sandman, hang in there.

and depth of sleep based on one's physical and psychological states and genetic and environmental factors, as well as one's own sleep history.

Why sleep? What's the purpose? Research into sleep deprivation investigates the function of sleep. Deprived of sleep, experimental animals will die within a few days, no matter how well fed, watered, or housed they are. In human subjects, sleep deprivation for many days produces fatigue, memory loss, and irritability (although resulting long-term psychological or physiological damage has not been confirmed). On rare occasions, loss of sleep can provoke psychotic episodes character- ized by screaming, crying, incoherent muttering, and hallucinating. Fragmentary delusions and paranoid thoughts are more common. Sound inviting? As we said before, insomnia sucks.

Dr. William Dement, a sleep researcher at Stanford University, sug- gested that sleep is so important to human survival that it should be considered the fourth vital sign — after pulse, respiration, and tem- perature. We are inclined to agree with him. But unfortunately, sleep is rarely considered to be an important part of the history taken and physical exam performed by physicians. If problems are acknowledged, the proffered remedy too often only consists of a prescription for sleep- ing pills. What many doctors do not realize is that there are behavioral remedies that are safe, effective, and *all natural*.

Nicotine

Regardless of what you may have heard in congressional testimony, nicotine is a highly addictive, poisonous alkaloid found in tobacco. "Poisonous" means that it kills people. Death usually occurs gradually over the course of many years. But nicotine is only one of over 4,000 known toxic poisons found in cigarettes. To name just a few, acetalde- hyde is a free radical that is linked to accelerated aging. Carbon mon- oxide and nitrogen oxide decrease the oxygen-carrying capacity of the blood. The tar of tobacco smoke contains polynuclear aromatic hydro- carbons, which have been implicated in up to 80% of all cancers. Heavy metals such as arsenic, cadmium, lead, and radioactive polonium sup- press the body's immune system and, like acetaldehyde, act as free radicals. Yuk.

Every year, 50,000 Americans die of cigarette-related deaths. One out of every six deaths in the United States is linked to smoking. Smoking increases the risk of high blood pressure and atherosclerosis (forma- tion of fatty deposits in arteries), which lead to heart disease, peripheral

Cigarette Smoking

Cigarette smoking is deadly. Statistically speaking, each cigarette you smoke shortens your life by eight minutes. Smoking is the single most preventable cause of death. Over two decades ago, the Surgeon General of the United States began to issue a warning on all cigarette packs:

WARNING: Smoking may be hazardous to your health.

More recently, the message got even stronger:

SURGEON GENERAL'S WARNING: Smoking Causes Lung Cancer, Heart Disease, Emphysema, And May Complicate Pregnancy.

There's no confusing this message. But maybe the next one will be even more direct:

*SURGEON GENERAL'S **FINAL** WARNING: You haven't been listening, have you? NOW PUT DOWN THOSE NASTY CIGA-RETTES THIS INSTANT!*

The good news is that if you are a smoker and succeed in quitting, your body's level of toxic carbon monoxide and nicotine will rapidly decrease. You will notice that your stamina and senses of smell and taste improve. After 7 to 10 years of not smoking, your risk of having a heart attack or developing cancer approaches that of people who have never smoked. If you try unsuccessfully to quit, there is compelling evidence that a diet rich in antioxidants (vitamins C, E, B complex, and beta-carotene) may protect your body from some of the hazards of smoking.

If your efforts to quit have not succeeded, by all means don't despair. Of those who have quit, almost all made many unsuccessful attempts before they finally succeeded. And remember that just because you smoke does not make you a bad person, regardless of the increasingly hostile attitudes held by society toward smokers. Shame and guilt are not only unkind, they are also extremely ineffective methods of helping people to quit. But by far the best way to protect yourself is to never start in the first place. When that alleged friend offers you that first cigarette, *just say no!*

vascular disease (diminished blood supply to the arms and legs), and cerebrovascular disease (diminished blood supply to the brain). Smoking also increases the risk of lung diseases such as emphysema and chronic obstructive pulmonary disease. According to the American Cancer Society, cigarette smoking unequivocally causes 30% of all cancers. Specifically, smoking increases your risk of developing acute leukemia and cancers of the mouth, pharynx, larynx, stomach, pancreas, colon, rectum, anus, genitals, bladder, cervix, kidney, and lung. In addition, smoking is a risk factor associated with osteoporosis, low-back pain, lumbar disc herniation, and failed spinal fusion.

Alcohol

Alcohol (chemical name ethanol) is an intoxicating, potentially addictive substance obtained by fermentation of carbohydrates with yeast. Alcoholic beverages supply calories (seven calories per gram) but little or no nutrients. Alcohol abuse is the cause of many accidents and multiple medical and social problems.

Two ounces of hard liquor per day is associated with elevated blood pressure. More than three ounces per day is associated with actual hypertension. Heavy drinking increases one's risk of hemorrhagic stroke as well as cardiomyopathy, esophageal varices, cirrhosis of the liver, bleeding disorders, osteoporosis, pancreatitis, neuropathy, and impotence. Drinking just one beer a day can add 54,000 calories to your diet or 16 pounds to your waistline over the course of a year and contributes to obesity. Alcohol ranks third among congenital conditions associated with mental retardation. The list goes on and on.

High alcohol consumption has also been linked to a number of cancers, most notably to cancer of the mouth, pharynx, larynx, esophagus, digestive tract, liver, rectum, bladder, lung, and breast. Many studies have observed a synergistic effect between alcohol and cigarettes in regard to cancers of the mouth, throat, and esophagus. That is, the effect of using both substances is not merely additive but rather is multiplicative. People who have one to three drinks a day run a 60%

higher risk of developing oral cancer than do nondrinkers. Add cigarettes and the risk escalates.

The Nurses' Health Study found that women who drink only moderately (one to two drinks per day) have a 50% higher rate of breast cancer compared to those women who were nondrinkers. Heavy drinking doubles or triples the risk of colorectal cancer.

As hazardous as heavy drinking is for one's health, there is some indication that moderate use of alcohol may actually have a beneficial effect on the heart. Study after study has linked light or moderate drinking with a reduction in heart disease. Moderate drinkers have been found to have less heart disease than both nondrinkers and heavy drinkers. Some scientists believe that this benefit is due to the improvement in the ratio of good cholesterol (high-density lipoprotein, or HDL) to bad cholesterol (low-density lipoprotein, or LDL). It may also be the result of an anticoagulant effect on the platelets. Another consideration is that moderate alcohol intake can reduce stress, which is a major risk factor in heart disease.

In addition, some studies indicate that red wine is a highly effective antioxidant. What is an antioxidant? An antioxidant is a substance that prevents or limits oxidation. When metal is exposed to oxygen, it rusts. When butter is exposed to oxygen, it becomes rancid. This process of oxidation can also occur in the body. Unstable oxygen molecules, called free radicals, are responsible. They combine with healthy molecules and cause damage ranging from cosmetic to life threatening. Furthermore, free radicals break down skin tissue, making it look older than it is, while increasing the risk of cancer and heart disease.

With regard to individuals suffering from chronic pain, it is important to be aware of the potential interactions of alcohol with other medications. Drinking alcohol while taking aspirin or nonsteroidal anti-inflammatory drugs (e.g., ibuprofen) may cause stomach problems such as gastritis or ulcers. Alcohol taken in combination with acetaminophen (Tylenol®) or narcotic medications (e.g., Percocet®, Vicodin®, or Lorcet®) that contain acetaminophen may cause serious liver damage. Alcohol slows the clearance of many drugs from the body, thereby prolonging and strengthening their effect. For example, alcohol taken in combination with sedatives such as barbiturates and tranquilizers may result in excessive and prolonged sedation.

We have found that a considerable number of people with chronic pain use alcohol, alone or in combination with other drugs, in an attempt to cope with their condition. Some have done so because their pain has been undermedicated and/or otherwise undertreated. Unfortunately, alcohol is a poor substitute for adequate pain management and may lead to other serious health and social problems.

With good reason, doctors continue to warn against anything more than moderate drinking, if at all. Moderate drinking is defined as one drink per day or less for women and two drinks or less for men. One drink is a can of beer (12 ounces), a glass of wine (5 ounces), or 1½ ounces of hard liquor (80 proof). And remember — don't drink and drive.

Ergonomics

Ergonomics, or human engineering, is an applied science concerned with designing and arranging the things people use in such a way as to maximize efficiency and safety. As it relates to the spine, ergonomics plays an important role in maintaining proper alignment and reducing the fatigue that can be experienced with repetitive movements and activities.

Traditionally, furniture and equipment have been designed to fit the average person. But it so happens that God created a motley crowd to roam the earth. And everybody isn't average. Some people are "real big," and some people are "real small." If you happen to be one of those individuals who departs markedly from the norm, you may have experienced some frustration as a result. Just ask a professional basketball player how he feels when he goes shopping for a new car and has to shoehorn himself into the driver's seat of the average size vehicle. In case you were wondering, a lot of those guys are driving trucks.

Always remember: designing and arranging your environment based on sound ergonomic principles is essential to maximize efficiency and safety and minimize musculoskeletal stress and strain.

Social and Emotional Support

In Chapter 1, we discussed the power of validation. It is truly incredible how much better people feel when they perceive that others understand and care about their circumstances. We see it all the time. "Snapshots" of people taken before and after experiencing validation of their pain are like night and day. The simple act of validation has saved lives. Many lives. It is amazing how something as simple and low-tech can achieve such startling results and make such a difference in people's lives. Although securing social and emotional support is not likely to cure the pain condition, it almost always dramatically improves one's resolve to pursue — and follow through with — effective treatment. Often the biggest challenge one faces is finding such a support system. Investigate whether there is a support group in your area that focuses on problem solving and emotional validation of the pain experience. Avoid groups that never get past simply grumbling about their difficulties. The most useful groups will provide a good blend of emotional support and useful information about coping with chronic pain. For information about groups in your area, check the yellow pages or contact:

The American Chronic Pain Association
P.O. Box 850
Rocklin, CA 95677

Realistic Goal Setting

Want to know how to avoid chronic frustration? Stop setting unrealistic goals. We can't count the number of chronic pain sufferers we have met who carry all of their old, prepain standards for personal performance with them. One woman, who was in tears and suffering greatly,

Ergonomics Tips

Fortunately, recognition of the range of human individuality is beginning to find its way into workstation design and automobile engineering. However, people with chronic pain have needs that require special ergonomic accommodations. Specific ways in which you can improve your home and work environment include the following:

♦ When standing for long periods of time, change your body position every few minutes to decrease stress on the muscles supporting your spine. It is helpful to shift your weight alternatively from one foot to the other. It is also beneficial to use a step stool and to alternate between propping up first one foot and then the other.

♦ The importance of wearing quality shoes that provide good arch support and cushion cannot be overemphasized, especially if you work on a concrete floor all day long, day after day.

♦ When lifting, keep your feet apart to increase your base of support. Spare your back muscles by raising the object while keeping it close to your body and by lifting with your legs.

♦ Pushing an object is less stressful than pulling. Pulling may strain back muscles or, worse yet, herniate a disc. Alternatively, pushing allows you to use powerful leg muscles. So when you have the option, *push, don't pull.*

♦ When driving long distances, use a lumbar support or a rolled-up towel for your low back. Because driving imparts a constant vibration to the spine, it is important to stop every hour or so to walk around and to stretch those back muscles.

♦ Most people are surprised to learn that you can strain your back while sitting. As a matter of fact, disc pressure in a sitting position far exceeds that in a standing position. Sitting in a forward flexed position increases disc pressure to almost twice that of a stand-

told us that she could not afford to take time away from her household and family duties to participate in a coordinated program designed to help her feel and function better. Yet, she was unable to take care of ing position and can overstretch spinal ligaments. Sitting in an upright position minimizes the load on the spine. An ergonomically designed chair supports the back at its weakest area, the low back, and promotes good sitting posture, which protects the back from fatigue and injury. If your job is sedentary and you sit eight hours a day, it pays to invest in a good chair. At the very least, you should buy a lumbar support or roll up a towel to support your lower back. The seat pad should be short enough to allow a few inches behind the knee area so that the vessels and nerves that pass behind the knee will be free of pressure. The armrests should be close enough to your torso so that you do not have to lean to the side to reach them. The seat back should be able to tilt back about 10 degrees. The proper height and width of the seat back depend on the size of the individual. It should be slightly wider than the torso and provide lateral support with slightly curved sides. The optimal seat back has an adjustable lumbar support. The chair should have casters so that you can turn and roll easily. You should not have to jerk the chair to properly position it. Plastic mats may be placed over carpet to facilitate movement.

♦ Don't sit too long. It is advisable to get up and move around every hour or so to avoid maintaining a static position for an extended period of time.

♦ One of the most common ergonomic mistakes made in the workplace is to make employees perform tasks at improper work heights. This puts them at a mechanical disadvantage and leads to unnecessary wear and tear on the musculoskeletal system. The proper work height is the level at which the worker does not have to flex or extend his or her neck to do the task on the tabletop. If you work at a computer, the monitor should be at a height that does not require raising or lowering your head when looking at the screen or the keyboard. The top of the screen should be about eye level.

things at home the way she used to. Her plan was to push herself even harder to get things accomplished. Of course, this led to increased pain, sleeplessness, debilitation, and more profound feelings of depression and despair. She needed help in readjusting her self-expectations. Unfortunately, she was so caught up in them that she never did permit herself to get the help she needed.

Setting realistic goals is not always easy. Starting an exercise program is a good example. We often find that people with chronic pain overdo it at the beginning. They carry with them the memory of what they used to do, and this serves as an unspoken guide to what they now *should* do. Guess what happens. They feel like failures after they push themselves too hard and hurt more. They erroneously infer that increased pain must signal further injury. They are, in a sense, punished for their efforts and become fearful of exercising in the future. If they do attempt it again, they are less likely to succeed the next time, and before you know it, they become disgusted with themselves and conclude that they will never get better. This sets up a vicious cycle in which fear of exercise leads to further deconditioning, inactivity, and pain. Quality of life takes a beating. There's a better way.

As discussed in Chapter 10 (Active Physical Interventions), set realistic goals based on your *present,* not past, physical condition. Don't set yourself up for failure. If you have had multiple back surgeries, training for the Olympic bungee-jumping competition is probably not a good idea. But swimming a gradually increasing number of laps in a pool or walking a little farther each day over the course of several weeks may be very realistic as well as beneficial. Make copies of the exercise progress record form provided in Appendix B, and use it to plan and carry out a new exercise program. Above all, don't forget to incorporate the use of positive reinforcement.

Positive Reinforcement

We cannot overemphasize the importance of incorporating positively reinforcing activities into your life. With chronic pain, the balance of positives to negatives in life gets out of whack. This makes it difficult to cope with the many problems that arise. Choose your friends carefully. Maintain a positive mental attitude. Concentrate on the things that you *can* do rather than the things that you *can't* do. Pursue hobbies and activities that you enjoy. These things *will* make a difference. It's your life. Make the most of it.

When working toward a goal, don't berate yourself for falling short of success. Readjust your strategy and/or your expectations for change. Punishing yourself only serves to weaken behavior. It is through reinforcement that behavior and motivation become strong. So reward yourself for good behavior. Don't be too hard on yourself. If you smoke a cigarette or fail to exercise for a few days, don't dwell on it. Just keep looking ahead. Persist, but be patient. It takes time to regain confidence. But it will be through positive reinforcement that your performance and self-confidence will return.

Relaxation Techniques

When we talk to our patients about learning to relax, we often hear, "How can I relax with all this pain?" Good question. The fact is that it *is* possible to gain control over the body's responses to pain and other kinds of stress. And it feels better when this control is achieved. By relaxation, we are not talking about an add-on therapy. We are talking about learning how to change the balance of stress hormones circulating in the bloodstream. We are talking about how to increase the diameter of blood vessels. We are talking about reducing muscle tension and spasm. We are talking about adjusting physiological mechanisms that influence pain — all without drugs or any invasive procedures. We are talking about modifying human "software."

Learn to use relaxation techniques. There are many different approaches, including biofeedback, guided imagery, meditation, yoga, and progressive muscle relaxation. As with any skill worth acquiring, practice and consistency are essential. Remember: We want you in the driver's seat. Any tool that you can use to manage your pain has psychological as well as physiological benefits.

Volunteer

Sometimes by directly helping others, we indirectly help ourselves as well. This may be due, in part, to the fact that we are distracted from our own problems when we focus on the needs of others. And it may help us to place our own situation in perspective. Some people have to cope with chronic pain every day of their lives. Others have no food, shelter, or clothing. Still others may be grieving because they have lost a loved one through an illness or a tragic accident. No one has the market cornered on suffering. Whatever the reason, you may want to consider volunteering to serve your community through religious or other organizations.

Stop Fighting with Your Pain

Our cultural tradition dictates that if something stands in the way between us and what we want, we must fight it. We wage "war" on poverty, drugs, and cancer. How many times have you heard someone say, "I'm going to fight this cancer/illness/pain"? We hear it a lot. But, oddly enough, our patients have taught us that this is a big mistake. Instead, we tell people to *give up the fight*. "What?" they exclaim. "Give up the fight against pain? What kinds of doctors are you anyway? I thought you were here to help me."

Yes, our recommendation sounds counterintuitive, but it really is good advice. The initial assumption most people have is that in refusing to fight the pain, they would be raising the white flag out of despair — that the pain would succeed in forever making their lives miserable. But you know what? We have consistently observed that those who refuse to fight with their pain are far more likely to "win" than are their warring brethren. People with chronic pain who successfully come to accept its presence (even though they don't like it) notice a significant calming effect. Their nervous systems settle down. Stress hormone production and muscle tension decrease. Immune systems are strengthened. And they become better able to reach for the positive things in life. All of these factors result in reduced stress and strain on the mind and body. The natural consequence? Peace is restored. Pain and coping improve. So if you find yourself saying, "I'm going to beat this pain" — hit the brakes. Take a close look at what your mental attitude may be doing to you. There's a better way. Declare a unilateral cease fire and stop fighting. You really will notice a difference.

Prayer

People who have a strong religious faith tend to be healthier and re- cover from illness more quickly than those who do not. As noted in Chapter 9 (The Psychology of Chronic Pain and Illness), the research studies bear this out. Our clinical experience does too. And you know what? So does our personal experience. We have seen powerful things happen that we can attribute to nothing other than divine intervention. No kidding. We are convinced that there is more to our world than those things we can observe with our ordinary senses — *much more*. Explore your faith. Deepen it. And although you may not experience a miraculous cure, you will certainly experience a peace that you never thought possible in the face of chronic pain.

Validate Your Pain!

You are a whole person. You have a mind, a body, and a spirit. All three components interact with one another. A sick spirit will adversely affect the body and the mind and vice versa. All three need proper attention and nurturance. The information and ideas outlined in this book pro- vide proven guidelines for reaching your highest potential, despite odds that may sometimes seem overwhelming.

Together, we have covered a lot of territory in this book. Chances are, many of the issues addressed herein have connected with your own experience in maneuvering through the mine field of chronic pain management. It is not an easy journey, as our own patients have taught us. But armed with the principles presented in this book, it is one that can be successfully negotiated. As the saying goes, every journey begins with the first step. And in the journey to pain control and improved quality of life, the first step is crucial: *Validate your pain!*

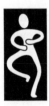

Checklist for
High-Quality Pain Care

High-quality care is about more that just professional credentials. In fact, we believe that, overall, having a doctor or therapist who has his or her head and heart in the right place is probably more important than an impressive resume. If he or she happens to have both, then you're in business.

What follows are questions relating to important elements to consider when evaluating members of your pain management team. We suggest that you make copies of this list and use it to rate each of your doctors and therapists. Rate as many of the 25 items as possible. Then total the number of "yes" and "no" responses. The more "yes" and the fewer "no" ratings, the better. Keep in mind that no one is perfect. But any items answered "no" should raise a red flag. More than a handful of "no" responses suggests that you need to start looking elsewhere for your care. Before you take this action, however, do your best to clearly communicate what you want from the doctor or therapist (feel free to use this checklist as a guide). This may help to move some of those "no" check marks over to the "yes" column.

Special Warning: In the unlikely event that your doctor gives you the "*I'm* the doctor — not you" or the "What medical school did *you* go to?" routine, forget the checklist. Wrap some garlic around your neck and run away fast!

PRACTITIONER CHECKLIST

TEAM MEMBER (Dr., Ms., Mr.): _____

Does he or she:	YES	NO
1. Treat you with respect?		
2. Seem to be a nice person?		
3. Seem to take your complaints and questions seriously?		
4. Make you feel comfortable in his or her presence?		
5. Give you the feeling that he or she is really concerned about you as a person?		
6. Conduct a thorough physical exam (if this is part of his or her role)?		
7. Give you feedback regarding diagnostic tests (X-rays, scans, lab tests)?		
8. Provide you with a firm opinion regarding what is wrong (diagnosis)?		
9. Talk with you about his or her treatment goals?		
10. Ask you about your treatment goals?		
11. Discuss a treatment plan and the various options that are available and not available?		
12. Discuss estimates as to treatment duration and cost?		
13. Include pain specialists from other disciplines in your treatment plan?		
14. Communicate regularly with other treatment team members?		
15. Address pain medication options — including narcotics?		
16. Use the term *physical dependence* rather than *addiction* when referring to narcotic pain medications?		
17. Seem to care if you understand and are satisfied with the diagnosis and treatment plan?		
18. Discuss your prognosis relative to the treatment plan and goals?		
19. Talk with you about your progress?		
20. Make modifications to the plan based on your response to treatment?		
21. Make an appropriate referral if things are not getting any better?		
22. Have a practice comprised mostly of people with chronic pain?		
23. Have a good reputation among doctors and patients?		
24. Have board certification in the appropriate specialty that was obtained via examination?		
25. Hold membership in professional organizations related to pain?		
TOTAL FOR EACH COLUMN		

Exercise Progress Record

Talk with your doctor and/or physical therapist about what specific exercises are appropriate for you. It is unlikely that your therapist has any experience with the behavioral management approach to exercise covered in Chapter 10 (Active Physical Interventions). We suggest that you talk with him or her about that information (or, better yet, provide a copy of this book). The key concepts and methods were developed at the University of Washington Multidisciplinary Pain Rehabilitation Center (the granddaddy of all chronic pain programs) and have been shown to produce impressive results with a minimum of complications. We have used this approach extensively and can attest to its efficacy.

Don't be put off by the apparent complexity of the form. Once you follow the steps a few times, it becomes easy as can be. Make a copy of the form for each exercise in your program. Have the forms with you while you exercise. Write down your performance after completing each exercise. Use the graphs to chart your progress. If you follow the steps, you will almost certainly see the graphs climb higher and higher. And most of all: *have fun*!

Exercise Progress Record   Exercise: _____

How to use this form: Use a separate form for each exercise in your routine. Write the exercise being measured in the space above.

(1) Obtain a *"behavioral baseline"* by doing this exercise until pain or fatigue starts to emerge. Then *STOP.* Record your repetitions, time, distance, etc. Don't push too hard. Do this for the first three days. Take the average of the three-day performance and multiply by 0.8 (80%). This will be your starting point.
(2) Establish an easy progression by *gradually* increasing the amount of exercise over time. Be at least 80% confident that you will be able to meet each daily goal when establishing your exercise targets.
(3) Write them down under the "Target" column. Record your actual performance upon completing each exercise session. Check the "Met Target" column if you succeeded.
(4) If you met fewer than 8 of the first 10 targets, you have set your rate of progress too high. Ease it back until you are successful at least 80% of the time.
(5) Graph your performance on the grid on the next page for a visual picture of your progress. It can be a great reinforcer.

Baseline Calculation:

(Day 1 _____ + Day 2 _____ + Day 3 _____) = _____

divide by 3 = _____ × 0.80 = | Baseline |

Progress Record

Session Number	Date	Target Reps; Time	Actual Reps; Time	Met Target
1				
2				
3				
4				
5				
6				
7				
8				
9				
10				
11				
12				
13				
14				
15				
16				
17				
18				
19				
20				

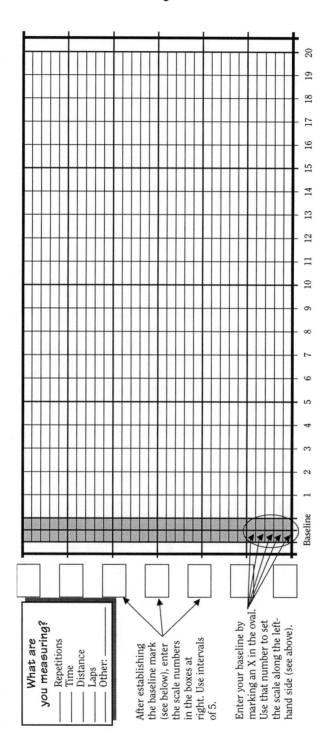

What are you measuring?
_____ Repetitions
_____ Time
_____ Distance
_____ Laps
_____ Other: _____

After establishing the baseline mark (see below), enter the scale numbers in the boxes at right. Use intervals of 5.

Enter your baseline by marking an X in the oval. Use that number to set the scale along the left-hand side (see above).

Baseline   1   2   3   4   5   6   7   8   9   10   11   12   13   14   15   16   17   18   19   20

Other Surgical
Interventions

Spinal Surgeries to Reduce Pain

Sympathectomy is the interruption of some portion of the sympathetic nervous system pathways. This may be accomplished by surgical or chemical means or by radio-frequency ablation (heat) or cryoneurolysis (freezing). Sympathectomy was first introduced as pain treatment because of the vascular effects of the procedure. Many patients suffering from ischemic pain due to arteriosclerosis and peripheral vascular disease experienced a reduction in pain following sympathectomy because of enhanced blood flow to the injured area. Upper thoracic sympathectomy — rarely done since the advent of effective long-acting antianginal medications and revascularization procedures — has been very successful in alleviating intractable angina (chest pain due to coronary artery disease) in most patients. Sympathectomy has also been found to be effective for a variety of other conditions, including postherpetic neuralgia, reflex sympathetic dystrophy, Raynaud's disease, phantom limb pain, and burning or dysesthetic (an unpleasant abnormal sensation produced by normal stimuli) stump pain.

Surgical sympathectomy for painful states involves three main sites: the heart, the abdominal organs, and the extremities. The probability that the procedure will be effective in alleviating the pain can be assessed in all three areas by performing a temporary pharmacological sympathetic block interspersed with placebo blocks. These blocks are

351

instrumental in establishing the crucial role that sympathetic overactivity plays in causing the pain. In addition, repetitive blocks may eliminate the pain and the need for surgical intervention. In a literature review of 500 patients who were treated with surgical sympathectomy, 85% reported excellent pain relief, 12% fair relief, and 4% no improvement. The 4% failure rate was believed to be most likely due to incomplete sympathetic denervation.

Sympathectomies can also be performed chemically by injecting phenol or absolute alcohol solutions into the targeted sympathetic pathway. This procedure requires the extensive experience, skill, and extreme care of an anesthesiologist to avoid serious complications. Chemical sympathectomy should be considered if sympathetic blocks provide significant pain relief, but only for the duration of the local anesthetic. Lumbar sympathetic chemical blocks can usually be performed to alleviate abdominal or leg pain with minimal risk of causing weakness by injuring the lumbar plexus. Stellate ganglion chemical blocks, on the other hand, are rarely performed to relieve arm pain because of the potential damage to surrounding structures in the neck.

Possible complications of sympathectomy include the following: postsympathectomy neuralgia, orthostatic hypotension (which usually resolves within 24 to 48 hours), pneumothorax (collapsed lung due to the abnormal accumulation of air in the pleural space), renal (kidney) impairment, and paralysis (due to injury to the artery of Adamkiewicz, which supplies the spinal cord). Misplacement of the needle into the intervertebral disc, epidural, and subarachnoid spaces during chemical sympathectomy has been reported, as well as accidental invasion of the aorta and vena cava. Although rare, the unwanted spread of the neurolytic solution to the lumbar plexus and spinal cord has caused sexual dysfunction and dysesthetic changes in the legs. For these reasons, most physicians choose to perform chemical blocks under radiologic guidance. Alternatively, they may opt for surgical sympathectomy or cryo- or radio-frequency ablation.

The decision regarding which method of sympathectomy to undergo is based on the severity of the disease, the patient's physical condition, and his or her attitude toward these techniques. Chemical, cryo-, and radio-frequency ablation produce sympathetic interruption for several months to years and are especially useful for older or debilitated patients suffering from cardiac or respiratory disease for whom anesthesia and surgery pose serious risks. In younger patients who are in good physical condition, surgical sympathectomy may be preferable.

Rhizotomy is a procedure in which the dorsal (sensory) roots of cranial or spinal nerves are interrupted within the spinal canal in order to alleviate pain. Like the sympathectomy, this may be accomplished surgically (dorsal rhizotomy), by chemical means (intrathecal or epidural alcohol or phenol), by radio-frequency (heat), or by cryoprobe (freezing). Unfortunately, these methods do not produce reliable long-term analgesia and expose the patient to the risk of additional damage to the central nervous system (brain and spinal cord).

Although motor fibers are spared (thereby avoiding the risk of paralysis), complete severing of all the dorsal (sensory) roots to an extremity renders the limb anesthetic (devoid of sensation) and virtually useless. In addition, many have pain recurrence within four to six months because of nerve regeneration. For these reasons, total dorsal rhizotomy to a functional limb should not be performed.

Midline or bilateral pain requires bilateral dorsal rhizotomy. In the sacral area, this may lead to loss of anal and bladder sphincter control. This serious complication renders pain relief by this technique impractical and inadvisable in most cases.

Rhizotomy was reported in some early studies to be effective for chronic, intractable lumbosacral radicular pain. However, the study with the longest follow-up reported unimpressive results. As defined by (1) patient satisfaction and (2) report of 50% or greater sustained pain relief, there were no instances of long-term success.

Radio-frequency (heat) rhizotomy of the glossopharyngeal and vagus nerves to relieve severe excruciating cancer pain in the throat and larynx has been reported to be successful. The same procedure on the sensory root of the trigeminal nerve is highly effective for relief of severe cancer pain in the anterior (front) two-thirds of the head. The disadvantages of the procedure are that it produces loss of all sensation, is frequently followed by uncomfortable dysesthesias, and carries the risk of keratitis (inflammation of the cornea) because of the loss of the corneal reflex (closure of the eyelid when the cornea is touched).

Complications of surgical rhizotomy include wound infection, meningitis, hemorrhage, spinal cord infarction or mechanical trauma with ensuing paralysis, and cerebrospinal fistula. Unless extreme care is used, chemical rhizotomy tends to result in unwanted spread of the neurolytic agent. Because of the undesirable side-effect and complication profile and the high failure rate, rhizotomy is rarely done today.

Epidural adhesiolysis is a procedure used in the treatment of failed back syndrome in which there is epidural fibrosis and adhesions. Guided by fluoroscopy, a needle is inserted at the lower end of the spine (caudal block through the sacral hiatus, that is, the opening of the tailbone) into the epidural space, and a catheter is then threaded. A dye is injected that reveals defects, an expected finding in patients with epidural fibrosis. Then a mixture of steroid and local anesthetic such as lignocaine (a cousin of Novocain® used in the dentist's office) is injected to decrease inflammation, swelling, and pain. Following this, a highly concentrated solution of sodium chloride (10%) is injected to dissolve the fibrosis and adhesions. So far, research indicates that only a small number of patients experience even short-term relief from pain, and most of these individuals suffer a recurrence of pain within a few months of this treatment.

Chymopapain injection or *chemonucleosis* is a procedure in which chymopapain, an enzyme, is injected into the nucleus of a bulging disc in order to break down its protein and decompress the nerve root. The procedure was approved by the Food and Drug Administration for use in the United States in 1982. It was used widely in the mid-1980s but fell out of favor for two reasons: because of allergic reactions to the chymopapain and because of serious and unpredictable neurological complications, including paralysis.

Today, chymopapain injections are rarely done in this country. However, they are frequently done in Canada and Europe to treat radicular symptoms due to herniated disc. The reported success rate is up to 80% in properly selected patients.

Cordotomy is a procedure in which the spinothalamic tract within the spinal cord is severed in order to interrupt the conduction of painful messages traveling to the brain. The operation is most effective in alleviating sharp or aching pain and is less effective for treating burning, crawling, dysesthetic pain. It may be useful in treating unilateral pain (pain on one side of the body), whether it is due to cancer or a benign process. Patients with bilateral or midline pain must undergo bilateral cordotomies in order to obtain relief from pain. The surgery is ineffective in alleviating pain above the level of the fourth cervical vertebra. Therefore, patients with pain in the upper neck and head are best treated by other methods.

Cordotomy is extremely effective in bringing about pain relief in 80 to 90% of cases. It interferes only with pain and temperature sensation and does not result in the potentially disabling loss of touch and position sense brought about by dorsal rhizotomy. The risks associated with this procedure are considerably greater for a bilateral cordotomy compared to a unilateral cordotomy and include permanent bladder dysfunction, respiratory problems, and unilateral weakness. The major drawback is that pain often recurs over time due to nerve regeneration. By two years, only 40% of patients report continued pain relief.

Brain Surgeries to Reduce Pain

Hypophysectomy is the surgical removal or destruction of the pituitary gland. This gland is composed of two lobes: the anterior lobe and the posterior lobe. The anterior lobe excretes several important hormones that regulate the proper functioning of endocrine organs, such as the thyroid gland, ovaries, and testicles. It plays a vital role in the growth, maturation, and reproduction of the individual. The posterior lobe of the pituitary gland is a reservoir for antidiuretic hormone (which causes retention of water when the body signals that it is dehydrated) and oxytocin (which stimulates milk ejection in breast-feeding mothers and contraction of the uterus). The posterior lobe releases these hormones as needed. The pituitary gland is located at the base of the brain and is attached by a stalk to the hypothalamus, from which it receives important neural messages and instructions.

The purpose of a hypophysectomy is to alleviate diffuse pain caused by widespread metastasis to the bone from hormonally dependent cancers of the breast or prostate. The procedure may be successfully performed on patients with inoperable cancer in a number of ways: with the use of alcohol injection, cryo (cold) or thermal (hot) lesions, or open surgery.

Over 80% of patients experience excellent postoperative pain relief that lasts 3 to 12 months. Potential complications include death, injury to the nearby hypothalamus, visual loss, oculomotor deficits (pertaining to eye movements), drainage of cerebrospinal fluid from the nose (rhinorrhea), and meningitis. Virtually all patients undergoing hypophysectomy require hormone replacement therapy postoperatively.

Hypophysectomy, while used less often today compared to the 1980s, has not fallen into disrepute or disuse. The operation is performed on selected patients with hormonally dependent, metastatic cancer whose pain is unrelieved by oral medications, including narcotics, and who are not suitable candidates for other methods of pain control.

Thalamotomy is a surgical technique by which specific groups of cells in the thalamus of the brain are destroyed. The thalamus is the relay station for sensory messages, including pain. The goal of this procedure is to alleviate pain that is diffuse in distribution. It may also be performed to relieve tremor and rigidity in Parkinson's disease.

In an analysis of 150 cases reported in the literature with different types of central pain (pain due to a lesion of the central nervous system, that is, the brain or spinal cord), up to 36% of the patients reported good pain relief following thalamotomy at the expense of a 27% complication rate. Used in the treatment of phantom limb pain, the short-term success rate was only 20%. Long-term follow-up of these patients revealed an even lower success rate. In patients with nociceptive pain (pain due to mechanical, chemical, or thermal stimuli at the peripheral nerve endings), the initial success rate was much higher, 60 to 70%. In cancer pain, a subgroup of nociceptive pain, the initial success rate following thalamotomy was higher still, about 80%. However, that success rate dropped rapidly to 30% by the end of the first year. Possible complications of the operation include infection, intracerebral hemorrhage, and neurological impairment, including hemiparesis (weakness on one side of the body) and dysesthesias (unpleasant, abnormal sensations produced by normal stimuli).

Thalamotomy has never enjoyed widespread use in the United States for relief of chronic pain because of its poor long-term success rate. This is most likely due to the nervous system's ability to reorganize itself after injury. Nevertheless, thalamotomy may play a beneficial role in the management of cancer pain in patients with short life expectancy, especially when the involved areas are the head and neck or widespread metastasis.

Deep brain stimulation is the electric stimulation of discrete, deep-seated regions of the brain via implanted electrodes for the purpose of alleviating chronic pain. It has been utilized as a method to produce analgesia since the 1970s and is a viable option for patients unwilling to undergo destructive procedures. There are two general target sites: the periaqueductal-periventricular gray (PAG/PVG) region and specific sensory nuclei of the thalamus (VPM/VPL). Stimulation of the PAG/PVG is most effective in relieving nociceptive pain. For example, it has been used successfully in patients suffering from pain due to cancer and failed back syndrome. Success is defined as 50% or greater long-term reduction in pain. Both endogenous opioid- and nonopioid-dependent mechanisms of pain relief have been identified.

Stimulation of the thalamus seems to selectively reduce neuropathic pain. It has been found to be most effective for deafferentation pain (pain due to the destruction or interruption of sensory nerve impulses) such as phantom limb and stump pain following amputation.

The PAG/PVG electrode insertion technique involves CT- or MRI-guided surgery via a burr hole drilled into the skull. This is performed preferably under local anesthesia, but general anesthesia may be indicated in especially anxious patients. For thalamic (VPM/VPL) targets, the patient must be awake and cooperative during exploration of the target area with a stimulating and recording electrode.

Potential complications of deep brain stimulation include intracranial hematomas (2%), transient neurological deficits (8.5%), infection (6 to 12%), lead migration (9 to 10%), and component breakage (8 to 12%). The procedure is an effective, nondestructive treatment for patients with diffuse, intractable, nociceptive and/or deafferentation pain.

Other Surgeries to Reduce Pain

Peripheral nerve stimulation has been used for the treatment of pain since 1965. Initially, many technical and clinical complications were associated with the procedure. For example, equipment malfunction and electrode migration frequently occurred. In addition, scar formation caused by direct contact between the nerve and the cuff containing the electrodes often led to constriction of the nerve and more pain. Because of this, flat electrode arrays were developed and fascia (a sheet or fibrous band of tissue) was placed between the nerve and the stimulator. This approach fortunately proved to be much more stable and clinically effective and was associated with fewer complications.

Peripheral nerve stimulation has been used successfully to treat neurogenic pain in the arms, legs, and thorax (intercostal nerves). The best candidates are patients who suffer from pain in a single nerve distribution. However, some carefully selected patients with multiple nerve lesions have undergone successful implantation. Clinical syndromes that have been effectively treated by this means include reflex sympathetic dystrophy, causalgia (burning pain, often accompanied by trophic skin changes, due to injury to a peripheral nerve), plexus avulsion, and entrapment neuropathies. Clinical selection criteria include chronic intractable pain which is unresponsive to other therapies, temporary relief with local anesthetic, no psychological contraindications including drug habituation, and a successful screening trial.

Potential complications of peripheral nerve stimulation include bleeding, infection, nerve injury, poor pain relief, and equipment failure. Because of improvements in equipment and surgical technique, fewer than 5% of implanted systems now require mechanical revision.

Neurectomy is the surgical removal of a part of one or more peripheral branches of the cranial or spinal nerves. While it was the first neurosurgical procedure used to alleviate chronic pain, it no longer plays a significant role in pain management.

The advantages of neurectomy include the ease and safety of the operation, which can be done under local anesthesia, and the predictable loss of function. With the exception of the trigeminal nerve (which supplies the muscles of mastication and the sensation of the face and cornea of the eye), functional regeneration of the severed nerve does not occur as long as the two ends of the nerve are widely separated. Neurectomy can be expected to produce complete loss of sensation in the area previously supplied by the nerve.

The disadvantages of the procedure far outweigh the advantages. Most peripheral nerves are mixed and, as such, contain both motor and sensory fibers. Therefore, loss of sensation is accompanied by undesirable weakness. Furthermore, not only is the sensation of pain eliminated, but all other sensations as well, including light touch, temperature, and pressure. Several long-term problems can also be anticipated. Adjacent intact sensory nerves sprout branches into the anesthetic area, thereby decreasing the size of the region of pain relief. If the original anesthetic area is small, the sensory loss may actually disappear within a matter of months, only to be replaced with the original painful sensation. In addition, changes in the central nervous system can lead to a new pain syndrome called denervation hypersensitivity or anesthesia dolorosa. This is a very distressing complication for which there is no reliable treatment. Finally, whenever a peripheral nerve is resected, a neuroma (a tumor growing from a nerve) is formed. Although not all neuromas are painful, those that occur in areas of the body where pressure is frequently applied often cause pain. For these reasons, it is advisable to avoid neurectomy as a method of treatment for chronic pain because few long-term successes can be anticipated and the complication profile is undesirable.

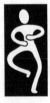

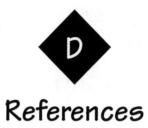

References

Carette, S. 1995. Fibromyalgia 20 years later: What have we really accomplished? *Journal of Rheumatology* 22, 4:590–594.

Chino, A.F. November 1993. Childhood abuse: A precursor to fibromyalgia? Poster presented at the meeting of the American Pain Society, Orlando, FL.

Corcoran v. United Healthcare, Inc. 1992. 965 F.2d 1321. 5th Cir.

Deardorff, W.W. and J. Reeves II. 1997. *Preparing for Surgery: A Mind–Body Approach to Enhancing Healing and Recovery.* Oakland, CA: New Harbinger.

Deardorff, W.W., H.S. Rubin, and D.W. Scott. 1991. Comprehensive multi-disciplinary treatment of chronic pain: A follow-up study of treated and non-treated groups. *Pain* 45:35–43.

Fordyce, W.W. 1976. *Behavioral Methods for Chronic Pain and Illness.* St. Louis: CV Mosby.

Guildenberg, P.L. and R.A. DeVaul. 1985. *The Chronic Pain Patient: Evaluation and Management.* Basel: Karger.

Kuttner, R. 1998. Must good HMOs go bad? *New England Journal of Medicine* May 21 & 28.

Melzak, R. and P.D. Wall. 1965. Pain mechanisms: A new theory. *Science* 150: 971–979.

Nurses' Health Study. 1995. Referenced in *PDR's Family Guide to Nutrition and Health.* Montvale, NJ: Medical Economics.

Perry, S. and G. Heidrich. In Melzack, R. *Tragedy of Needless Pain.*

Portenoy, R. and K. Foley. 1986. Chronic use of opioid analgesics in non-malignant pain: Report of 38 cases. *Pain* 25:171–186.

Porter, J. and H. Jick. In Melzack, R. *Tragedy of Needless Pain.*

Saal, J. 1990. *Physical Medicine and Rehabilitation: State of the Art Reviews* 4, 2.

Sarno, J.E. 1984. *Mind Over Back Pain.* New York: Warner.

Sarno, J.E. 1991. *Healing Back Pain: The Mind–Body Connection.* New York: Warner.

Sarno, J.E. 1998. *The Mind–Body Prescription.* New York: Warner.

Spiegel, D., J.R. Bloom, H.C. Kraemer, and E. Gottheil. 1989. Effect of psychosocial treatment on survival of patients with metastatic breast cancer. *Lancet* ii:888–891.

Tennant, F.S. Jr. and G.F. Uelman. 1980. Prescribing narcotics to habitual and addicted narcotic users: Medical and legal guidelines in California and some other western states. *Western Journal of Medicine* 133:539–545.

Tennant, F.S. and G.F. Uelman. 1983. Narcotic maintenance for chronic pain: Medical and legal guidelines. *Postgraduate Medicine* 73:81–86.

Waddell, G., J. McCulloch, E. Kummel, and R. Venner. 1980. Nonorganic physical signs in low-back pain. *Spine* 5, 2:117–125.

Website http://www.consumerwatchdog.org.

Yuan, H. 1994. *Spine Letter* 1, 6:1.

Zenz, Strumpf, and Tryba. 1992. *Journal of Pain Symptom Management* 7: 69–77.

Zimbardo, P. 1969. The human choice: Individuation, reason, and order versus deindividuation, impulse, and chaos. In Arnold, W.J. and D. Levine (eds.). *Nebraska Symposium on Motivation.* Lincoln: University of Nebraska Press. 237–308.

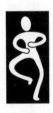

Index

A

abdominal muscles, 33
abdominoplasty, 276
ablation, 351, 352
ABT-594, 128, 170
acetaminophen, 127, 128, 129, 130, 131, 157, 162, 163
 alcohol and, 335
acupuncture, 42, 201, 235–239
 chi, 236
 immune response and, 238
 meridians and, 236
 NIH position statement, 237, 238
acute pain, *see* pain, acute
addiction, 105, 107, 108, 109, 110, 111–113, 115, 117, 118, *see also* narcotic medications
 benzodiazepine, 152, 153
 morphine, 273
 pseudo-, *see* pseudoaddiction
aerobic exercise, 42, 207–210
 benefits of, 208
alcohol, 334–336
Alexander, Franz, 86, 87
alkaline phosphatase, 47
allodynia, 144
alpha-2-adrenergic agonists, 164–165
alprazolam, 150–151
alveoli, 209
Alzheimer's disease, 170
amantadine, 158
Ambien®, *see* zolpidem
Amerge®, *see* naratriptan hydrochloride
American Cancer Society, 334
American Chronic Pain Association, 337
American College of Rheumatology, 91
American Pain Society, 91

American Psychiatric Association, 150
amitriptaline, 139, 143, 155
amphetamines, 128, 156–157
amylase, 47
analgesia, patient-controlled, *see* patient-controlled analgesia
anatomy of pain, 21–43, *see also* specific topics
 central nervous system, 39–40
 Gate Control Theory, 41–43
 nervous system, 35–39
 spine, 29–35
Anderson, Bob, 207
anesthesia, 266, 268, 282–283
anesthesia dolorosa, 359
anion, 254
annulus fibrosus, 32
anticonvulsants, 127, 128, 146–148
antidepressants, 42, 127, 128, 138–142, 143, 155
antihistamines, 128, 154, 155, 164
antinuclear antibody, 48
antipsychotic medications, *see* neuroleptics
antispasmodics, *see* muscle relaxants
anxiety, 3, 19, 191, 194, 221
 history taking and, 46
 medications for, 149, 151, 153, 166
 pain gate and, 42, 184
arachnoiditis, 52, 53, 146, 147
arm pain, 60
arrogance, 71
arteries, 209
arterioles, 210
arthritis, 30
 bone scan and, 56
 defined, 23, 24
 gouty, 49

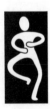